THE
PRIMAL
BLUEPRINT

MARK SISSON

The Primal Blueprint

Library of Congress Control Number: 2008941735

Library of Congress Cataloging-in-Publication Data
Sisson, Mark, 1953–

The Primal Blueprint:
Reprogram your genes for effortless weight loss, vibrant health, and boundless energy / Mark Sisson

ISBN 978-0-9822077-0-3
1. Health 2. Weight Loss 3. Diet 4. Physical Fitness

Editor:	Brad Kearns
Design/Layout:	Jason Saito, Weston Graphics
Project Manager:	Aaron Fox, Primal Nutrition
Text Consultant:	Catherine Fisse
Copy Editor:	Laura R.Gabler
Index:	Leoni McVey
Consultants:	Rudy Dressendorfer, PhD, R.P.T, Bradford Hodgson, Walter Kearns, M.D., Reagan Smith, Jennifer Zotalis

For more information about the Primal Blueprint, please visit primalblueprint.com
For information on quantity discounts, please call 888-774-6259

Publisher: Primal Nutrition, Inc.
23805 Stuart Ranch Rd. Suite 145
Malibu, CA 90265

DISCLAIMER

The ideas, concepts and opinions expressed in this book are intended to be used for educational purposes only. This book is sold with the understanding that author and publisher are not rendering medical advice of any kind, nor is this book intended to replace medical advice, nor to diagnose, prescribe or treat any disease, condition, illness or injury. It is imperative that before beginning any diet or exercise program, including any aspect of the *Primal Blueprint* program, you receive full medical clearance from a licensed physician.

Author and publisher claim no responsibility to any person or entity for any liability, loss, or damage caused or alleged to be caused directly or indirectly as a result of the use, application or interpretation of the material in this book. Sorry, but that's what my lawyers forced me to say in order for me to be able to offer you my insights. If you do not agree with this disclaimer, you may return the book to the publisher for a full refund.

ACKNOWLEDGMENTS

My editor Brad Kearns made a tremendous contribution in the preparation and editing of this manuscript. His extensive writing experience and insights on health and fitness were invaluable to the creation of the final product. Aaron Fox, my ace general manager and webmaster at MarksDailyApple.com, was a brilliant strategist, researcher and project manager for the *Primal Blueprint*. MarksDailyApple.com staffers Bradford Hodgson and Reagan Smith offered excellent insights to help improve the text and provided extensive research and fact-checking support. Catherine Fisse's unique and often devil's advocate viewpoint helped me present a clear and focused message. The outstanding copy editing skills of Laura R. Gabler helped get this book to the finish line triumphantly. Devyn Sisson made Dad look good with her cover photography. The design talents of Jason Saito of Weston Graphics, are on display with the interior text layout. Brett Geoghegan and the staff at The Brand Garage designed the cover. Don Derenthal designed the Grok and Korg figures.

The provocative insights and opinions of numerous authors and bloggers have inspired me, among them: Loren Cordain (author of *The Paleo Diet*), Jared Diamond (author of *Guns, Germs and Steel*), Dr. Michael and Dr. Mary Dan Eades (authors of *Protein Power*), Gary Taubes (author of *Good Calories, Bad Calories*), and bloggers Art DeVany at arthurdevany.com, Peter at *Hyperlipid,* and Stephan at *Whole Health Source.* For an expanded list of my favorite books and web sites, and a comprehensive index of books, newspaper and magazine articles, research papers, and Internet links that were utilized in the research and preparation of this text, please visit MarksDailyApple.com

Olympic triathlon Gold and Silver Medalist Simon Whitfield has shown that the power of living primally can indeed apply to high level endurance athletics. Dr. Walter Kearns' consultations helped me present the medical and scientific material in an organized, factually accurate, and easy to understand manner. My wife Carrie and children Devyn and Kyle keep me grounded and balanced when my primal obsessions threaten to take over my days and nights! I owe you guys a vacation…and this time I'm coming along too!

TABLE OF CONTENTS

Chapter 4: Primal Blueprint Law #1: Eat Lots of Plants and Animals

Welcome from Mark

The doctor of the future will give no medicine, but instead will interest his patients in the care of the human frame, in diet, and in the cause and prevention of disease.

—**Thomas Edison**

Disclaimer, part II: this book was written at knifepoint.... Okay, not really. But my frequent discourses on all matters primal over the past two and a half years at my blog MarksDailyApple.com have prompted unceasing requests for more, as in, "Hurry up and finish the book!" I owe a tremendous debt of inspiration and enlightenment to those readers and the dynamic contribution they have made to the *Primal Blueprint*. This work represents the culmination of my primal philosophy, which has taken shape over the past 20 years through extensive research and life experience. I'm not a scientist or doctor; I'm an athlete, a coach, and a student on a lifelong quest for exceptional health, happiness, and peak performance. I have an insatiable curiosity about what we need to do to achieve such goals and a growing mistrust of the answers that have been heaped upon us by the traditional pillars of health "wisdom" (Big Pharma, Big Agra, the AMA, the FDA, and other government agencies), the health and fitness profiteers glorified by Madison Avenue, and even the know-it-all multilevel marketer next door.

In its essence, *The Primal Blueprint* is my effort to distill the information I've studied from the world's leading evolutionary biologists, paleontologists, geneticists, anthropologists, physicians, nutritionists, food scientists, exercise physiologists, coaches, trainers, and scientific researchers into a concise list of behavior laws that have promoted optimal gene expression and indeed survival over the course of human evolution. While the book you are holding is a product of the new millennium, the behavior laws are as old as the dawn of mankind; they merely reinform us about the fundamentals of health that seem to have been forgotten, or misinterpreted, in the modern world.

I do not have any agenda besides improving your health, fitness, and overall enjoyment of life. I am not beholden to any employer, government agency, professional licensing board, or sponsor or to any other higher power that might result in the filtering of my message. I *am* an opinionated guy and not afraid of a challenge. However, I strive to maintain an open mind and will modify my position based on feedback from others, whether from experts, ordinary health enthusiasts, or the publication of new research. I simply don't trust many of the major elements of *Conventional Wisdom* (a recurring term throughout the book, akin to a yellow highway hazard sign) that we have blindly accepted as gospel for decades.

In my case, the mistrust has been well earned over the past 35 years of trying to do "the right thing" (another recurring theme) by diligently following Conventional Wisdom. For several years of my youth, I ran in excess of 100 miles a week with a single-minded focus toward competing in the 1980 U.S. Olympic Marathon Trials. At my peak, I was considered by many to be a picture of health: 6 percent body fat, a resting heart rate of 38 beats per minute, and a marathon time of two hours, eighteen minutes that had placed me fifth in the national marathon championships.

While I reached some notable heights during my endurance career, I also experienced some devastating lows. Soon after my best marathon performance, the monumental physical stress of my training regimen and the state-of-the-art "high-energy" diet that fueled it resulted in a succession of serious overuse injuries, illnesses, and burnout. While I looked like a picture of health, I was really one of overstress and inflammation. I was the fittest guy my friends knew, yet I suffered from recurring bouts of fatigue, osteoarthritis in both of my feet, severe tendonitis in my hip joints, stress-related gastrointestinal maladies, and six or more upper respiratory tract infections each year.

Most people have traveled a less extreme path than I, yet nearly all of us have experienced similar results following the Conventional Wisdom of our time: weight-loss efforts doomed to a 96 percent long-term failure rate, workout programs leading to fatigue and increased appetites for sugar, and medications that exacerbate the underlying cause of pain while barely alleviating symptoms (not to mention the unpleasant side effects).

I applaud your efforts and desires to do the right thing, and I deeply empathize with your frustration in trying to succeed amidst a whirlwind of conflicting and confusing advice. My goal with the *Primal Blueprint* is to expose much of the lucrative health and fitness industry as ethically and scientifically bankrupt. I will peel back the many layers of marketing blather, folk wisdom, and manipulative dogma and replace it with 10 simple *Primal Blueprint* behavior laws modeled after the evolutionary success of our ancestors.

Pause and reflect on the following simple statement for a moment, for it is the most powerful and compelling rationale for living according to the *Primal Blueprint:* Human beings prevailed despite incalculable odds by adapting to the selective pressures in their environment over thousands of generations. Our primal ancestors were lean, strong, smart, and productive, which enabled them to reproduce, rule over more physically imposing members of the animal kingdom, and exploit virtually every corner of the earth. This is no mean feat, yet Conventional Wisdom has essentially dismissed the legacy of our ancestors in favor of quick fixes.

Today at the age of 55, I feel healthier, fitter, happier, and more productive than ever. I am no longer a marathon or triathlon champion (nor do I want to be), but I maintain a weight of 165 pounds with 8 percent body fat. I eat as much delicious food as I want, am not beholden to regular meal times or even regular meals, exercise just three to four hours per week (instead of the 20 to 30 I put in back in the day), and almost never get sick. My personal clients (ranging from world-champion triathletes to ordinary citizens just trying to lose a few—or a lot of—pounds), as well as thousands of readers at MarksDailyApple.com, report similar life-altering benefits from following the *Primal Blueprint*. Now it's your turn.

> *The **Primal Blueprint** is the centerpiece of a vibrant community of people connected by the Internet and committed to living their lives to the fullest potential, challenging the status quo, and not being afraid to try something **old**.*

Your Way or the Highway

My intention in this book is to show you the immense personal power you have to control your health and fitness destiny and to give you the tools to reprogram your genes, reshape your physique, and enjoy a long, healthy, energetic, and productive life. The *Primal Blueprint* principles are wonderfully simple, practical, and inexpensive, and they require minimal, if any, sacrifice or deprivation. Unlike many of the gimmicky diet and exercise books that have graced the best-seller shelves in recent decades, the *Primal Blueprint* is intuitive and easy to follow—not for 14 days or 30 days or eight weeks but for the rest of your life.

I recognize and appreciate real-world concerns like lack of time, budget issues, motivational challenges, dysfunctional social circumstances, eating disorders, ingrained bad habits, and other powerful influences that can sabotage the picture-perfect diet plan served up by the celebrity of the moment. On numerous occasions, I've felt the disappointment of taking a plunge with my heart and soul into a new diet or athletic training regimen, only to fall well short of the ambitious goals I had set. Adding insult to injury, I often discovered later that I'd been given bad advice—by my government (thanks to the tainted influence of special interests), Madison Avenue, or a less-than-knowledgeable coach, peer, or professional expert. Few things in life are more frustrating!

With the *Primal Blueprint*, there's no need for trepidation. This is not a regimented program where I shove my agenda down your throat and cajole you to go against your own common sense or pleasure-seeking human nature. My experience with Marks-DailyApple.com has taught me the value of the collaborative approach to health and well-being. Whenever I'm in a position to raise an interesting theory or discussion point that might be considered contrary to Conventional Wisdom, I immediately have thousands of readers with the ability to contribute freely to the discussion. Many of these readers are forward-thinking doctors, scientists, researchers, or coaches whose valuable input and suggestions I could not have otherwise easily solicited. This interplay often forces me to substantiate—or at times significantly modify—my position. It always requires me to adapt my message to resonate with real people and their real-life experiences. The philosophical positions and practical guidelines that shape the message of this book have been heavily battle-tested, scrutinized, refined, and finally approved by thousands of "Primal" enthusiasts (as well as skeptics) at MarksDailyApple.com.

You see, the *Primal Blueprint* is more than just a book. It's the centerpiece of a vibrant community of people connected by the Internet and committed to living their lives to the fullest potential, challenging the status quo, and trying something *old*. I encourage you to participate at MarksDailyApple.com. Share your experiences with the program and connect with an audience that can relate to you in a way that goes beyond what a book or even a paid trainer can offer. Every day, I augment the foundation of the *Primal Blueprint* with easy-to-read, hard-hitting but lighthearted commentary on all manner of healthy lifestyle topics, including delicious recipes, workout tips and videos, evaluation of the latest research, and an extensive library of bite-sized inspiration and reminders to keep you eating, exercising, and living to your potential.

In this book, I detail a basic framework of diet, exercise, and lifestyle guidelines that you must observe to be successful. However, making the pieces fit comfortably into your own life is best left up to you. I strongly support you making allowances for, adjustments to, and occasional deviations from the *Primal Blueprint* based on your particular real-life concerns and constraints. You'll encounter many references to my *80% Rule* in the book (I detail the concept in this section's sidebar), which basically means you can chill out and enjoy your life rather than invite the additional stress and anxiety that comes from a perfectionist approach or an overly strict regimen. After all, our ancestors had to adjust constantly to their unpredictable environment and have given us the tools to do the same. That's the *Primal* part. The word *Blueprint* in the title connects us to the familiar analogy of construction plans that provide the foundation for action but are often altered during the actual construction project. A program that allows you to go with the flow frees you to listen more deeply to your own intuitive knowledge, which is far more expert than any outside resource.

The fact that you are in control will give you the most powerful source of motivation you can imagine—instant and ongoing direct feedback that the *Primal Blueprint* is working. No more exercising until exhaustion or obsessing about the arduous restrictions common to popular weight-loss programs. The *Primal Blueprint* is a way of life that is attainable for everyone, not just the socialites in Palm Beach or the gym rats in Venice Beach. It's time to pursue your own unique peak performance goals and enjoy your life to the absolute maximum, carrying on a tradition that humans have pursued for tens of thousands of years. Thank you for agreeing to take this journey with me. Let's have some fun and get Primal!

Mark Sisson
Malibu, CA
April 2009

P.S. The length of this book may intimidate you, and indeed extensive discussion was had about whether this book should be a more abbreviated overview of the 10 *Primal Blueprint* laws to kick-start lifestyle change. However, the 20-year journey that has resulted in this culmination of my Primal philosophy does not allow for any shortcuts. If you are not the type to hunker down and blitz through the entire book in a few sittings, you have the option to review the "In This Chapter" and "Chapter Summary" sections that precede and close each chapter, respectively, and dive into areas of particular interest to you. However, if you're like me, the more you read about our evolutionary history and our straying modern ways, the more you'll just want to go back to the beginning....

Striving For Perfection With the 80% Rule

I believe that if you are aligned with the *Primal Blueprint* 80% of the time, you will experience great success and likely build momentum toward being even more compliant, with less effort, as time proceeds. Since this admonition is potentially controversial ("Sisson offers a cop out!"), I'd like to further explain the spirit of the rule. Hopefully, you will feel comfortable with my approach, and - more importantly – with yours!

The 80% Rule is not a license to make less than a full commitment to the *Primal Blueprint* – that is, to strive for a "B" grade as your ultimate goal. As my kids have heard me say from time to time on the topic of schoolwork, "If you make a half-assed effort half the time, you'll get a quarter of results...and it will be twice as hard!" This is particularly true in the important example of moderating your intake of processed carbs and getting off the sugar high-sugar crash cycle that we will cover in great detail shortly. Even a couple of steps out onto a slippery slope aren't so easy to recover from!

Throughout the book, you will notice a fairly aggressive tone when I assert the risks that following Conventional Wisdom can pose to your health, and the urgency with which you must change your mentality and behavior to protect and nurture your health, fitness and overall well being by following the *Primal Blueprint*. What I suggest is that you strive for 100% success - total compliance for the *Primal Blueprint* guidelines and zero tolerance for the unhealthy foods, exercise and lifestyle habits that are prevalent today. With that in mind, please realize a couple of things:

- Many of the benefits of a strict and disciplined "healthy" lifestyle can be compromised by a perfectionist mentality.
- The forces of hectic daily life (cultural traditions, convenience and fast pace) will divert you from your ideal often, and that this is perfectly okay (just make smart adjustments!). Strive for 100% with the understanding that your efforts will probably get you to 80%.

I'm a big believer in enjoying life, and indeed this has been my overpowering inspiration for developing the *Primal Blueprint*. Remember that the program presented here was inspired in part by assorted dead ends and disappointments, such as my aforementioned experience with physically unhealthy endurance training and competition. My desire to enjoy more regulated energy levels, and eliminate symptoms of digestive distress and sub-par immune function was a driving force in my discovery and implementation of Primal-style eating. If the *Primal Blueprint* urged that you eat bugs and mud ten times a day, it might be emotionally and psychologically harmful, and therefore a bad idea – even if it were technically deemed "healthy" to your physical body.

The 80% Rule exists because I understand how difficult lifestyle change can be. I want you to make an honest and devoted effort, but I never want you to feel discouraged that you aren't measuring up to arbitrary standards created in your mind or by society. In the Conclusion, I discuss at length how process-oriented goals that emphasize effort and enjoyment of the experience are far healthier than the more common mentality of obsessing about results. Consider the familiar example of failed weight loss efforts triggering self-destructive eating habits. If millions of dieters altered their goals from losing weight at any cost (struggling, suffering, engaging in deprivation, restriction, and obsessive/compulsive calorie counting) to simply enjoying meals more by choosing healthy, great-tasting *Primal Blueprint* foods, and not stressing about portion sizes, regimented meal guidelines, or what the scale says every day, success rates would skyrocket. I think legendary basketball coach John Wooden captured the spirit of the 80% Rule well with this quote: "Perfection is impossible. However, *striving* for perfection is not. Do the best you can under the conditions that exist. That is what counts."

> *Perfection is impossible. However,* **striving** *for perfection is not. Do the best you can under the conditions that exist. That is what counts."*
> —**John Wooden**

INTRODUCTION

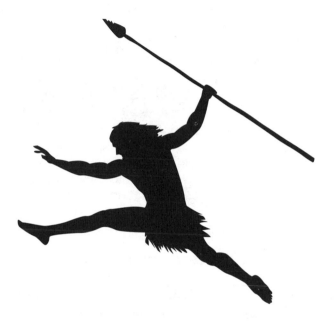

What Is Going On Here?

Conventional Wisdom vs. The Primal Blueprint

In the *Primal Blueprint* (PB), we will challenge and reframe these major elements of Conventional Wisdom (CW). Consider these alternatives with an open mind; we will discuss each in detail throughout the text.

Grains – wheat, rice, corn, bread, cereal, pasta, etc.

 CW: "Staff of Life" – foundation of healthy diet. 6-11 daily servings recommended by US Government and numerous other experts. Provides main source of energy for working muscles. Choose whole grains for more nutritional value, and extra fiber.

 PB: "Worst mistake in the history of the human race" (UCLA evolutionary biologist Jared Diamond). Drives excess insulin production, fat storage, and heart disease. Allergenic, immune-suppressing, nutritional value inferior to plants and animals. Whole grains possibly worse due to offensive pro-inflammatory, immune and digestive system disturbing agents – especially excessive fiber.

Saturated Animal Fat

CW: Limit intake. Heart disease risk factor. "Eating fat makes you fat." Replace saturated fats (meat, lard, dairy) with PUFA's (polyunsaturated fatty acids) like vegetable oils.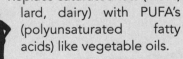

 PB: Little or no association with heart disease risk. (Framingham and Nurses Health studies). Should be major dietary calorie source (from animal foods). Drove human evolution/advancement of brain function for two million years. Promotes efficient fat metabolism, weight control and stable energy levels. Major risk factor for heart disease is actually Metabolic Syndrome, driven by excess PUFA's/insufficient Omega-3's, high carbs/excess insulin and overly stressful lifestyle.

Cholesterol

CW: Strictly limit intake. Elevated levels = elevated heart disease risk. Take statin drugs and eliminate animal foods (especially eggs) 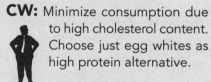 if total is 200 or over. Consider pre-emptive statin therapy if family history of heart disease.

PB: Essential metabolic nutrient, little or no relevance to heart disease risk (Framingham and Nurses Health Studies). Only dangerous when oxidation and inflammation occur (from poor diet and exercise habits). Statins can have disastrous side effects and minimal, if any, direct benefit.

Eggs

CW: Minimize consumption due to high cholesterol content. Choose just egg whites as high protein alternative.

PB: Zero correlation with heart disease or cholesterol levels. Yolk extremely nutritious, whites minimally so. Enjoy in abundance.

Fiber

CW: Important dietary goal, derive mostly from grains. Improves gastrointestinal function, lowers cholesterol, speeds elimination, helps control weight by minimizing caloric intake.

PB: Incidental fiber from vegetables and fruit is optimum. Excess fiber (from grain-based diet) contributes to nutrient deficiency by inhibiting nutrient absorption. Also hampers gastrointestinal function and elimination.

Meal Habits

CW: Three squares (or six small meals) daily to "keep flame burning". Skipped meals = slowed metabolism, lower energy levels, sugar cravings and future binging risk.

PB: Eating frequency is a personal preference, but *it's all about insulin*: control production and even sporadic eating habits will sustain energy without regular meals (it's in our genes!). Intermittent Fasting is a great catalyst for weight loss.

continued

Cardio Workouts

CW: Centerpiece of fitness program. Promotes cardiovascular health and weight control, minimizes heart disease and cancer risk. Minimum 30 minutes, three times per week (but more is better) of sustained efforts in medium to difficult intensity zones (happens by default - keeping up with class/ group or trying to jog instead of walk).

PB: Frequent medium to difficult sustained efforts (aka "Chronic Cardio") = overstress, fatigue, burnout, injury, accelerated aging, and increased disease risk. Ineffective for weight loss: calories burned through Chronic Cardio simply increase appetite, particularly for sugar. Slow down for better health and peak performance!

Strength Training

CW: Focus on form and deliberate work/return rhythm. Lift to failure in sequence through numerous stations (takes about an hour for a complete workout), includ- ing isolating body parts to get desired size, toning and "cuts".

PB: Emphasize explosive movements over deliberate pace. Conduct full body, functional exercises to de- velop *Primal Fitness* (broad athletic competence with optimal strength-to-weight ratio). Finish most sessions in 30 minutes or less. Occasional "Primal" max efforts (including sprints) promote optimal gene expression, hormone flow and organ function = delay of aging process.

Weight Loss

CW: Achieve with high complex carb/low fat diet, regimented meals, portion control and Chronic Cardio exercise program. Severe calorie restriction coupled with overly stressful exercise effective for those "fit into the dress by June" emergencies. Bottom Line: It's all about "calories in, calories out"…and lucky genes!

PB: Driven by high fat/moderate protein/low carb diet, intuitive, sporadic meals, and exercise and Primal Exercise Laws. Don't worry about portion control, regimented meals, fanatical exercise or even family genetic predisposition. Calorie restriction with extreme exercise leads inexorably to long-term failure. Bottom line: *It's all about insulin* to enjoy effortless lifelong weight control.

Play

CW: Ah, brings back fond memories of childhood. Who has time these days?

PB: Outdoor, active, unstructured fun is an integral component of overall health and balanced lifestyle, and scientifically proven to increase work productivity.

Sunlight

CW: Avoid the sun to prevent skin cancer! Lather up with SPF 20, 30, 40, 50 – all you got!

PB: Get adequate sun to avoid skin (and other) cancers! Vitamin D synthesis promotes healthy cellular function. Cover up with clothing, find shade or go inside after sufficient daily exposure is achieved.

continued

Prescription Drugs

CW: Relieve pain, speed healing, prevent/cure disease, and address genetic frailties. Everyday use can enhance quality of life (Viagra, etc.).

PB: Mask/exacerbate underlying causes, compromise homeostasis and thus health, and produce disastrous side-effects. Simple lifestyle changes can replace vast majority of pills. Wonderful in case of emergencies only!

Footwear

CW: Sturdy, cushioned shoes minimize injury, improve comfort. Custom orthotics can provide additional support and protection.

PB: Get Primal - go barefoot! Perpetual use of "big" shoes weaken feet, increase injury risk and increase pain throughout lower extremities.

Goals

CW: Be specific and measurable. Helps you stay motivated and focused. "Consistency is key". Missed workouts = guilt, weight gain, and lost fitness.

PB: De-emphasize specific, results-oriented goals (potential to discourage – a la weight loss failure or "post-marathon blues"). Stay motivated by focusing on fun, and release attachment to outcome. Consistency = over-stress. Vary routine to minimize stress and improve adaptive response by genes. Missed workouts drive recovery, improvement and freshness.

Americans will always do the right thing—after they've exhausted all the alternatives.
—**Winston Churchill**

I'm going to ask you to forget most everything you thought you knew about diet, exercise, and health. There is a distressing amount of *flawed Conventional Wisdom* that confuses, misleads, manipulates, and complicates even the most devoted efforts to do the right thing: eat healthfully, exercise effectively, control weight, and avoid today's incredibly common health conditions like obesity, arthritis, indigestion, insomnia, diabetes, heart disease, and cancer.

In the *Primal Blueprint*, you will learn why eating a low-fat diet rich in grains like wheat, rice, bread, pasta, and cereal can easily make you fat and malnourished. You'll learn why millions of joggers and gym-goers put in the time and effort to lose weight yet routinely compromise their health and accelerate the aging process as a direct result of their devotion to fitness. You'll learn why cholesterol level and saturated fat intake are *not* the major risk factors for heart disease that we have been led to believe and why a relatively high-fat diet promotes health and longevity. I'll show how weight loss does not have to involve the suffering, sacrifice, and deprivation we've been conditioned to accept but instead is a matter of eating the right foods (plants and animals), avoiding the wrong foods (processed carbs—including grains—and trans and partially hydrogenated fats), and exercising strategically, for far fewer hours than you might assume, to reach your desired fitness goals.

All the answers are found in a set of 10 simple, logical diet, exercise, and lifestyle behaviors that I call the *Primal Blueprint*. Modeling your 21st-century life after our primal hunter-gatherer ancestors will help you greatly reduce or eliminate almost all of the disease risk factors that you may falsely blame on genes you inherited from your parents. Unfortunately, too many of us narrowly define genes as largely unalterable inherited traits—height, body type, eye color, physical or intellectual abilities, and "family history" health conditions and diseases. While some genes are indeed responsible for traits that are largely unaffected by lifestyle, many more play a bigger role in your health than you might realize. As coming chapters explain in detail, your genes—guided by what you eat, how you move, and even how you think—are the traffic cops that direct the functioning of every single cell in your body, every moment of every day.

Whatever you throw at them, your genes are going to respond in an effort to promote survival and, beyond that, homeostasis (the balanced and synchronistic

> *Instead of falling victim to your genetic vulnerabilities, you can control how your genes express themselves in constantly rebuilding, repairing, and renewing your cells.*

functioning of all systems in the body). After all, this is the essence of human evolution. From a philosophical perspective, the *Primal Blueprint* does not presume to declare a right versus wrong way to live your life. Your body will still valiantly pursue homeostasis and survival when you sit on the couch downing Cheetos and Dr. Pepper. I am merely presenting the steps you can take to reprogram your genes to trigger *desirable gene expression* and achieve—as the cover suggests—"effortless weight loss, vibrant health, and boundless energy." By following the *Primal Blueprint* laws, you can be the best that your genes allow you to be. What better definition of *vibrant health* is there?

The idea that we can reprogram our genes through lifestyle behavior constitutes the central premise of this book. It also represents a clear departure from today's fatalistic Conventional Wisdom, which suggests that our genes, for better or worse, determine our destiny and that we have little say in the matter...unless prescription drugs or the Human Genome Project can come to the rescue. True, you might have a genetic tendency toward accumulating excess body fat or a family history of type 2 diabetes, but you'll be more likely to see these traits expressed when you make poor lifestyle choices and send the wrong signals to your genes. Instead of falling victim to your genetic vulnerabilities, you can control how your genes express themselves in constantly rebuilding, repairing, and renewing your cells. Briefly, here are the most critical, life-altering elements of the *Primal Blueprint*:

Ramp Up Your Fat Metabolism by eliminating processed carbohydrates from your diet to minimize your body's insulin production. This means eliminating not only sugars and sweets but grain products, including wheat, rice, pasta, and corn (yep, corn is a grain, not a vegetable). A diet that emphasizes meat, fish, fowl, nuts, seeds, and colorful natural carbs, such as vegetables and fruits, is the primary way to improve your general health, control your weight, and minimize risk of heart disease, cancer, diabetes, arthritis, and other diet-influenced medical conditions. If you are carrying excess body fat, it will disappear virtually effortlessly when you focus on eating the delicious, filling, nutritious foods that have sustained humans throughout the course of evolution for two million years.

Optimize Your Exercise Program by engaging in a genetically desirable blend of frequent, low-intensity energizing movement (walking, hiking, easy cardio), regular short, intense strength-training sessions, and occasional all-out sprints that help improve body composition and delay the aging process. This strategy is far superior to the Conventional Wisdom approach of following a consistent schedule of frequent medium-to-high–intensity sustained workouts, such as jogging, running, or cycling; cardio machines; or group classes. That workout plan—which I refer to derisively as *Chronic*

Cardio—places excessive and prolonged physical stress on your body, which inevitably leads to fatigue, injuries, compromised immune function, and burnout. Sometimes, less really is more.

Manage Stress Levels with plenty of sleep, play, sunlight, fresh air, and creative outlets and by avoiding trauma that often arises from stupid mistakes. Rebel against the tremendous cultural momentum toward sedentary lifestyles, excessive digital stimulation, and insufficient rest. Honor your primal genes by slowing down and simplifying your life. Your ancestors worked hard to survive, but their regular respites from stress gave them the peace of mind and body that are so highly coveted today.

Is Dying of Old Age Getting Old?

As you will soon discover, our genes were not only designed through evolution to keep us healthy, but they desperately *want* us to be healthy. Today, with the hectic pace of the high-tech modern world, we struggle with how to do the right thing by our genes. The ensuing failure creates a level of frustration and confusion that causes many of us, whether overtly or deep down inside, simply to give up. Experience teaches us how difficult it is, if not impossible, to be lean, fit, energetic, and healthy following Conventional Wisdom. Instead, we succumb to the forces of consumerism designed to placate our pain with silly shortcuts, comforts, conveniences, and indulgences. Consequently, the popular "Hey man, life is short!" rationalization becomes a self-fulfilling prophecy.

The consequences of eating processed foods, exercising excessively (or, conversely, being inactive), and making poor lifestyle decisions work in concert against our genetic mandate for health. At the very least, we can experience excess body fat storage, subpar fitness results, aching joints, gastrointestinal problems, frequent minor illnesses, sugar cravings, energy level swings, and recurring fatigue. Sounds bad enough as it is, but continuing to mismanage your genes with bad choices over years and decades will likely result in obesity, diabetes, heart disease, cancer, and/or the vast majority of degenerative conditions requiring a doctor's care or medication. A huge percentage of all doctor visits today are a direct consequence of lifestyle choices that are misaligned with the environmental and survival conditions that shaped our primal genetic makeup.

These consequences are painfully obvious to most everyone, and our collective interest in doing the right thing has driven a booming fitness industry, incredible advancements in medicine, much greater awareness of healthy foods and lifestyle choices, sharp declines in smoking, and sharp increases in restaurants offering salad bars and smoothies. Ironically though, the collective health of America—and other Western countries that have adopted our fast-paced culture—is worse than ever. A study released in 2008 by Johns Hopkins University suggests that by the year 2030, 86 percent of all

> *Physician and author Dr. Deepak Chopra asserts that organs and tissues have the ability to last 115 to 130 years before they fail due to aging.*

adults in the United States will be overweight or obese (up from the current estimate of 65 percent); what's more, a National Institutes of Health conference report stated that "our trends predict that *all* Americans will be obese by 2230!"

We reluctantly accept as fact that the normal human life span consists of growing up to reach a physical peak in your early 20s, followed by an inevitable steady decline caused by the aging process. Under this faulty assumption, we allow ourselves to gain an average of one and a half pounds of fat per year starting at age 25 and continuing through age 55[1] (we also lose half a pound of muscle per year, resulting in adding a pound a year in the wrong places as we age). Our last decade or two (until we reach the average life span of about 78 years)[2] is usually characterized by inactivity, excess body fat, assorted medical conditions, and a host of prescription drugs to alleviate the pain and symptoms of chronic disease. Twenty-seven percent of us will die from cardiovascular disease, and another 23 percent will die from cancer.[3]

I know that 100 percent of us will die from something, but personally, I'd prefer dying from old age. Physician and author Dr. Deepak Chopra estimates that perhaps only 1 percent of us will check this box when we check out and further asserts that organs and tissues have the ability to last 115 to 130 years before they fail due to aging. Of the one trillion dollars America spends annually on health care, the Centers for Disease Control and Prevention (CDC) estimates that 70 percent of that is spent on lifestyle-related chronic diseases, such as obesity, diabetes, and heart disease. A surprising number of people accept all this as a normal part of life, believing that some of us are just fortunate to have "good genes" and the rest must cross their fingers against bad luck.

Sure, millions of modern citizens contributing to these woeful statistics are completely disconnected from what's required to be healthy. It might be hard for you even to relate to this segment of humanity that hasn't a clue. However, even the most health conscious among us often struggle. Despite a sincere commitment to do the right thing by Conventional Wisdom, we have experienced widespread failure to lose that last 5, 10, or 50 pounds. Injuries, fatigue, and burnout plague exercisers ranging from weekend warriors to professionals. We reflexively turn to prescription drugs to treat symptoms of distress, even though most conditions are minor and easily corrected by simple dietary and lifestyle changes. In the process, we interfere with normal gene-driven metabolic processes and thwart our innate ability to heal naturally—paving the way to one day join the masses on the wrong side of the stats.

The story is sad, but the good news is that your destiny for the most part is in your hands. By the time you complete this book, you will understand the big picture and all the necessary details of how to eat, exercise, and live in order to reprogram many of your genes to favor optimal gene expression. In the process, you will take control of your own body and your own life. This is really the only sensible way to counter the tremendous momentum pushing us away from health, balance, and well-being in our hectic modern world.

Be Like Mike—Your Genes Don't Have To Be Your Destiny

If I pop off at this point in the journey and say something like, "It follows that a condition like arthritis is mainly caused by bad diet and insufficient exercise," I might get a predictable comeback like, "Actually, Mark, rheumatoid arthritis runs in my family. My mother and grandmother both suffered from it." This type of family lore passed through the generations does have a measure of truth to it—you may indeed be predisposed to arthritis, breast cancer, or other conditions that have strong genetic influences. However, it is more likely that some of your lifestyle choices (perhaps learned from your parents) have programmed your genes to respond in unfavorable ways, rather than some unseen hand of fate slapping you simply because you "chose your parents" unwisely.

We now know that you have far more influence on how your genes shape and mold you than anyone believed possible as recently as a decade ago. Accepting this reality might just turn a potential genetic nightmare into the best thing that ever happened to you. A heightened awareness of elevated genetic risk for heart disease, diabetes, or cancer has inspired many to take an alternate route and forever avoid these undesirable "fates."

Researchers from the Max Planck Institute of Evolutionary Biology in Germany studied height variations among different hunter-gatherer cultures and discovered that body size can be related directly to population density; those living in large settlements are smaller than those living in wide open tundra, savanna, or desert regions. Combine this finding with the extensive research confirming that differences in nutrition can influence height, and it's clear that lifestyle factors can significantly affect things that we generally believe to be hard wired. Evidence from identical twins raised apart with disparate lifestyle practices, and enjoying consequently varied levels of health, casts further doubt on the "genetic destiny" school of thought. A recent intensive study of identical twins concluded that poor diet and lack of exercise were far greater predictors of which ones would get diabetes than was heredity.

Experts in quantum physics and epigenetics are going even further, taking the buzz phrase "mind-body connection" out of woo woo land and into mainstream science. Dr. Bruce Lipton, Ph.D., a cell biologist, a medical school professor, and author of the acclaimed *The Biology of Belief*, leads a burgeoning field of scientific study (coined "new

continued

biology") asserting that our DNA is controlled by signals from outside our cells, *"including the energetic messages emanating from our thoughts."*

Certainly, depression is known to suppress immune function via hormones arising from negative thoughts. Is it preposterous to consider a basketball player growing to six feet six inches (even though his two brothers and father did not reach six feet), simply because he spent so much time and energy focused on being a basketball player—and needing to be tall—that he essentially willed himself to grow? Lipton would argue that it's not only possible, but that comparable things happen, in one form or another, to each of us. Basketball legend Michael Jordan might also be amused with the question, because these facts are from his family. After being famously cut from his high school varsity team as a sophomore, he sprouted four inches in a single summer!

Surely you can relate to people who, without a second thought, blame a life of health problems and excess weight on genes. And surely we can all reference people with happy, positive dispositions who in turn seem to have more energy, less illness, and better health than average. Lipton declares, "It has been statistically established that one third of all medical healings (including surgery) are derived from the placebo effect as opposed to intervention....We have all been endowed with an innate healing ability that has been with us since the evolution of our species...."

> *Genes (good or bad) + bad attitude + bad lifestyle behaviors = bad news.*
>
> *Genes (good or bad) + good attitude + good lifestyle behaviors = good news.*
>
> *Your genes don't have to be your destiny!*

Chapter Endnotes

[1] *Physiology of Sport and Exercise*, by Dr. David Costill and Jack Wilmore.

[2] The Central Intelligence Agency's World Factbook reports that the 2008 U.S. overall life expectancy at birth is 78 (75 for males; 81 for females).

[3] The 2008 American Heart Association "Heart Disease and Stroke Statistics," available for download at americanheart.org, reported that in 2004, 869,000 deaths were attributed to heart disease and 550,000 to cancer. 2005 CDC stats indicate the percentage references, but recent headlines suggest cancer has surpassed heart disease as the number one killer. cdc.gov/nchs/data/nvsr/nvsr56/nvsr56_10.pdf

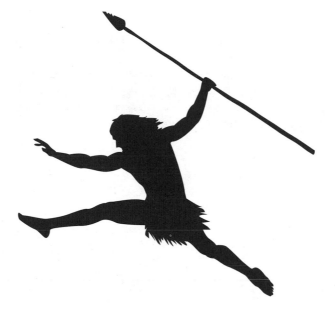

CHAPTER 1

The Ten Primal Blueprint Laws

("Commandments" Was Already Taken)

In This Chapter

I introduce the "re:evolutionary" premise that we should model our diet, exercise, and lifestyle behaviors after our primal ancestors from 10,000 years ago, adapting them strategically to the realities of high-tech modern life. The inexorable technological progress of civilization has led us ever farther astray from the dietary habits and active, stress-balanced lifestyles that allowed our ancestors to prevail under the harsh competitive circumstances of evolution. However, we are genetically identical (in virtually all respects relevant to human health) to our hunter-gatherer ancestors, owing to the fact that evolution ground to a halt when the major selection pressures of starvation and predator danger (eat or get eaten!) were eliminated. Thus, we can achieve effortless weight loss, vibrant health, and boundless energy by living according to the *Primal Blueprint*.

Genes are more than just the largely inalterable inherited traits that we typically associate the term with. They are the traffic cops that direct the function of all the cells in your body, at all times. The central premise of this book is that your genes don't have to be your destiny, that you can "reprogram" them with healthy lifestyle behaviors and thereby make even strong genetic predispositions to disease, excess body fat, and other adverse health conditions irrelevant.

The 10 *Primal Blueprint* laws are:
1. Eat Lots of Plants and Animals
2. Avoid Poisonous Things
3. Move Frequently at a Slow Pace
4. Lift Heavy Things
5. Sprint Once in a While
6. Get Adequate Sleep
7. Play
8. Get Adequate Sunlight
9. Avoid Stupid Mistakes
10. Use Your Brain

Nothing in biology makes sense except in the light of evolution.
— **Theodosius Dobzhansky**

The quote by Dobzhansky was also the title of a famous 1973 essay in which the noted evolutionary biologist and devout Russian Orthodox Christian acknowledged that, whether or not you believed in the existence of a higher power, you could not begin to understand even the simplest concepts in biology unless you understood how evolution had worked to shape and differentiate the genes of every single one of the several million species on the planet.

Within the past hundred years, tens of thousands of anthropologists, evolutionary biologists, paleontologists, epigeneticists, and other scientists have worked diligently to piece together a fairly detailed interpretation of the environmental and behavioral factors that directly influenced our development as a species. As a result, we now have a very good picture of the conditions under which we emerged as *Homo sapiens*.

Some seven million years ago, hominids (our prehuman ancestors) split from apes and branched out into various new species. Then, about two million years ago, the humanlike species *Homo erectus* began to take charge of the food chain with their large brains, upright stature, skilled use of tools and fire, and organized hunter-gatherer societies. Over time, *Homo erectus* branched into various species and subspecies (*Homo neanderthaensis*, *Homo habilis*, *Homo sapiens*, and others). Most researchers believe that the modern *Homo sapiens* species evolved in Africa between 200,000 and 100,000 years ago, prevailing over all other *Homo erectus* subspecies. Then, about 60,000 years ago, a small number of modern humans left Africa and began their great migration across the planet. Recent archaeological findings strongly support this "out of Africa"[1] theory: that the entire human population of the planet, amazingly, can trace their origins to a small pool of intrepid *Homo sapiens* in Africa. There were only an estimated 2,000 to 5,000 African humans at that time, and some scientists believe that only about 150 people crossed the Red Sea to begin the migration. Talk about six degrees of separation!

"Are We Not Men? We Are Devo!" (Devo album cover, 1978)

I hope you are sitting down to absorb one of the most critical—and quite possibly mind-blowing—tenets of the *Primal Blueprint*:

*Our primal ancestors were likely stronger
and healthier than we are today.*

"How can this be?" you ask. It's all about survival of the fittest. The human body is the miraculous result of millions of years of painstaking design by evolution. Through natural selection involving countless small genetic mutations and adaptations in response to a hostile environment, our ancestors were able to prevail over unimaginably difficult conditions and opponents and populate all corners of the earth.

Many anthropologists suggest that the human species reached its evolutionary pinnacle (in terms of average muscularity, bone density, and brain size) about 10,000 years ago. After that, we started to take it easy and get soft. Our physical decline was a natural consequence of a couple of things. First, we had already spent thousands of generations leveraging our increasingly proficient brain function to manipulate and tame the natural environment (with tools, weapons, fire, and shelter) to our advantage. The second factor was perhaps the most significant lifestyle change in the history of humanity: the gradual advent of agriculture. When humans began to domesticate and harvest wheat, rice, corn, and other crops as well as livestock (this happened independently around the globe, beginning about 10,000 years ago in the Mediterranean Fertile Crescent; North America was one of the last areas to adopt agriculture, about 4,500 years ago),[2] the ability to store food, divide and specialize labor, and live in close civilized quarters eliminated the main selection pressures that had driven human evolution for two million years—the threats of starvation and predator danger captured in the familiar term *survival of the fittest*.

> *The development of agriculture and civilization caused humans to become smaller and sicker, leading to a dramatic decline in life expectancy.*

When humans no longer faced these constant selection pressures, evolution essentially ground to a halt in conjunction with the flourishing of civilization. Consequently, many researchers assert that today we are genetically identical to our primal ancestors (at least for our purposes here, relating to human health; I'll explain more later and also in the *Primal Blueprint* Q&A appendix at MarksDailyApple.com). This idea that human DNA—the genetic "recipe" for building a healthy, lean, thriving human that resides in each of our 60 trillion cells—is almost exactly the same today as it was 10,000 years ago has been most notably promoted by the work of Dr. Boyd Eaton, chief anthropologist at Emory University in Atlanta and author of *The Paleolithic Prescription*, and the late James V. Neel, founder of the University of Michigan's Department of Genetics, and supported by hundreds of other leading anthropologists, evolutionary biologists, and genetic researchers.

While our primal ancestors made the most of their genes (remember, they had no choice; the alternative was to starve or become some other creature's dinner!), we have fallen far short. The development of agriculture and civilization caused humans to become smaller (including our brain size) and sicker (originally due to contagious diseases and other repercussions of civilization). Today, our inferior diet, exercise and lifestyle behaviors are what diminish our quality and span of life.

Human life expectancy 10,000 years ago was about 33 years. While not too impressive by 21st-century standards, primal man actually lived longer than his civilized successors all the way into the early 20th century! Average life expectancy reached a low of 18 during the Bronze Age (~3300–1200 B.C., Ancient Egypt, etc.), rose only slightly to a range of 20-30 through Classical Greek (~500-300 B.C.) times, the Roman Empire (~0-500 A.D.), and the Middle Ages (~700-1500), and was still only between 30 and 40 as late as the early 20th Century. Around that time, medical advancements (antibiotics, hospital and community sanitation, decreased infant mortality rates, etc.) helped life expectancy skyrocket.

What's more, fossil records show that primal humans who could steer clear of fatal misfortune could enjoy long lives of excellent health and fitness (that's cool for us; for them it was a necessity). Remarkably, some could live to be as old as 94![3] Among present-day hunter-gatherers (e.g., Ache, Hadza, Hiwi, and !Kung—groups that have almost no modern conveniences or medical care) it is not uncommon to see strong, healthy folks living well into their 80s. More than a quarter of the Ache people of Paraguay make it to 70. Moreover, 73 percent of Ache adults die from accidents and only 17 percent from illness. Think about the extraordinary implications of hunter-gatherer longevity: with no medications or medical care of any

> *The human species reached its evolutionary pinnacle about 10,000 years ago. After that, we started to take it easy and get soft.... Hence, the Ultimate Human award goes to **Grok,** my nickname for the prototypical preagricultural human being.*

kind, a massive lifelong struggle for food, clothing, and shelter completely devoid of any modern comforts, primal humans (and modern humans living primally) can still live to what even us softies consider old age. Obviously, they're doing a lot of things right!

Of course, the civilization-driven decline in life expectancy didn't matter in a pure evolutionary context. As long as civilized humans made it to reproductive age and had children, they could pass their genes along to the next generation without penalty. No one will argue that moving beyond survival of the fittest is a bad thing, but the sober reality is that today's technological age is enjoyed by the fattest, laziest humans in the history of humanity. Hence, the Ultimate Human award goes to *Grok*, my nickname for the prototypical preagricultural human being. Grok[4] is the central character of both this book and my blog. He's a lean, strong, healthy, character whom you will grow to love.

Unlike Grok, who ruled the planet with little more than a spear and a thatched hut in his portfolio, even the most impoverished humans of the last several thousand years, extending up to the present day's Third World inhabitants, have not really "competed" genetically. The presence of the most rudimentary modern influences, such as grain consumption, food storage, permanent shelters, and basic firearms and other weapons, all suppress the true Darwinian survival of the fittest playing field that allowed Grok to thrive. Sure, being a math whiz or a natural athlete may significantly influence your path through life and give you a competitive edge in pursuits to which you are inclined, but these genetic attributes no longer provide a survival advantage in the evolutionary sense. Tour de France legend Lance Armstrong has a genetically superior cardiovascular system, but he could have easily cruised through life as a candy-chomping, video-gaming fat kid and still have reproduced successfully (although he would have had much less chance of flying in private jets or palling around with rock stars and world leaders...) due to lack of selection pressure for human endurance in the modern world.

In fact, considering all the comforts and medical advancements of modern life, we could easily argue that we currently exist in a state of *devolution*. For the most part, this is great (many of us have suffered illnesses or traumas over the course of our lives that would have killed us a century ago, let alone 1,000 or 10,000 years ago). However, we must be vigilant not to let the advantages of modern life compromise our health (e.g., hitting the pharmacy instead of the gym to address your back pain).

The virtual halting of evolution means that each and every human living today is still subject to the same evolutionary-based laws for healthy living that drove the original design process of Grok. The challenge is in applying the *Primal Blueprint* laws to modern life. How do we leverage the lessons and benefits of natural selection against the pressures of a complex modern society bent on promoting consumerism and quick fixes over the pursuit of health? How do we reprogram our ancient genes to recapture excellent health? We simply have to ask ourselves, "What would Grok do?"

A SNiPpet About Evolution

Contrary to the *Primal Blueprint* assumptions, you might have read articles suggesting that humans are continuing to evolve. It appears from all the research that, yes, based on sheer population numbers and cultural interbreeding, there have been far more random mutations (what scientists call *genetic drift*) in the human race over the past several thousand years than in equivalent years prior. Almost all of these minor differences (adult lactose tolerance in direct descendants of herders being one arguable exception) have had no impact on the basic ways we all metabolize food, respond to exercise, or otherwise deal with challenges of our environment. Obviously, when any animal population goes from a million worldwide 10,000 years ago to six and a half billion as we have today, the range of small nonlethal genetic differences will be significant. However, these differences are largely an artifact of an exploding population—not of natural selection or functional adaptations.

In fact, there are now thousands of documented traceable single nucleotide polymorphisms—SNPs (pronounced "snips")—proving how "different" we all are. SNPs are like minor spelling errors within the written instructions (nucleotides) of genes that quite often have little or no effect on the final protein product for which the gene encodes. But the mere existence of all those differences within our vast population doesn't mean we are "evolving" in the sense of moving in a better direction vis-à-vis either health or natural selection.

Part of what we are dealing with here is a semantic issue: how is the term *evolved* best used in the context of the *Primal Blueprint?* On the one hand, *evolution* can mean "the changes seen in the inherited traits from one generation to the next"—pretty simple. On the other hand, most anthropologists discuss evolution in the more Darwinian context of "favorable heritable traits that become more common in successive generations of a population while unfavorable traits are selected out." I look at evolution in terms of how natural selection acted on our ancestors to favor the strong and healthy and weed out the sick, weak, or unfit. But as mentioned earlier, when you remove the primary selection pressures (with unlimited calories, shelter, vaccines, and antibiotics), suddenly anyone who can reach puberty and procreate has "evolved" successfully, even if later years are full of discomforts and disease. This is important, for it means that any and almost all nonfatal products of random mutation or genetic drift (i.e., SNPs) are incorporated into the genome without penalty—and passed on to the next generation.

Many of the recent reports on so-called accelerated evolution suggest that more harmful SNPs than beneficial ones are appearing. As a result, we have a litany of documented SNPs that predict greater risk for certain diseases. You can even spend $3,000 and have a test that identifies many of your risky SNPs. But having these slight genetic "misspellings" doesn't guarantee that the possessor will get a particular disease. All that happens is that the possibility increases somewhat that if you don't play your cards

continued

right, you might develop the condition. Worse yet, some geneticists have suggested recently that your lifestyle behaviors could adversely affect future generations (e.g., transferring a predisposition for obesity to your offspring thanks to a maladaptive grain-based diet).

I suppose one could argue that we are in a midadaptation phase in our evolution toward withstanding processed carbohydrate intake or inactivity. However, because we haven't fully adapted, we still suffer from the ill effects (some people are affected far more than others, but all are affected negatively in some way). Presumably, we could wait another thousand generations to see if we fully adapt to overemphasizing sugars and grains, but I don't wish to be sick and fat in the meanwhile. I say, when in doubt, adhere to the same type of diet and lifestyle (environment) that surrounded the original design process of Grok—the *Primal Blueprint!*

You Have to Fit Your Genes to Fit into Your Jeans

In order to begin to understand the concept of reprogramming your genes, it will help to understand what they actually are and how they work. Each of your 50 or 60 trillion cells contains a nucleus with a complete set of DNA instructions divided into handy subsets called genes. There are approximately 20,000 different genes located on the long strands of DNA in each cell. These DNA strands are further organized into 23 pairs of chromosomes with which you may be familiar. In any given cell, only a small fraction of the total number of genes is actively involved in carrying out the main "business" of that particular type of cell. Depending on environmental signals, genes trigger the manufacture of certain specific proteins and enzymes to perform the various tasks required of them. For example, the beta cells in your pancreas manufacture insulin but don't grow bigger when you lift weights, and liver cells can synthesize nutrients, but they don't grow new bone tissue. And yet each cell has the entire "recipe" for a human residing on the DNA.

> *Genes don't know—or care—whether these environmental signals promote or compromise your health; they simply react to each stimulus in an effort to promote your immediate survival.*

Perhaps the most important thing to understand is that genes are not self-determining. They do not turn on or off by themselves but do so only in response to signals they receive from their immediate environment. It's as if they are programmed by the environment to respond accordingly. As we begin to talk about reprogramming your genes, you will begin to understand the power you have to influence certain genes to turn on and others to turn off.

Genes actively control cell function all the time, so the overall health and survival of your body is primarily dependent on which genes get turned on or off in response to their immediate environment. Genes don't know—or care—whether these environmental signals promote or compromise your long-term health; they simply react to each stimulus in an effort to sustain your short-term survival, as they have been designed to do by evolution and molded by the precise behaviors of our ancestors. Sprint or lift weights, and the biochemical "by-products" from that specific activity turn on certain genes that repair and strengthen the exercised muscle. Do too much exercise, and other genes promote excessive production of catabolic hormones, leading to prolonged inflammation and hindered recovery. An allergic reaction represents your body's (misdirected) genetic response to a perceived airborne or ingested threat. An autoimmune disease is often a genetic overreaction of that same system caused by unfamiliar foods (see Chapter 5). Type 2 diabetes typically develops after prolonged periods when your genes are trying to protect you from the dangers of eating too many carbohydrates.

In a profound example our genes' ability to switch on and off, researchers studying the link between smoking and lung cancer have discovered that tobacco smoking causes *hypermethylation* (a complete or partial deactivation) of a single gene known as MTHFR. Turning off MTHFR triggers an opposite effect—*hypomethylation* (systemic dysfunction)—in many other genes, setting the stage for further cancer development.

The idea that the environment influences whether genes are turned on or off is not a new one. In 1942 geneticist and evolutionary biologist C. H. Waddington first coined the term *epigenetics* to describe how genes might interact with their surroundings to create a unique individual. Today the study of epigenetics is one of the fastest growing subdisciplines of genetics. Moreover, the burgeoning field of *nutrigenomics* has identified hundreds of ways that nutrients (foods or supplements) impact gene expression. You may be familiar with the direct influence folic acid has on reducing neural tube birth defects, which is why all pregnant women are advised to take supplemental folic acid. This is but one small example of the powerful influence diet can have on reprogramming genes.

An Australian study suggested that human genes are adversely affected by sugar ingestion for two weeks (genetic controls designed to protect the body against diabetes and heart disease are switched off as an acute reaction to eating sugar) and that prolonged poor eating can cause genetic damage that can potentially be passed through bloodlines! On an even grander scale, research shows that certain cells within the body called mesenchymal stem cells can become bone cells, fat cells, muscle cells, or even cancer cells in adults, depending upon the environmental signals they receive.

Clearly, your lifestyle behaviors can either destroy or support many aspects of your health and can often be far more relevant than inherited predispositions to allergies, di-

abetes, or even more serious conditions. Not to make light of the serious genetically influenced health challenges that many face over their lifetimes, I would argue that we are
all predisposed to heart disease, cancer, arthritis, and today's other leading lifestyle-related health problems if we mismanage our genes with the wrong diet, exercise, and
myriad other lifestyle behaviors.

Obviously, you cannot grow your kids seven feet tall simply by feeding them healthy
food and making sure they get plenty of sleep; we all have profound limitations in how
our genes can express our unique individual potential. For confirmation, just take a look
at the physical marvels in the Olympic 100 meter dash or on an NFL or NBA roster, col-
lections of the most physically gifted athletes on the planet. These athletes might be one
in a million genetically, but their specific behaviors have resulted in
optimal gene expression. The choices they have made—the foods they've eaten, how they've
trained, even how they've thought—have all helped them make the most of their natu-
ral-born talents to rise to the top of very competitive arenas. This is all you ought to be
concerned with—making the most of your own genetic recipe to enjoy a long life of excellent health and peak performance through the 10 *Primal Blueprint* laws.

The chapters that follow will explore in great detail the rationale, benefits, and practical suggestions for living according to the 10 simple *Primal Blueprint* laws. These laws
represent the specific behaviors that led directly (shaped by two million years of evolution) to the genetic recipe for a healthy, lean, fit, happy human being. Almost nothing
has changed in this recipe since preagricultural times—except the way we have unwit-
tingly chosen to program our genes for less-than-optimal health. By understanding how
these behavioral laws shaped our genome, we can reprogram our genes to express themselves in a direction of health. And when I say simple laws, I really mean it. If you read
just this following section and never opened the book
again, you'd have all the information you need to live
a long, healthy, disease-free life. Here then is a brief description of the laws of living 10,000 years ago and a
quick primer on how to adapt them to a healthy 21st-
century lifestyle.

> "*We are **all** predisposed
> to disease if we
> mismanage our genes.*"

Primal Blueprint Law #1: Eat Lots of Plants and Animals

 Plants and animals encompass everything our ancestors ate (from a huge list of individual foods) to get the protein, fats, carbohydrates, vitamins, minerals, antioxidants, phenols, fiber, water, and other nutrients necessary to sustain life, increase brain size, improve physical fitness, and support immune function. Ironically, the primal human diet differs greatly from what Conventional Wisdom recommends. Because the various diet camps passionately argue conflicting positions to a confused public, it's essential to reflect on how profoundly important and logically sound it is to model our diets after the diets of our ancestors, whose bodies evolved to survive, reproduce, and thrive on these foods. Talk about a lengthy and severely scrutinized (as in, "life or death") study protocol!

Primal humans across the globe ate widely varied diets due to environmental circumstances, such as climate, geography, seasons, and activity level. Notably, they also ate sporadically—mostly due to the lack of consistent availability of food (not a big issue in the developed world these days, eh?). Consequently, we became well adapted to store caloric energy (in the form of body fat, along with a little bit of muscle and liver glycogen) and burn it when dietary calories were scarce. You may be disturbed out about possessing the genetic trait to store extra food calories efficiently as fat. However, by simply eating the right kinds of foods, you can leverage this bank account "savings and withdrawal" mechanism to your advantage—maintaining ideal body fat levels and stabilizing daily appetite and energy levels. *Hint:* it's all about moderating your insulin production.

Today similar principles apply for healthy eating. Focus on quality sources of animal protein (organic, free-range, or wild sources of meat, fowl, and fish), an assortment of colorful vegetables and fresh fruits, and healthy sources of fat (nuts, seeds, their derivative butters, certain oils, avocados, etc.). Realize that a significant amount of Conventional Wisdom about healthy eating is marketing fodder that grossly distorts the fundamental truth that humans thrive on natural plant and animal foods or that relies on gimmicks to support dogma of questionable validity. For example, eating at particular intervals (three squares or six small meals a day), combining food types at meals, severely restricting certain nutrients, following purification or detox diets, getting colon cleanses, replacing meals with processed formulas, striving for specific calorie ratios, aligning food choices with your blood-type, or keeping score of your portions and weekly treat allowances are all gimmicks that have no credibility in the context of evolutionary biology.

Furthermore, regimented programs are virtually impossible to enjoy and stick to over the long term, because they run counter to human nature. We humans thrive on eating an ever-changing variety of natural foods that satisfy and nourish us, in times and amounts that fluctuate according to moods, environmental circumstances, activity level, and many other factors. I suggest you enjoy eating as one of the pleasures of life and reject everything you've ever heard mandating when and how much you should eat. Instead, eat when you are hungry and finish when you feel satisfied. Realize that natural foods are intrinsically the most delicious, because they satisfy your cravings and distinct tastes, stabilize mood and energy levels, and promote health and well-being.

Primal Blueprint Law #2: Avoid Poisonous Things

The ability of humans to exploit almost every corner of this earth was partly predicated on consuming vastly different types of plant and animal life. Primal humans developed a keen sense of smell and taste, along with liver, kidney, and stomach function, to adapt to new food sources and avoid succumbing to poisonous plants that they encountered routinely when foraging and settling new areas. For example, the reason we have a sweet tooth today is probably an evolved response to an almost universal truth in the plant world that anything that tastes sweet is safe to eat.

While we have little risk of ingesting poisonous plants on walkabouts today, the number of toxic agents in our food supply is worse than ever. By *toxic* I mean human-made products that are foreign to your genes and disturb the normal, healthy function of your body when ingested. The big offenders, including sugars and sodas, chemically altered fats, and heavily processed, packaged, fried, and preserved foods, are obvious.

What's less accepted and therefore more insidious as a dietary "poison" are processed grains (wheat and flour products, such as bread, pasta, crackers, snack foods, baked goods, etc., as well as rice, corn, cereals, etc.). You heard right—these staples of diets across the globe are generally inappropriate for human consumption for the simple reason that our digestive systems (and our genes) have not had ample time to adapt to both the unfamiliar protein structure of grains and the excessive carbohydrate load of all forms of cultivated grains, including even whole grains. Essentially, the advent of grains and civilization has eliminated the main thing that's made humans healthy: selection pressure to reach reproductive age—and to care for ourselves, and others, beyond!

Ingesting grains and other processed carbohydrates causes blood glucose levels to spike (both simple and complex carbs get converted into glucose—at differing rates—once they enter the body; we'll use the accurate term *blood glucose* to convey what many call *blood sugar*). This spike is a shock to our primal genes, which are accustomed to natural, slower-burning foods. Your pancreas compensates for this excess of glucose in the bloodstream (too much glucose is toxic to the body—hence the importance of timely insulin shots for diabetics) by secreting excessive levels of insulin. While insulin is an important hormone that delivers nutrients to muscle, liver, and fat cells for storage, excessive insulin released in the bloodstream causes glucose to be removed so rapidly and effectively that it can result in a "sugar crash": mental and physical lethargy and (because the brain relies heavily on glucose to fuel it) a strong craving for quick replacement energy in the form of more high-carbohydrate food. This leads to a vicious cycle of another ill-advised meal, another excessive insulin response, and another corresponding blood glucose decline.

Because insulin's job is to transport nutrients out of the bloodstream and into the muscle, liver, and fat cell storage depots, its excessive presence in the bloodstream inhibits the release of stored body fat for use as energy. Insulin's counterregulatory hormone, glucagon, accesses carbs, protein, and fat from your body's storage depots (muscle, liver, fat cells) and delivers them into the bloodstream for use as energy. When insulin is high, glucagon is low. You don't have fuel in your bloodstream, so your brain says, "Eat now! And make it something sweet so we can burn it immediately!" Unfortunately, the mobilization of stored body fat has been humans' preferred energy source (and weight-control device) for a couple of million years. It's as simple as this: you cannot reduce body fat on a diet that stimulates excessive—or even moderately excessive—levels of insulin production. Period.

> *The mobilization of stored body fat has been our preferred energy source (and weight-control device) for a couple of million years. It's as simple as this: you cannot reduce body fat on a diet that stimulates excessive levels of insulin production.*

Beyond the weight-loss frustrations, overstressing your insulin response system over years and decades can lead directly to devastating general system failure in the form of type 2 diabetes, obesity, cardiovascular disease (thanks to vascular inflammation, peripheral oxidative damage, and other insulin-related troubles we will learn more about later), and diet-related cancers. Chapter 5 will explain in detail that even whole grains (brown rice, whole wheat bread, etc.) are not particularly healthy, because they still trigger excessive insulin production and can interfere with mineral absorption as well as displace the far more nutritious plants and animals from being the caloric emphasis of your diet.

Primal Blueprint Law #3: Move Frequently at a Slow Pace

 Grok spent several hours each day moving about at what today's exercise physiologists might describe as a very low-level aerobic pace. He hunted, gathered, foraged, wandered, scouted, migrated, climbed, and crawled. This low-level activity prompted his genes to build a stronger capillary (blood vessel) network to provide oxygen and fuel to each muscle cell and readily convert stored fat into energy (fat is the main fuel used for low-level aerobic activity). His daily movement also helped develop strong bones, joints, and connective tissue. What Grok did not do was deplete his energy and muscle glycogen supply with sustained efforts that were even moderately taxing. This counterintuitive behavior could have left him vulnerable to a predator, starvation, or some other misfortune.

Today most of us either are too sedentary or conduct workouts that are too stressful and misaligned with our primal genetic requirements for optimum health. The exercise gospel for decades has been to pursue a consistent routine of aerobic exercise (jogging, cycling, cardio machines, group classes, or any other sustained effort), supposedly leading to more energy, better health, and weight control. However, too many lengthy workouts at elevated heart rates (between 75 percent and 95 percent of maximum) can put you at risk of exhaustion, burnout, injury, and illness. The high-carbohydrate diet required to perform these workouts day-in and day-out only adds to the problem. At the extreme—such as with the overtrained marathon runner or ironman triathlete—a commitment to fitness can actually accelerate the aging process.

Overexercising is a common scenario when you consider how our active population has such strong focus, dedication, and willpower to push through signs of fatigue. Our bodies are simply not adapted to benefit from chronic aerobic exercise at intense or even mildly uncomfortable heart rates nor to slog through exhausting circuits of resistance machines several days a week. The mild to severe difficulty of these Chronic Cardio or strength workouts overtaxes the stress response (commonly referred to as the fight-or-flight response) in your body. Here, your pituitary gland tells your adrenal glands to release cortisol into your bloodstream. Cortisol is a powerful stress hormone that is critical to a variety of physical functions and energy production. The spike of cortisol in the bloodstream from a stressful event increases respiration, heart rate, blood circulation, and mental focus and even converts muscle tissue into glucose for quick energy. This is a great example of how we abuse a system that was genetically designed to respond to emergencies, such as Grok facing a predator.

Even today the fight-or-flight response is highly desirable and effective in the face of true danger or peak performance stimulus, such as a modern Olympic athlete crouching in the starting blocks or an emergency worker summoning superhuman strength for a rescue effort. Unfortunately, when the stress response is triggered repeatedly (by the constant hectic pace of modern life coupled with workouts that are too long, too difficult, or too frequent), your adrenal glands can so overproduce cortisol that they eventually become fatigued and release less-than-normal levels of cortisol and other hormones critical to many aspects of health. Thyroid hormones and testosterone also decrease from prolonged stress, resulting in a decline in energy levels, loss of lean muscle tissue, a suppressed immune system, and the general condition best described as burnout.

The uplifting—but actually catabolic ("breakdown")—effect of cortisol in the bloodstream is the reason many people feel fantastic for about four to eight weeks following a severe exercise and diet program. Initially buoyed by the short-term performance-enhancing effect of high cortisol levels, they will typically crash and burn when the adrenals become exhausted by unrelenting stress. This "cortisol story" is an extremely important factor in balancing fitness with health (no, they are not the same!) and enjoying a long, disease-free life. I discuss the subject in further detail in many areas of the book and also in the Q&A at MarksDailyApple.com.

Regarding weight-loss goals, the notion of burning calories through chronic exercise to lose weight has proven to be flawed. Overexercising increases your appetite, particularly for quick energy carbs to address your chronic depletion of stored energy. This pattern of stressful exercise and extra eating results in a body fat stalemate—not a good return on investment for all that hard work!

What our genes truly crave is frequent movement at a slow, comfortable pace: walking, hiking, easy cycling, or other light aerobic activities with a heart rate range of 55 percent to no more than 75 percent of maximum. These efforts are far less taxing than the typical huffing and puffing, struggling and suffering exertion level that we've been conditioned to think leads to fitness. Find ways every day to move more often—walking (even across parking lots, instead of cruising for a close space; take the stairs instead of the elevator—it all adds up over a lifetime!), hiking, swimming, easy cycling, or anything else that moderately elevates heart rate. Strive to accumulate two to five hours per week of low-level exercise. More is better as long as you have the time and can resist the temptation to "go hard." If possible, make an effort to go barefoot frequently to develop natural balance, flexibility, and leg strength.

Primal Blueprint Law #4: Lift Heavy Things

 Grok's life demanded frequent bursts of intense physical effort—returning gathered items (firewood, shelter supplies, tool material, and animal carcasses) to camp, climbing rocks and trees to scout and forage, and arranging boulders and logs to build shelter. The biochemical signals triggered by these brief but intense muscle contractions prompted improvements and adaptations in muscle tone, size, and power.

Today, following a strength-training program featuring natural, total-body movements (squatting, lunging, push-ups, pull-ups, etc.) helps you develop and maintain lean muscle mass, increase metabolism to maintain low levels of body fat, increase bone density, prevent injuries, and enjoy balanced hormone and blood glucose levels. An approach of short-duration (always under an hour, but often lasting only 10-30 minutes), high-intensity workouts—conducted fairly regularly but without excessive regimentation (always aligned with your energy levels)—will produce superior results to a routine of going to the gym too often for workouts that last too long. The latter is a recipe for fatigue and undesirable gene expression. You can enjoy extraordinary benefits doing as little as two focused, intense 25-minute sessions per week, with minimal risk of overtraining or mental burnout.

Primal Blueprint Law #5: Sprint Once in a While

In a primal world where danger lurked around every corner, Grok's ability to run was a strong indicator of whether he would live long enough to pass those superior genes down to the next generation. Whether he was dashing off to avoid a charging herd of mastodons or running down small game for dinner, Grok's occasional sprints triggered gene expression within fast twitch muscle that enabled him to sprint a little faster the next time. That which didn't kill Grok made him stronger. Take that, Nietzsche!

Today occasional maximum effort sprints help increase energy levels, improve athletic performance, and minimize the effects of aging by promoting the release of testosterone and human growth hormone (these are beneficial for women as well as men). Once a week (or more frequently if you are an experienced athlete), when energy and motivation levels are high, choose a simple, brief session and go all out! Examples include sprints on hills, grass, or beach; plyometric drills; and intervals on a stationary bike. We'll detail many other options in Chapter 6.

Primal Blueprint Law #6: Get Adequate Sleep

Our ancestors' activity and sleep patterns were shaped by sunrise and sunset. Days started early (they actually caught the worm…and ate it!), and after the sun went down, it was safer to huddle together and rest. Furthermore, hunter-gatherers required plenty of downtime to repair and rejuvenate from their active lifestyles. Studies of modern hunter-gatherers suggest it wasn't always an uninterrupted eight hours either. It's likely that Grok slept together with his family or a small tribe, sharing a night watch for predators and tending to the needs of crying babies. The occasional afternoon nap was also available when the urge hit, with no guilt about what else he should really be doing.

Today, with life exponentially more hectic and stressful than at any time in human history, adequate sleep and restoration are widely neglected. The causes are modern distractions including digital entertainment, ingestible toxins (e.g., sugar, alcohol, and prescription and over-the-counter medications), and, of course, the ubiquitous alarm clock. It's critical to create calm, relaxing transitions into bedtime and then obtain sufficient hours of sleep such that you wake up naturally (no alarm, except occasional special circumstances) refreshed and energized.

Adequate sleep helps the immune system function optimally and promotes release of the key hormones that enhance brain and endocrine function. Go to sleep at the same time each night after a calm, deliberate wind down—no television, heavy exercise, big meals, or other high stimulation before bed. Your sleep requirements will vary according to lifestyle circumstances (and, of course, sometimes you have to compromise perfect sleep… you can't delay an airplane flight if you miss your alarm). Don't be afraid to take naps when your afternoon energy levels lull. The world will not miss you while you grab a few quick winks, and you will refresh the optimum balance of brain chemicals to increase productivity when you get back at it.

Primal Blueprint Law #7: Play

Our ancestors spent hours every day involved in social interaction not related to their core "careers" of securing food and shelter and caring for their young. Studies of modern hunter-gatherers, such as the !Kung Bushmen of the Kalahari Desert in Africa, reveal that they generally work far fewer hours and have more leisure time than the average 40-hour-plus modern worker. Anthropologist Marshall Sahlins's popular theory of the "original affluent society" argues that hunter-gatherers are able to achieve affluence (indeed a more literal definition than the consumerism-tainted one that we are familiar with) by desiring little and meeting those desires in daily life.

Once the day's catch was complete or the roots, shoots, nuts, and berries had been gathered, it was time for Grok to play. Youngsters would chase each other around and wrestle, vying for a place higher up in the tribe's social strata. Primal humans might also have practiced spear- or rock-throwing for accuracy, chased small animals just for sport, or spent relaxing time hanging out and grooming each other. The net effect of their play was to support family and intergenerational bonding, unwind from frequent life-threatening stress, and also keep their bodies primed for the physical challenges of daily life.

Today *play* is a four-letter word. We still pick Blackberries in our spare time, but now they're on a Web site and they come with various calling plan options and messaging features. The unrelenting stimulation of modern life, combined with the consumerism mentality of the free market economy, makes play more important than ever—yet more difficult to schedule. Take some time every day to unplug from the office or daily chores and have some unstructured fun. Particularly if you have children, you can model that play is a lifetime endeavor—and learn a few things from them while you're at it! Besides being fun and socially redeeming, play offers biochemical benefits in the form of endorphins released into the bloodstream and provides a healthy balance to the excessive mental strain and endless stimulation thrust upon us in the digital age.

Primal Blueprint Law #8: Get Adequate Sunlight

Cavemen weren't really men (or women) who lived their lives in caves all the time. They spent most of the day outdoors pursuing their various survival tasks. Regular sun exposure allowed Grok to manufacture plenty of vitamin D, which is critical to healthy cell function. Adequate vitamin D is nearly impossible to obtain from diet alone, and we cannot manufacture it without sufficient exposure to sunlight.

Today getting adequate sunlight—and hence vitamin D—is nowhere near a given, what with our penchant for spending much of our time in confined spaces, such as cars, offices, and homes. Experts believe a variety of serious health problems result from this relatively abrupt change in human lifestyle (sound familiar?). Besides the critical vitamin D requirement (while burning is certainly not healthy, a slight tan indicates that you have adequate vitamin D exposure), natural sunlight also has a powerful mood-elevating effect, which can enhance productivity at work and comfort with interpersonal relations.

Getting regular sunlight implies that you are spending time outdoors, appreciating open space and breathing fresh air. The net effect of taking time to enjoy these positive environmental surroundings (perhaps during your daily moderate exercise sessions!) is an excellent stress-balancer to being in confined spaces with artificial light and stale air. Your cells become truly energized on a biochemical level when you obtain regular doses of sunlight, fresh air, and open space.

Primal Blueprint Law #9: Avoid Stupid Mistakes

Our ancestors required a keen sense of observation and self-preservation to avoid danger. They were always scanning, smelling, and listening to their surroundings, ever aware of potential danger and what immediate action they might need to take. Whether it was running from a saber-toothed tiger, dodging a falling rock, eluding a poisonous snake, or just avoiding a twisted ankle from a careless step, hypervigilance and risk management were premium skills honed to perfection every day. Even a twisted knee or sprained ankle could spell death to anyone who couldn't run away from danger or effectively hunt food. It's likely that stupid mistakes from brief, careless lapses in judgment were a strong factor in diminishing the life expectancy of our exceptionally healthy ancestors.

Today vicious tigers are not a life-threatening safety concern, but we humans obliviously or carelessly (can you say, "multitasking"?) find ways to invite pain and suffering of a different nature into our lives. Buckle your seat belt; don't drink, text, or phone and drive; and be prepared and hypervigilant when you go backpacking in the wilderness, descend a steep hill on your 15-pound racing bike, or use a blowtorch, chain saw, or tile cutter. Devote a little more attention and energy to risk management in your daily choices so you can enjoy a long, happy life and pass your own superior genes to the next generation

Primal Blueprint Law #10: Use Your Brain

One of the most important things that separates humans from all other animals is intellectual ability. The rapid increase in the size of our brains over just a few thousand generations was the combined result of optimum dietary choices (including high levels of healthy fat and protein—see Law #1) and a continued reliance on complex thought—working the brain out just like a muscle. The best proof of this is the fact that hunter-gatherers all around the world developed language, tools, and superior hunting methods independently.

While you might argue that we use our minds plenty to navigate and make a buck in today's world, the reality is that many of us are stuck in unfulfilling or rote jobs or are otherwise disconnected from continued intellectual challenge and stimulation. Numerous studies of general intelligence qualities identify curiosity as one of the most profound markers and nurturers of intelligence. Opportunities for intellectual stimulation are everywhere in daily life. Commit to some personal challenges, such as learning a new language, playing a musical instrument, or taking an evening college class. Research indicates that risk of devastating mental conditions including depression, dementia, and Alzheimer's can be reduced by keeping your brain active as well as your body.

Learn Them, Know Them, Live Them!

Law #1: Eat Lots of Plants and Animals. Enjoy the natural, satisfying foods that fueled two million years of human evolution.

Law #2: Avoid Poisonous Things. Avoid processed foods (sugars, grains, and chemically altered fats) that are foreign to our genes and make us fat and sick.

Law #3: Move Frequently at a Slow Pace. Enhance fat metabolism and avoid burnout by keeping active but taking it easy.

Law #4: Lift Heavy Things. Short, intense sessions of functional, full-body movements support muscle development and delay aging.

Law #5: Sprint Once in a While. Occasional all-out sprints trigger optimal gene expression and beneficial hormone flow.

Law #6: Get Adequate Sleep. Avoid excessive digital stimulation and sync with your natural circadian rhythm for optimal immune, brain, and endocrine function.

Law #7: Play. Balance the stress of modern life with some unstructured, physical fun!

Law #8: Get Adequate Sunlight. Don't fear the sun! Adequate sun exposure helps synthesize vitamin D to ensure healthy cellular function.

Law #9: Avoid Stupid Mistakes. Cultivate hypervigilance and risk management to avoid the stupid mistakes that bring "avoidable suffering" to modern humans.

Law #10: Use Your Brain. Engage in creative and stimulating activities to nurture your mental health and overall well-being.

That's It

Aside from—ahem—the reproductive act, I challenge you to name any other significant behavior that shaped our genes and today plays a critical role in our health and well-being. Could it really be this simple? Could the prevention of and cure for obesity, diabetes, heart disease, physical decline, most cancers, and the general overstressed existence of the modern human be contained in a list of ten *Primal Blueprint* laws? While you may be able to find detractors to extract bits and pieces of this blueprint and offer up a critical view, the premise is absolutely unassailable: our genes are suited for a hunter-gatherer existence, because that is how we *Homo sapiens* have evolved and spent the great majority of our time on earth.

The same genes that can get the signal to turn against you to develop heart disease, diabetes, atherosclerosis, high blood pressure, high cholesterol, arthritis, and everything else on the list of conditions that might afflict you and your loved ones can also be triggered to unlock your potential to enjoy more energy, a leaner, fitter body, a substantial slowing of the aging process, and a low risk of illness, injury, and burnout. The secret is to do the right thing: follow lifestyle habits that promote desirable gene expression and avoid those that promote negative outcomes.

That statement alone—to do the right thing—is no revelation. The revelation here is how easy, natural, and fun the lifestyle behaviors are that will help you build your ideal body. Now you can enjoy natural, delicious, nutrient-dense foods that promote good health and effortless weight management by moderating insulin production. Now you have permission to back off from uncomfortable workouts and regimented schedules and instead enjoy an active lifestyle with regular low-intensity aerobic movement punctuated by occasional brief and very intense efforts. You can even hang out in the sun and take a nap in the name of health!

You will notice the benefits of the *Primal Blueprint* program in a matter of days, not weeks or months. Your genes are active all the time, either helping you build, regenerate, and maintain homeostasis or unintentionally tearing you down. It's all based on the environmental signals you provide them: food choices, activity levels, and even your thoughts. Hence it is critical to understand the impact on your genes—and overall health—when you select what food to eat, workout to do, or pill to swallow.

> *When I wrote The Origin of the Species, and for some years afterwards, I could find little good evidence of the direct action of the environment; i.e., food, climate, etc., independently of natural selection. Now there is a large body of evidence.*
> —**Charles Darwin**

Chapter Summary

1. Grok: Survival of the fittest drove two million years of evolution to create the ultimate human being…10,000 years ago! *Grok* is the nickname for our primal human lifestyle role model, who was stronger and healthier than us. Soon after Grok's time, the advent of agriculture across the globe eliminated the main selection pressure on humans: starvation. With agriculture and civilization making selection pressure irrelevant for thousands of years up to the present day, evolution ground to a halt, and we have gone soft as a consequence. However, because our DNA is virtually identical to Grok's, we can adapt his evolutionary-based lifestyle behaviors into our 21st-century lifestyle to pursue optimum health. The overall functioning of your body is primarily dependent on how your genes respond to their immediate environment. The *Primal Blueprint* is an instruction manual consisting of 10 simple behavior laws that trigger our genes to build a healthy, energetic, happy, lean, strong, bright, productive modern human.

2. Diet: Eat natural sources of plants and animals and avoid processed foods (sugar products, grains, chemically altered fats and other processed foods). Grains, while a global food staple long believed to be healthy, should be avoided because they stimulate an excessive release of insulin and are far less nutritious than vegetables, fruit, nuts, seeds, and animal foods. A diet emphasizing grains inhibits fat metabolism, precludes us from eating more nutritious plant and animal foods, and also paves the way for serious disease.

3. Exercise: Move frequently at a slow pace (walking, jogging, hiking), lift heavy things (regular strength-training sessions that are intense and brief), and conduct occasional all-out, short-duration sprints to stimulate growth hormone release, build muscle, reduce fat, and delay the aging process.

4. Lifestyle: Get adequate sleep (restores muscles and rejuvenates the brain), find time in your busy schedule for unstructured play (relieves stress and improves emotional and mental well-being on a chemical level), get adequate sunlight (stimulates production of important vitamin D and helps balance the negative effects of spending excessive time confined indoors, avoid stupid mistakes by practicing hypervigilance and risk management for today's hazards, and use your brain for creative, passionate outlets to balance the often repetitive or intellectually rote elements of your existence.

5. Blueprint for Success: The *Primal Blueprint* laws are simple and intuitive, unlike many elements of Conventional Wisdom that suggest you have to struggle and suffer to attain your fitness and weight-loss goals. You will notice the benefits of *Primal Blueprint* living immediately—more stable energy, better immune function, more enjoyable eating and exercising—as your genes direct your cells to function optimally at every moment.

Chapter Endnotes

[1] **Origin of Man**

   The "out of Africa" theory is also known as the Recent Single-Origin Hypothesis (RSOH), Replacement Hypothesis, or Recent African Origin (RAO) model. The theory, originally proposed by Charles Darwin in his *Descent of Man*, modernized by Christopher Stringer and Peter Andrews, and strongly supported by recent studies of mitochondrial DNA, says that anatomically modern humans evolved solely in Africa between 200,000 (first appearance of anatomically modern humans) and 100,000 years ago, with members leaving Africa 60,000 years ago and replacing all earlier human populations, including *Homo neanderthalensis* and *Homo erectus*.

[2] **Origin of Agriculture**

   Dr. Jared Diamond, evolutionary biologist, physiologist, and Pulitzer Prize–winning professor of geography at UCLA, is the author of *Guns, Germs and Steel: The Fates of Human Societies*, which discusses the advent of agriculture and its effects on civilization and human health. Chapter 5 of *Guns, Germs and Steel* details agriculture's origin (including which crops were cultivated) in several locations around the globe.

   The Emergence of Agriculture by Bruce Smith details the great transition of humanity from a hunter-gatherer lifestyle to agriculture and thus civilization. *Guns, Germs and Steel* and Richard Manning's *Against the Grain* detail the negative aspects of humankind's shift to agriculture, blaming it for large-scale disease, imperialism, colonialism, slavery, and an inexorable progression to global warfare. All this thanks to the abuse of "free time" resulting from the specialization of labor and the importance of power—over resources, humans, and geography—previously irrelevant in the largely egalitarian hunter-gatherer societies.

[3] **Primal Human Life Span**

   The estimate of 94 years is from Dr. Richard G. Cutler, molecular gerontologist and longevity expert, who has produced more than 100 papers on the subject. Dr. Cutler was a research chemist at the Gerontology Research Center at the National Institute on Aging, National Institutes of Health for 19 years. Dr. Cutler's estimate of "maximum lifespan potential" from *Homo sapiens* 15,000 years ago of 94 is actually higher than the corresponding figure attached to modern humans of 91! The estimate is derived from laboratory analysis of skeletal material, with particular emphasis on the ratio of body weight to brain size. Other factors involved in making accurate life span calculations are age of sexual maturation to life span ratio (a 5:1 ratio is common among humans) and rates of caloric intake and expenditure.

[4] **Grok**

   In Chapter 2 we talk about Grok as the patriarch of a primal family. However, in the interest of political correctness and ease of reading, you can view Grok as a not-necessarily gender-specific euphemism for primal ancestor(s) whom we aspire to emulate in lifestyle behaviors. For example, "Grok never ate sugar, and neither should you."

CHAPTER 2

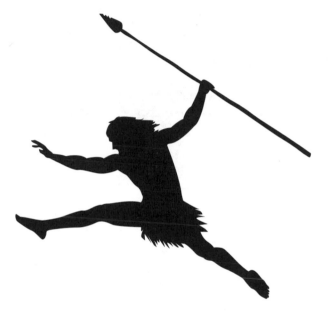

Grok and Korg

From Indigenous to Digital: One Giant Step (Backward) for Mankind

In This Chapter

We will examine the contrasting daily lives of Grok and his primal family with their modern-day antithesis, the Korg family. No, not to see who can travel 20 miles quicker (the Korgs' SUV beats Grok's bare feet with a few hours to spare…although the story might be different if it were a footrace!), but to examine the benefits of adapting primal behaviors to the modern world and the damage caused by living in conflict with our genetic predisposition to be fit, healthy, and happy.

The extremely unhealthy saga of the Korgs might seem embellished, but it's actually a statistically accurate indicator of many lifestyle trends today: hectic schedules compromising quality family time; processed foods emphasized in place of natural foods; prescription drugs used in place of lifestyle change; digital entertainment replacing physical activity; and overly stressful exercise programs that cause even the most devoted to fail with weight loss and fitness goals.

While the story is distressing, the good news is that with some simple, enjoyable lifestyle modifications, the momentum can turn immediately in the direction of better health (including freedom from dependence on prescription medications), higher energy, successful long-term weight loss, and a more enjoyable life for you and your family.

A man's health can be judged by which he takes two at a time—pills or stairs.
                                                                    —Joan Welsh

As we contrast a day in the life of our primal and modern families, we must refrain from the common knee-jerk rationalizations about the superiority of today's technological world. While infant mortality rates and death from tiger attacks are way down (notwithstanding that 2007 taunting incident at the San Francisco Zoo), it is sobering—pardon the pun—to consider that motor vehicle accidents (heavily influenced by alcohol use) are the leading cause of death for youth ages 15 to 24, followed by suicide and homicide. While no one is arguing that we should disavow our worldly possessions and go back in time to mud huts and spears, we must take a hard look at our lifestyles and absorb some powerful lessons offered by the legacy of our ancestors.

Livin' Large 10,000 Years Ago

Your impression of primal life might be negatively colored by sensationalized portrayals of precivilization humans as filthy, grunting savages dwelling in caves or by the harrowing vision of man potentially meeting his doom in the jaws of a beast or by the fangs of a snake. Unpleasant camping experiences (you know—too many mosquitoes, strange night noises, or no hot showers) might add to a dark vision of what it might have been like to live in hunter-gatherer times. Indeed, life was rough in many ways—much time and energy was devoted to getting food and other basic essentials that we take for granted. However, in many other ways—including the most simple and fundamental areas necessary for a healthy, happy life—Grok actually had it pretty good.

Ten thousand years ago, a time period coinciding with the ending of the last major ice age, the continent of North America was populated with small bands of hunter-gatherer tribes. Many theorize that this migration (probably driven by the tracking of big game herds) originated from Russia and moved very slowly eastward over dozens of generations across the Bering Land Bridge (which became submerged about 10,000 years ago) and then south into Canada and the United States. These tribes typically numbered 10 to 30 people comprising nuclear or extended families. While the average human life expectancy was about 33 in Grok's time,[1] if Grok had been able to avoid misfortune by accident, predator, or illness, his life expectancy would have increased dramatically.

Shortly after Grok's time, the advent of agriculture drastically changed the nature of human life on earth and caused numerous markers of human health to steadily decline as previously mentioned. Matt Ridley, author of *The Agile Gene*, reports that average brain size in 50,000 B.C. was 1,567cc for males and 1,468cc for females. Strange as it may seem, average brain sizes today are 1,248cc for males and 1,210 for females, with the onset of the shrinkage closely related to the advent of agriculture.

Grok's Walk

Grok and his longtime mate have two children, a 12-year-old boy and a one-year-old girl. Two other children didn't make it past infancy, a traumatic yet unavoidable part of life that the couple likely mourned deeply but from which they quickly moved on. Grok and his small band of 20 relatives live in what is now known as the great Central Valley of California. It's a cool, moist climate supporting vast pine forests, owing to the lower mean temperatures of the era (mean earth temperatures have continued to rise over the last 10,000 years).

The gathering of berries and other fruit, leafy greens, primitive roots, shoots and other vegetation, nuts, and seeds provide the bulk of Grok's food supply. Grok probably enjoys fish from nearby rivers, and hunts a variety of small mammals, such as beaver, rabbit squirrel, and mole. He might score occasional big game (mammoth, mastodon, bison, bear, lion, saber-toothed tiger, wolf, deer, and moose), but these animals are nearing the end of their era. He also enjoys the rich nutrition offered by various juicy, high-protein insects (remember, I said we'll strive to model *most* of Grok's lifestyle behaviors...).

Naturally, we'll start our day with Grok's family at sunrise. They awaken easily to the sound of birds chirping and begin their morning routine amidst the ageless singsong babble of a one-year-old. First things first—time to put together the morning meal. Grok's mate provides the baby the most nutritious food ever known to humankind—breast milk. The baby will begin to eat solid food within a few months but will continue to rely heavily on breast-feeding for three years. This not only will provide nutrition for physical growth but will give her immune system a head start dealing with potential health issues her mother has already overcome.

Grok's son will also enjoy a power breakfast. Because it's now late summer, special treats abound in the form of fat grub worms and local berries in their narrow ripening window. The current bounty is a far cry from the severe reduction in their caloric intake the previous winter, caused by unusually heavy rains. Fortunately, Grok and his family had been able to tap into their genetic ability to efficiently mobilize their stored body fat and make up for the caloric deficits in their diet. The family had also adapted to their winter circumstances by sleeping more and reducing their daily activity level.

The son gladly handles the chore of picking a basket of berries and quickly returns to camp. After breakfast, they turn their attention to preparing items for their daily endeavors: tidying up woven storage receptacles, sharpening rudimentary weapons like spears, and packing food rations (mostly nuts and seeds) for their planned journey. Today they are going for a long walk, heading east toward the Sierra foothills to gather more berries and perhaps score some small game. Everyone is eager—even though the temperature will be warm and the walk will be longer than their typical daily wanderings—because they will get to enjoy a cool dip in a river at the midpoint of their journey.

After a nutritious breakfast, the family heads out, mother carrying the baby and the preteen keeping busy harassing squirrels with rocks. Arriving at the river, they feast on more berries and a few freshwater clams, sip clean water, and blissfully bathe, splash, and jump off rocks into the crystal clear and brisk river. Grok's occasional brief exposure to cold water offers more than fun.[2] He doesn't know it, but this activity is considered a "natural" healer that helps boost immune function and antioxidant defense, decreases inflammation and pain, and increases blood flow and lymphatic function, something particularly therapeutic for tired muscles.

After his splash, Grok lounges on a sunbaked rock. His eyes gradually begin to shut, and he nods off for a power nap. As soon as his eyes fully close, positive hormonal changes occur in Grok's body.[3] Humans have adapted to obtain great benefits from even brief naps. One reason is the need for continued vigilance at nighttime against predators or other dangers made uninterrupted sleep difficult. Another is because the relaxed pace of primal life lends itself to afternoon shut-eye opportunities. Grok quickly drifts into the deepest, most restorative "delta" sleep cycle. Stress hormone levels are moderated and his brain chemicals are rebalanced, allowing him to wake up 20 minutes later refreshed and relaxed. The daughter takes the opportunity to doze off for far longer, even as she is hoisted up into her carrying sling as the family heads off.

Clad in skirts made of plant fiber and animal skin, the family moves effortlessly in bare feet over undulating terrain and makeshift animal trails. The ground is covered with rock and plant debris, including sharp burrs discarded by native plants, but they deftly cruise along for hours without so much as a cramp or stubbed toe. Even at 12, Grok's son has already developed excellent cardiovascular endurance, muscle strength, and balance. And because a physically challenging life is routine to him, he probably doesn't moan or complain about the length of the journey or the boredom factor ("Are we there yet?"). After all, no video games await indoors.... The parents pause on numerous occasions to teach him about native plant life, point out animal markings, and dispense other environmental lessons that will serve him well and keep him safe as he grows to assume ever-more challenging and valuable hunter-gatherer responsibilities.

Typical of humans 10,000 years ago, Grok and his family are of similar height and weight (but with more muscle and less body fat) to a modern family. Grok sports a single-digit body fat percentage and the well-balanced physique of today's Olympic decathlete. Pardon the expression, but Grok's mate, by today's standards, would probably qualify as a "hottie". Her ac-

> *Typical of humans 10,000 years ago, Grok and his family are of similar height and weight (but with more muscle and less body fat) to a modern family.*

tive lifestyle gives her striking attributes of a ballerina, a gymnast, and an ironman triathlete rolled into one enviable primal physique.

While Grok initially had planned to return to their permanent settlement that same evening, he chats briefly with his mate to discuss a spontaneous change of plans—to rest for the day and camp out. Because expectations and complexities are so minimal in Grok's life, the family easily goes with the flow of significant decisions like these without a second thought—this despite being unprepared for an overnight stay. It simply means a couple hours' additional work to gather up materials and construct a temporary shelter, build a fire, and get some dinner. No worry—they are safe together and accepting of every circumstance nature brings them.

Grok and his son head out for a quick hunt. We'd be surprised how primitive their weapons are, but the duo are able to leverage their extraordinary intelligence and instinct about the natural world to quickly procure a couple of rabbits for dinner. Walking back to camp, their celebratory banter is rudely interrupted by the appearance of a brown bear, drawn by the smell and wishing to make an unfair trade of lives for rabbits. A surge of fight-or-flight hormones flood the bloodstreams of Grok and his son. Grok immediately delivers a stream of detailed instructions to his son (back up slowly, maintain eye contact, etc.). His son nods calmly, naturally stifling his instinct to scream or run in the interest of survival. Grok, seemingly fearless in the face of this menacing creature, calmly lays the rabbits down on the ground and carefully joins his son in deliberate retreat. The bear issues a couple of loud roars just to be sure everyone knows who's boss, gathers his "kill," and moseys along. For good measure, Grok and his son take off on a dead sprint for 60 seconds, until they are safely out of the predator's sight.

Twenty minutes later, the fight-or-flight chemicals have worn off, the father-and-son debriefing is complete, and Grok arrives back at camp with empty hands and, most likely, a smile and shrug of the shoulders. This gesture epitomizes the requisite disposition for the uncertainty of primal life. It's a coping mechanism we have hardwired into our genes: "Don't worry, be happy."

Grok's mate has discovered some leafy green vegetation that they will eat raw or cook briefly over the campfire with a few wild potatoes. A computer analysis of the nutrient content of the food they consume, even without the rabbits, over the course of a typical month (a sufficient time period to account for the feast-or-famine realities of primal life and our graceful genetic ability to deal with it effectively) would reveal optimum levels of carbohydrates, protein, fat, vitamins, minerals, fiber, antioxidants, and other elements they need to sustain a lifetime of exceptional fitness and vibrant health. Similarly, if we were to draw Grok's blood for laboratory analysis, this primitive human would likely come up a big winner by today's health standards: he would be free of disease markers such as high C-reactive protein levels (indicative of undesirable systemic

inflammation); he would possess ideal levels of cholesterol, triglycerides, blood glucose, and insulin; and he
would be free of common modern-day nutrient deficiencies.

After dinner, the family lingers around the campfire
for perhaps an hour or two, relaxing, telling stories, and
winding down the day as the sun sets. This routine of
quality family time in the evening is likely more than
today's average working parents spend with their children in an entire week (families average 19 minutes together per day of time free from television and other
distractions).[4] As the sun sets, Grok and his family are
ready for a good night's sleep.

> " *Don't bother about
> being modern.
> Unfortunately it is the
> one thing that,
> whatever you do, you
> cannot avoid.*
> —**Salvador Dalí** "

The American Dream—Unplugged
(Or Should We Say, "Plugged In?")

Our modern family, the Korgs (Korg is Grok spelled backward—fitting when
you consider the Korgs' dramatic departure from Grok's simple, healthy lifestyle),
live where Grok did in California's Central Valley, in what is now known as Stockton. Stockton is a medium-sized, middle-income community located on the Sacra-
mento River delta, only an hour's drive from the metropolitan San Francisco Bay Area,
which has a population of some seven million. The Korgs—and thousands of other
families like them in bedroom communities outside the Bay Area proper—believe they
have the best of both worlds: an "easy" commute to Bay Area salaries combined with
affordable housing (Stockton's median home price is several hundred thousand dollars
less than most comparable homes in the Bay Area), less congestion, and good recreational, educational, and cultural opportunities. Ken Korg's two hours a day in the car
seem like a routine cost of living the American Dream.[5]

An Alarming Morning

Waking up naturally with the sun? Not the Korgs. Ken's wife, Kelly, is up and out of
the house when it's still dark, heading to the gym for a 6:00 A.M. Spinning class. It's a
struggle for her to get her butt onto the bike seat for that class three days a week, but Kelly
knows that her only chance to get a workout—or, for that matter, to enjoy some personal
time—is before the family stirs and the responsibilities pile up. Besides, Kelly has struggled all her life with her body weight and would dearly love to drop the 20 or more pounds
suggested by her physician to get her body mass index (BMI) into the healthy range.

When the alarm clock emits its digital chirping bird signal (very similar to Grok's; you can also choose breaking waves or wind chimes!) in the darkness of 5:15 A.M., an immediate stress reaction initiates throughout Kelly's body. Even the benign digital birds jolt her abruptly out of a restful sleep cycle and stimulate a mini fight-or-flight response by spiking her cortisol levels. Rising in the dark further disrupts her circadian rhythm (since a variety of hormones and brain chemicals are sensitive to light and dark cycles), resulting in a stressful start to Kelly's day—ironic in that her early-morning workout is part of her sincere commitment to become more healthy.

The rest of the Korg family avoids Mom's cortisol spike, but due to a host of other factors, they have their own issues waking up. Ken is already awake when his alarm sounds at seven o'clock, but his mind and body are in no hurry to get up and out of bed. Part of his situation is psychological—he is not terribly excited to face an hour on the freeway. Other factors in his body's slug imitation are the medications he's taking and the previous night's late dessert—a generous slice of cheesecake made with 60 grams of processed carbohydrates, partially hydrogenated vegetable oil, and assorted unpronounceable chemical preservatives.

Ken's cheesecake spiked his blood glucose just as he was attempting to fall asleep, interfering with the release of melatonin that naturally triggers sleepiness. Instead of spending the first hour in bed drifting into ever deeper cycles of sleep, Ken was fidgeting and twitchy because of the excess blood glucose in his system. Besides the glucose coursing through his veins, Ken's brain waves were jacked up from spending the final 90 minutes of his evening watching television. Even though he was exhausted and thus attempting to wind down after a long day, the fast-moving, flickering images on the screen (often violent or otherwise arousing) caused irregular stimulation to Ken's retina. This type of stimulus is transferred directly to the brain via the optic nerve and disturbs the normal function of the hypothalamus, the control center for many vital body functions, including the initiation of proper sleep patterns.[6]

Alas, Ken is one of more than 30 million Americans to hold a prescription for sleep medication,[7] which he reaches for on occasions like these. The quick-acting sleep medication combined with the eventual heavy insulin release to counter the cheesecake has Ken dead to the world within 20 minutes of taking the pill. Seven hours later, the effects of his Ambien pill are still pronounced; he feels sluggish and groggy instead of naturally refreshed and energized.

Nevertheless, it's time to get the Korg clan moving, so he drags himself out of bed and heads over to the bedrooms of his 14-year-old son and six-year-old daughter. Rousing them is not an easy task. Kenny Korg is experiencing his greatest need for sleep since infancy, and, like most modern teenagers, he isn't getting enough.[8] Kenny is also affected by a couple of other common adolescent conditions: drowsiness during the day and a delayed circadian phase, which has him naturally wanting to stay up later and wake up later. Kenny would feel fantastic with a regular afternoon power nap, but of course napping isn't cool, so he usually fights his body's need by ingesting a caffeine-laced energy drink or soda. He effortlessly stays up late playing computer games or cruising MySpace and texting his friends. Because he often doesn't power down until 11 P.M. or midnight, the 7 A.M. alarm comes far too early for him to feel rested and energized.

Young Miss Cindy Korg has her own troubles waking up. The mind-numbing effects of the cherry-flavored antihistamine/decongestant/cough suppressant/analgesic over-the-counter medication her mom had given her the previous evening are still lingering after a fitful sleep. She wakes up groggy, with blocked sinuses, but must rally to get to school on time. Cindy's third upper respiratory tract infection this year was chalked up to "the bug that's going around." However, bugs are always going around; it was really her suppressed immune system—weakened by the ever-present processed carbs and sugars in her diet—that prevented her from easily containing the virus after the first contact.

Kelly, always wanting to do the right thing as a mother, unknowingly prolonged Cindy's ordeal by giving her a common cold "remedy" that was intended to ease her suffering but that interfered with her daughter's natural defenses. Pounding the cough syrup every four hours for a few days likely doubled the time required for complete recovery by quelling the mild fever that was her primary defense against the virus, blocking the production of mucus intended to drain the virus into the stomach (where it can easily be killed by stomach acid), drying out the sinuses so she could breathe easier (but causing them to swell to the point that she can't breathe out of her nose at all this morning), and suppressing a productive cough that might have kept her up at night but would have allowed her lungs to expel the virus-laden mucus. These "symptoms" were actually Cindy's potent gene-based natural defenses—all thwarted by modern medicine.

Cindy's tendency to get sick more often than other kids her age is partly due to immune-suppressing dietary factors but also may be strongly associated with Kelly's choice to stop breast-feeding her after only three months. Tired of waking up every few hours at night or having to interrupt her workday to pump breast milk and having been sold on the benefits of infant formulas by TV and magazine ads, Kelly made the switch at least a year earlier than many progressive pediatricians would have recommended. Simply by the mother coming in contact with the baby's skin and picking up any pathogens on the body, the mother's immune system manufactures the antibodies and immune cells required to resist infections. She then passes those antibodies and lymphocytes ("natural killer" white blood cells) to the baby through breast milk. For that reason, many cultures breast-feed for two or three years. At any rate, Cindy finally summons the strength to get dressed and head downstairs.

Kelly bursts through the door as the family is shuffling around trying to get ready for the day. She's chipper and energized from her 50-minute class, which had elevated her heart rate to 85 percent of maximum or higher for most of that time period. The intensity of the effort has released a flood of stress hormones into her bloodstream, so she's on a "runner's high" (due to the effects of natural painkilling endorphins) as she greets her family. Kelly quickly sticks three waffles into the toaster. Trying to shop healthy, she always chooses whole grain waffles for her family. (I'll detail in the Chapter 5 sidebar "The Holes in the Whole Grain Story" why whole grains can even be considered *less healthy* than refined.)

Kelly dutifully cracks open a can of Slim-Fast meal-replacement drink. Main ingredients: skim milk powder, sugar, fructose, and cocoa, along with plenty of chemicals, synthetic vitamins, and vegetable oils—not much nutrition but plenty of simple carbs (38 grams) to raise blood glucose temporarily and stimulate an insulin surge. The "good" news: it contains only 240 calories. A minute later, the Korgs' power breakfast is ready: orange juice and whole grain waffles with some DNA-disturbing margarine and "low-sugar" maple syrup (made with artificial sweeteners[9] and woefully far removed from the sweet nectar that flows out of a hole drilled in a Vermont maple tree).

Kelly's second shake at lunch will result in a total of only 480 calories consumed since seven o'clock the previous evening—a period of 17 hours. While our bodies are adept at supplying adequate energy through intermittent food consumption (such was the reality of daily life for Grok), Kelly's high-intensity dawn workout coupled with the energy demands of her busy day make it not a good time to skimp on healthy food. As a consequence, her body's genetically programmed mechanisms (the same used by Grok in wintertime or when facing starvation) will attempt to slow down her metabolic rate to conserve fat stores and send a powerful signal to the appetite center in her brain to consume excessive carbohydrate calories (to quickly replace lost muscle glycogen and protect against this perceived starvation).

Unlike Grok, Kelly's calorie-restriction efforts will not result in the burning of stored body fat, because the frequent insulin spikes after her high-carb shakes, eating binges, and even "healthy" American meals can inhibit fat burning and, in fact, (with high-insulin eating habits followed over time) produce metabolic changes that make it increasingly difficult to mobilize stored fat for energy. This condition is obviously affecting Kelly, such an active, disciplined person failing so miserably to reduce body fat. The net effect of Kelly's punishing (elite athletes spend a substantially lower percentage of total exercise time at elevated heart rates than Kelly)[10] early-morning workouts and devoted calorie restriction is a reduction in muscle mass (which further lowers her metabolic rate and certainly doesn't improve her body image), an increase in body fat (due to the binge eating and slowed metabolic rate), and recurring fatigue, mood swings, and frustration.

The sting of failure is intensified every time Kelly sees her peppy neighbor Wendy, who has dropped eight pounds in two weeks since following her new multilevel marketing-driven cleansing diet. Upon further examination of these remarkable results, however, it's evident that the eight pounds consist almost entirely of water and muscle tissue. Wendy's severe calorie-restriction program kicks into gear a fight-or-flight response mechanism known as gluconeogenesis (Latin for "sugar" + "new" + "make"), where her muscle tissue is converted into glucose to supply her energy needs. The depleted state of her muscles results in significant water loss, considering that every gram of stored glycogen binds with four grams of water in the body. The eight pounds will return in a matter of days when exhaustion causes a return to normal, or supernormal, calorie intake.

"That Problem"...Among Others

Ken hates these first few minutes after Kelly gets home from her morning workout, because her energy level is such a stark contrast to the slow-moving household. On the flip side, Kelly is famous for shutting down around 8:30 P.M., after the stress hormone buzz wears off and insulin floods her system following dinner. With Ken's contrasting late-evening pattern, time for couple intimacy is virtually nonexistent. Furthermore, Ken has recently been experiencing "that problem" but is hesitant to share his concerns with anyone, let alone make an appointment with a physician to receive a prescription for Viagra. After all, Ken is still in his 40s and thinks Viagra is for old guys. Ken would be surprised to learn that about a third of all erectile prescriptions are dispensed to men under 50 and that use by men under age 45 tripled between 1998 and 2002.

Biochemically, Ken has several issues that contribute to his poor performance. The sustained high levels of cortisol in his bloodstream from his stressful lifestyle factors, such as inadequate sleep and job stress, suppress testosterone production, leading to diminished energy levels, weakened immune function, and, of course, reduced sex drive. His higher-than-optimum body fat levels and excessive insulin production from his high-carb diet and insufficient exercise also contribute to low testosterone, poor blood circulation, and other common-but-curable impotency factors.

Oh, almost forgot Ken's Lipitor (the world's best-selling drug with nearly $13 billion in sales in 2005), a statin medication he takes for "high" cholesterol that can cause muscle and liver problems, deplete CoQ10 (coenzyme Q10; a natural antioxidant and cofactor that is critical to cellular energy metabolism), and, yes, inhibit sexual performance. Ken only recently (and reluctantly, to his credit) started on Lipitor, at the behest of his doctor, who was concerned about his total cholesterol count of 205. Not in the high-risk range by any means, but enough for the doc to want to bring it down some, which the statins manage to do quickly. Unfortunately, statins also produce serious side effects,[11] mainly by blocking the production and flow of CoQ10 into cell mitochondria. This disturbance of mitochondria hampers the body's ability to generate normal amounts of energy (hence the common statin user complaint, "I feel tired and weak"), as well as fight free radicals and moderate inflammation. Furthermore, statins do not affect triglyceride (blood fat) levels or LDL (the so-called bad cholesterol) particle size (small, dense particles are worse), nor do they decrease risk of death in any women, in men over 65, or in men under 65 who have not had a heart attack.

Kelly, in turn, struggles with her self-esteem and body image, leading to reduced desire for intimacy. Furthermore, her stressful exercise regimen and poor nutritional habits interfere with healthy female hormone balance and contribute to the reduction of her drive.

Ken fills his commuter mug with coffee, hustles Cindy (with her cold medication hangover) into the car, and they depart. The first stop is four-tenths of a mile away at her elementary school.[12] It's four minutes until the tardy bell, and the front entrance is mobbed with a conga line of cars waiting to reach the drop-off zone. By the time Ken's car reaches its destination, Cindy is in a panic, as she will once again chase the tardy bell. Fear of a tardy slip may not be on par with a surprise visit from a bear, but the same fight-or-flight response occurs in Cindy as it did in Grok. The parting is anything but warm and comforting—a few choice words from the first grader and a quick admonishment in return from Ken: "Fine, maybe I'll just make you walk next time!" An excellent idea, considering the short trip from home to classroom by auto has taken six minutes, whereas even a leisurely walk (say, the pace that Grok and his family maintained for several hours, while trading off carrying a small child) from home to classroom would not have taken much longer.

Ken extracts his sedan from the campus swarm and soon begins his navigation of interstate freeways. As he drives up and over the small mountain range that marks the geographic boundary of the Bay Area, Ken spends his hour of "solitude" listening to talk radio—bouncing back and forth between sports and news talk—and taking several phone calls from friends or coworkers in the office. This constant and distracted stimulation to a brain still experiencing the effects of Ambien leads to mental fatigue before he even sets foot in the office. What's more, at the 40-minute mark of Ken's journey, he is suffering from heartburn and bloating (from his regular consumption of fried and fatty foods, dairy products, alcohol, sugars and desserts, sodas and other carbonated beverages, and substantial caloric intake before bed) as well as his typical recurring back pain (an affliction he shares with 60 to 80 percent of the general population).

Ken reaches into his briefcase and whips out his pill container, extracting a purple pill and a white capsule. The "healing purple pill" is Nexium (the third best-selling drug in the world with $5.7 billion in sales in 2005), which is used to treat the increasingly common condition known as gastroesophageal reflux disease (GERD) and its main symptom of heartburn. Nexium, classified as a proton pump inhibitor, blocks the production of hydrochloric acid in the stomach. This provides immediate relief for Ken's pain but seriously inhibits the digestive process, which relies on hydrochloric acid and other powerful acids to break down and assimilate nutrients from food.

Next is the white capsule Celebrex, a popular nonsteroidal anti-inflammatory (NSAID) prescription medication that reduces levels of hormonelike substances called prostaglandins that are part of a natural inflammation response occurring in Ken's body. He takes it to alleviate the back pain that accompanies the inflammation. He will pop another Celebrex this evening per the recommendation of his physician, who also suggested at his last visit that he schedule an appointment at a physical therapy clinic to obtain a customized back and core strengthening exercise routine. He's been meaning to schedule that but hasn't yet found the time.[13] Instead, Ken grabs some exercise here and there when the stars align and gaps open up in his schedule. Owing to his athletic youth, his competitive appetite is bigger than his physical condition. His forays into adult pickup basketball at the health club usually produce more tweaks and pulls than inspiration and motivation to pursue a regular, balanced total-body fitness program.

If Ken proceeds with the typical behavior pattern, he will use these prescription NSAIDs for years and neglect sufficient regular exercise. Down the road, owing to Ken's long-term use of such a powerful systemic anti-inflammatory medication, the drug's impact will diminish (at which point his doctor will probably put him on something stronger) and his body's natural ability to control all types of inflammation will have been steadily decimated. This will set the tone for a variety of serious health conditions to take root, including—owing to his poor diet and lifestyle habits—many cancers and heart disease. Yep, that's right—studies suggest a significant increased risk of heart attack when taking NSAIDs. Vioxx was a very popular NSAID taken by 80 million people worldwide from 1999 until 2004, when it was taken off the market due to concerns about side effects that increased heart attack risk. Celebrex sales skyrocketed as a result, until research suggested it posed similar risks. Celebrex sales then dropped sharply but steadily resumed to exceed $2 billion in 2006.

> "The idea on the medical horizon is that chronic inflammation is a root cause of degenerative disease. It is time for medical schools to improve nutrition education. If physicians are trained to use "food as medicine" they may not need to rely on drugs and their distressing side-effects to treat the inflammatory process.
> —Dr. Andrew Weil"

Spreadsheets and Chow Mein

After an hour and eight minutes of driving from the elementary school, Ken arrives at his office. He works as an accountant for a software company. The hours are regular (unlike many of his coworkers, who are selling or developing software and routinely working 10- to 12-hour days), and he makes a third more than he could in the same position in Stockton. Aside from the set hours and compensation benefits, the working conditions are challenging. Executives and division sales managers constantly enroll the accounting team in their hyperdrive, desperate mentality. They have a penchant for requesting ridiculously fancy presentations on short notice or strolling into Ken's office and literally breathing down his neck to obsessively review sales figures in the days counting down to quarterly close.

The perk of being able to leave promptly at 6:00 P.M. each evening is muted by the feeling of complete mental exhaustion that overcomes Ken as soon as he opens his car door in the parking lot. In his previous position (closer to home and for significantly less pay), Ken would take a leisurely lunch hour to eat a sandwich in the park or even join a coworker for a light workout at the gym. He'd return to work refreshed and proceed at a sensible pace through the afternoon hours, pausing often to share a laugh with coworkers. Lately, he has stayed at his desk to eat lunch, typically procured via a 40-second drive to a busy nearby intersection with numerous quick options.

Ken, inspired by Kelly's commitment, is also making a concerted effort to "do the right thing" and eat healthier. He eschews McDonald's and Burger King for Chinese buffet, which sounds healthier but is actually just as bad. He returns to the office armed with chow mein noodles and sweet-and-sour chicken, trying not to spill the mostly simple carbohydrate meal onto his spreadsheets. Laughter in the hallways has been replaced by the discernible buzz of anxiety, the unspoken fear that heads will begin to roll out the door if Ken's spreadsheets don't impress stockholders and executives. In contrast to the few brief moments of Grok's life-or-death encounter with a bear, Ken's workplace is essentially a daily nine-hour grind of unrelenting moderate stress. Ken and the rest of us would still choose the spreadsheets over being scared sheetless by a bear, but the impact of prolonged chronic stress is far more destructive to human health (and misaligned with our genes) than a pattern of brief intermittent stresses coupled with adequate downtime and a relaxed lifestyle.

The postlunch, insulin-driven sugar crash hits Ken hard, so he scarfs down one of the PowerBars Kelly had thrown into his briefcase (PowerBar Energize Tangy Tropical has 42 grams of carbs—25 of them sugar) and heads to the break room for his daily afternoon cup o' joe. Ken consumes two cups and one to two diet sodas each day, a total of about 250 milligrams of caffeine.[14] Not quite enough to classify him as an addict (actually, that's about the daily average for Americans), but it's definitely another substance, along with the several prescription and over-the-counter meds, that he is dependent upon to make it through his day.

Love, Money, and Insulin

Even while making a comfortable income by any reasonable definition, the Korgs are experiencing financial stresses familiar to many.[15] After paycheck deductions for taxes, 401(k), and, of course, the enticing employee stock purchase program (where 5 percent of his gross income is fed back to the monster), a third of his annual net goes to mortgage and related tax and insurance costs. Other healthy chunks go to car payments and insurance, groceries and dining out, medical expenses not covered by Ken's skimpy company policy, and the occasional whopper, such as two grand for a major surgery at the vet, two grand for Kenny Korg's class field trip to Washington, D.C., 800 bucks for Kelly's last-minute bereavement trip to the East Coast for a family friend's funeral, a C-note for a weight-loss "starter kit" that gung ho neighbor Wendy basically forced upon them (a 28 percent discount when buying an entire case!), and so on.

Kelly contributes to the family's bottom line running her own stimulating but stressful business as a freelance graphic designer. The flexible hours are great, although the healthy boundary between work and personal life often gets blurred. One favorite ritual is picking up her daughter from school every day and taking her out for a treat—carrying on a fond family tradition she and her sisters enjoyed with their mother. As Eric Schlosser details in *Fast Food Nation*, Kelly is cooperating with the food industry's institutionalized exploitation of American families that allows parents to replace quality time (particularly the nearly extinct family home mealtime, and the guilty conscience that goes with being too busy) with instant gratification—and therefore love—for their children.

The treat time coincides with Kelly's daily affliction of the afternoon blues, owing to her predawn wake-up call, the caloric depletion brought about by her crash diet, and the work/parent/personal health and fitness juggling act that is her life. The colorful, peppy, healthy lifestyle messaging inside the local Jamba Juice franchise helps Kelly rationalize about her impending insulin flash flood. She confidently orders up a 24-ounce Strawberry Surf Rider for herself and a 16-ounce Mango-a-go-go for her daughter. Cindy excitedly suggests adding a couple baked goods from the child's-eye-level display case to the tab. Ever vigilant, Kelly scans the choices to pick the healthiest and settles on a couple of reduced-fat blueberry-lemon loaves, "part of a complete breakfast—complement with a smoothie or fresh squeezed orange juice," says the Jamba Juice menu. Each loaf offers 290 calories, 73 percent of which come from processed carbohydrates (lead ingredients: sugar and flour) with virtually zero nutritional value and a guaranteed strong insulin response. Cindy finishes only half her loaf, but Kelly makes sure it doesn't go to waste.

The discipline of Kelly consuming fewer than 500 calories in the previous 19 hours is no match for a depleted brain and body. While the 24-ounce Strawberry Surf Rider will provide Kelly with some much deserved antioxidants and other healthy nutrients from the frozen fruit, 87 percent of its 490 calories come from sugar. Along with one and a half blueberry-lemon loaves, Kelly has ingested 925 calories (make that an even thousand, counting a few long pulls on her daughter's straw to try the Mango-a-go-go), including 187 grams of refined carbohydrates (that's more than the *Primal Blueprint's* recommended range of 100 to 150 grams for an entire day!). Her sugar/insulin roller coaster will again hamper her fat-burning efforts for hours after this onslaught and lead to fatigue and sugar cravings come dinnertime.

Young Cindy Korg's drink and half loaf send more than 100 grams of sugar into her little body, stressing her insulin system—and her immune system—yet again. The previous day, at a classmate's birthday party, she had consumed typical party fare of two slices of thin-crust cheese pizza (460 calories), a small slice of chocolate cake (235) with a small scoop of vanilla ice cream (150), some box juices with high-fructose corn syrup (she opened three over the course of the party and drank only half of the fluid [a typical ratio, as any parent who's hosted a birthday party can confirm] = 130 calories), and several assorted bite-sized candies from the take-home party favor bag (150 calories). Her total calories in the three-hour period came to 1,125, more than half in the form of simple sugar. That's enough to stimulate a significant insulin response in a 300-pound man, let alone a 55-pound child.

> *Studies suggest that overweight kids are highly likely to become overweight adults and consequently suffer from serious health problems and life-threatening diseases.*

Naturally (owing to family genes, her parents rationalize), young Cindy is already significantly overweight. Fortunately (from a psychological perspective only), unlike in past generations, her plump physique is shared by many of her fellow first graders.[16] While this certainly protects her self-esteem, it makes it difficult to change the popular chartered course of this young ship, sailing toward peril and doom. Studies suggest that overweight kids are highly likely to become overweight adults and consequently suffer from serious health problems and life-threatening diseases.

Kenny's World

We haven't heard much about the Korgs' teenage son, Kenny, which is appropriate because he is already emotionally disconnected from his busy family and pulled by the powerful force of peer influence in directions that create conflict with stable family life. In his early years, Kenny was naturally active and spent hours outside running and playing. Unfortunately, each passing preteen year saw more sedentary technological distractions commandeering his time and innocent backyard play being exchanged for competitive organized sports.[17]

While Kenny has some innate athletic ability, he lacks the naturally healthy aggression and competitiveness that allow young athletes to move to the front of the pack. Lacking time to connect with his son, Ken makes the common mistake of overpressurizing his son's athletic experience with misplaced emotion and "encouragement" that feels to his son like results expectations and criticism. By the time Kenny becomes a teen, he is finished with organized sports and deep into a new cultural phenomenon called MMORPG (massive multiplayer online role-playing games),[18] such as *World of Warcraft* and *Runescape*, where a player creates a digital persona and interacts with many others in a virtual world, often immersed for eight or 10 hours at a time. At school, he maintains grades that are decent yet below his potential, but he is incurring increasing reports of misbehavior in class. During a telephone conversation with the school counselor, the topic of attention deficit hyperactivity disorder (ADHD) is broached as a potential reason for Kenny's misbehavior.

Kenny's feelings of alienation are exacerbated at the dinner table that evening, when Ken peppers him with the exact same questions heard at the breakfast table about his son's decision to skip freshman basketball tryouts. The teen is naturally offended, unaware that one of the most common side effects of Ambien is short-term memory loss and that Ken truly has no recollection of the conversation from 12 hours prior (and some eight hours after popping the Ambien).

The exchange escalates into a blowout covering various pent-up resentments. Ken decides to make an appointment for his son to visit a psychiatrist. After two sessions, the shrink diagnoses Kenny with ADHD and promptly prescribes the amphetamine Adderall[19]—This despite growing controversy surrounding its overprescription to children who lack serious symptoms and a true clinical diagnosis, the potential link to serious cardiovascular side effects, and the high incidence of abuse among teenagers using the stimulant recreationally. (An estimated seven million American kids take stimulants prescribed for attention disorders, a 500 percent increase since 1991.)

It's more likely that emotional factors, lack of sufficient vigorous exercise, and poor dietary habits (sugar binges, regular caffeine intake, and lack of healthy fats) are to blame for Kenny's adverse classroom behavior. Unfortunately, Kenny now has another hurdle on the path to getting his mind and body back into balance for the challenging high school years ahead: the powerful effects of stimulant medication on his growing body.

When critiquing the particulars of kids and their exercise, sleep, dietary habits, and school high jinks, you might default to thinking, "What's the big deal?" Kenny and millions of his peers will continue their mildly objectionable ways, but they'll get through high school just fine (provided they heed *Primal Blueprint* Law #9, Avoid Stupid Mistakes). They'll go off to college and pull all-nighters fueled by pizza, Red Bull, and Top Ramen, then they'll unwind after exam pressure with lots of alcohol, more pizza, and maybe a few cupcakes at the Kappa Kappa Gamma bash. I don't think previous generations can claim they are unfamiliar with this routine.

It's true, young people are incredibly resilient, in case you've forgotten. With metabolism accelerated and the endocrine system flooding the bloodstream with peak levels of key growth and reproductive hormones, the raw (indeed, primal) energy of youth can often override any potential insulin-driven fatigue from a Red Bull buzz wearing off. We can all attest to the difference between being at our physical peak and being beyond it. At 55, I'm stoked to be able to (more or less) hang with my teenage son, Kyle, when we play Ultimate Frisbee (the official name of the game is simply Ultimate, given that Frisbee is a brand name and you can use any type of disc to play) till we drop. Then, while I'm sunk deep into the couch/ottoman licking my wounds and icing my strains, he'll grab an apple and his skateboard (and his helmet of course…remember Rule #9) and bust out the door to the next activity!

However, if we consider the concept that our genes—even young genes—are predisposed to all kinds of problems if we give them the wrong environment (and, hence, the wrong signals), we can conclude that it's just a matter of time until the fountain of youth runs dry. Remember in college those frat boys with six-pack abs drinking pony kegs every weekend? A decade later, you can find most of them with pony keg guts drinking six-packs every weekend. As a parent or an influential figure in a child's life (or perhaps an evolved young person reading the *Primal Blueprint*!), you can assert the importance of having a foundation of healthy lifestyle habits and a deep respect and understanding for how to get the best out of your body. This will pave the way for a future different from today's extremely disturbing one in which many experts predict a shorter life expectancy for children than for their parents—for the first time since…(Anybody? Bueller? Anybody?)… Since the advent of agriculture 10,000 years ago.[20]

"We Have Met the Enemy, and He Is Us"

This classic quote uttered by Walt Kelly's popular comic strip character Pogo captures the Korgs' plight perfectly: their well-intentioned efforts to do the right thing seem continuously sabotaged by cultural norms and misguided Conventional Wisdom. We are conditioned by the powerful forces of consumerism to pursue flawed solutions to our problems and ailments. The prescription drugs downed by Ken (and now Kenny, too), Kelly's overly stressful exercise routine and overly restrictive diet, the massive amount of unhealthy food ingested by the family on a daily basis, and the lack of simple, quality family time might be disturbing to read about, but they are absolutely the norm today.

If you felt the Korgs' tale was an appalling, melodramatic, and unrealistic example of a modern family, you have lifestyle reference points that are significantly more healthy and balanced than the average American family's. The references to the Korgs' daily routine, prescription drug use, weight-loss battles, eating and exercise habits, childhood obesity, teenage behavior challenges, and digital media use are provided in detail in the "Grok Chapter References" appendix.

As they say, your kids grow up—and you grow old—before you know it. A lack of awareness, lack of knowledge, and sometimes, sadly, a defiant, ignorant stance of disrespecting the essentials of health and well-being (including our genetic programming) tragically degrades the precious time families have together. This loss plays out every day and touches virtually every family in the modern world. It's time to stand up and take control of your health and well-being, to honor your genes by living according to the *Primal Blueprint*, and, finally, to reject many tenets of Conventional Wisdom that are flawed and hazardous to your health. In this book, we will do just that, further building momentum and crushing obstacles in our path as we march toward the ultimate expression of our human potential.

How Grok Probably Spent His Day

Hunting or gathering food . . . . 5 hours
Sleep, nap, rest, relax . . . . 10 hours
Habitat-, shelter-, basic human needs–related chores . . . . 3 hours
Leisure time consisting of play and family or group socializing . . . . 6 hours

Estimates derived from studies of the modern hunter-gatherer culture of the !Kung Bushmen in Africa.

How Ken Korg Spends His Day

Workplace . . . . 9 hours
Commute . . . . 2 hours
Sleep . . . . 6.7 hours
Television, computer, digital entertainment . . . . 4 hours [21]
Grooming, household chores, free time . . . . 2.3 hours
(components: leisure/educational reading: 24 minutes; meaningful conversation with child: 3.5 minutes)

Estimates derived from TV Free America in Washington, D.C., American Time Use Survey Summary (U.S. Department of Labor, Washington, D.C.), A.C. Neilsen Company, and Kaiser Family Foundation.

Chapter Summary

1. Grok's Lifestyle: Grok faced unimaginable hardships in primal life but in many ways enjoyed superior health to that of modern humans. While rates of infant mortality and death by predator or accident were far higher than today, if Grok were able to avoid such tragedy, he could enjoy robust health and supreme physical fitness into his 60s or 70s.

Grok's hunter-gatherer existence involved a diet of natural plants and animals, hours of low-level aerobic exercise every day, and occasional short bursts of maximum effort. Primal existence was simpler and slower paced, with life-or-death stressful events coming infrequently and lasting only briefly. This type of existence is more aligned with our genetic makeup than is the unrelenting stress of modern life.

2. Korg Lifestyle: Our modern suburban family, the Korgs, have diverged dramatically from the lifestyle basics modeled by Grok that are essential for good health. Long commutes, packed schedules, and excessive digital entertainment compromise family camaraderie. Financial pressures, insufficient sleep and downtime, extensive use of prescription drugs, poor dietary habits, and exhausting exercise programs lead to an excessively stressful modern existence and consequent health problems.

The Korgs' diet features excessive processed foods and insufficient nutritious foods. In particular, they eat too many simple carbs and grains that lead to excess insulin production. These dietary mistakes lead to assorted health problems, particularly undesirable body composition, beginning in childhood and continuing for a lifetime. Kelly Korg's well-meaning devotion to exercise and careful dieting does not lead to fat loss, because the workouts are too stressful and she regularly has excessive insulin in her bloodstream (from consuming too many carbs), which inhibits fat burning. Ken's lack of exercise, poor eating habits, work-related pressures, and reliance on prescription drugs to counter lifestyle errors make him tired and stressed and put him on the path to the eventual onset of serious disease. The Korg children are victimized by the disastrous cultural trends of today's youth, such as insufficient activity, excessive digital media use, high-insulin diets, and overpressurized athletic and academic experiences that lead to alienation and rebellion.

3. Your Family: It's critical to depart from these harmful cultural trends and create a different reality for you and your family. Modifying dietary habits to *Primal Blueprint* recommendations and placing limits on technology and jam-packed schedules in favor of relaxing family interaction will help reverse the appalling family dynamics characterized by the Korgs' story.

Chapter Endnotes

Grok Family References

[1]**Life Expectancy:** According to Wikipedia, life expectancy during the Paleolithic era (2.5 million years ago to 10,000 B.C) was around 33 years, factoring in the high rates of infant mortality. If Grok reached puberty, life expectancy increased up to age 39 and if he reached 39, he could expect to live until 54. And this was a ripped, energetic 54, not a guy struggling to hang on. The fatal hazards that befell Grok during his lifetime were entirely primitive: infections, accidents, and predators – not heart disease, diabetes or obesity.

The advent of agriculture and civilization caused life expectancy to drop significantly, reaching a low of 18 during the Bronze Age of 3,300 B.C. to 1,200 B.C.. Life expectancy remained low (between 20 and 30) through 1500 A.D. and then climbed only gradually, reaching ~30 in 1800 and ~40-50 in 1900 in the USA and Europe. The past century has seen a dramatic increase in lifespan in civilized countries, thanks mainly to medical advances that limit infant mortality and protect against disease plagues.

A 2004 study published by Rachel Caspari at the University of Michigan and Sang-Hee Lee at the University of California at Riverside revealed that a dramatic increase in human longevity that took place during the early Upper Paleolithic Period, around 30,000 years ago. The scientists studied dental information derived from molar wear patterns of *Australopithecines*, *Homo erectus* and *Neanderthals* and discovered a five-fold increase in the number of individuals surviving to an older age (defined by doubling reproductive age – so humans could become grandparents) around that time period.

The scientists speculated that "this trend contributed importantly to population expansions and cultural innovations that are associated with modernity." Elders could pass on critical life knowledge to younger generations, social networks and family bonds were strengthened and Grok could generally become a better parent by living longer.

"There has been a lot of speculation about what gave modern humans their evolutionary advantage," Caspari said. "This research provides a simple explanation for which there is now concrete evidence: modern humans were older and wiser."

[2] **Cold Water Benefits:** The healing properties of water have been recognized for thousands of years. Public baths were a common feature in ancient civilizations. The Romans, Greeks, Egyptians, Turkish, Japanese and Chinese all believed water was helpful for muscle recovery, sleep and immune protection. In the early 1800's Vincent Priessnitz, an Austrian farmer, pioneered the use of hydrotherapy as a medical tool. During the mid to late 1800's, a Bavarian monk named Father Sebastian Kneipp gained wide recognition for his water therapy work. He cured himself of pulmonary tuberculosis (a common and typically fatal condition referred to then as "consumption") by regularly plunging into the icy Danube River to stimulate his immune system. Kneipp wrote extensively on the subject of hydrotherapy and other natural healing topics, gaining notoriety that attracted people from across the world to visit his clinic.

Several studies support the historical anecdotes that cold water offers health benefits. One study conducted by the Thrombosis Research Institute at London's Brompton Hospital found that exposure to cold baths boosted sex hormone production, improved fertility, chronic fatigue conditions, immune function and blood circulation – reducing cardiovascular disease risk. Numerous studies indicate that the invigorating effect of cold water stimulates the release of endorphins by the autonomic nervous system. Anyone who has taken a plunge and emerged energized can attest to the powerful effects of cold water on the body.

[3] **Napping:** Data from the National Sleep Foundation suggests that "a well-timed afternoon nap may be the best way to combat sleepiness." Gregory Belenky, MD, Research Professor and Director of the Sleep and Performance Research Center at Washington State University, says naps can help make up for insufficient sleep, and that "it's even possible that divided sleep is more recuperative than sleep taken in a single block," noting how popular the afternoon siesta is in countries across the world. Dr. Mark Rosekind's studies with NASA pilots indicated that napping pilots had a 34% increase in performance and 54% boost in alertness that lasted for 2-3 hours. Harvard University studies show that 60-90 minute naps help the brain integrate new knowledge similar to nighttime sleep. A study published in the research journal *Sleep* suggests that naps ranging from ten to thirty minutes are optimal for improved cognitive performance and alertness

The Center for Applied Cognitive Studies says that "the length of sleep is not what causes us to be refreshed upon waking. The key factor is the number of complete sleep cycles we enjoy. Each sleep cycle contains five distinct phases, which exhibit different brain- wave patterns." Leading sleep researcher Dr. Claudio Stampi found that naps taken in the afternoon (a common low energy period in our circadian rhythms) were comparatively higher in the most restorative slow-wave sleep. During a 10-20 minute afternoon nap, your brain cells reset their sodium and potassium ratios, which are thrown out of balance after long periods of intense brain arousal, as in a typical busy day. "This is the main cause of what is known as 'mental fatigue'," the Center says about this nutrient imbalance. "A brief period in Theta (slow wave sleep) can restore the ratio to normal, resulting in mental refreshment."

[4] **Quality Time:** The Office of National Statistics "Time Use Survey" study indicates that today's average working parent spends nineteen minutes of digital distraction-free quality time per week.

Korg Family References

[5] **Commuting:** The Public Policy Institute of California reports that 18% of Californians commute over 45 minutes each way. 3.4 million Americans commute 90 minutes or more each way. The US Census reports that the average commute time nationwide is 25.5 minutes each way, with Californians commuting 10% longer than the national average. Tracy, CA, near the Korg's home of Stockton, had one of the longest average commute times in the state in 2000: 42 minutes each way.

In a United Kingdom survey of over 400 people by the International Stress Management Association, 44 percent said that rush-hour traffic was the most stressful part of their lives. A Hewlett Packard study of UK commuters found that blood pressure and heart rate were "higher than those experienced by fighter pilots going into combat and police officers facing rioting mobs."

A study by researchers at the New York University Sleep Disorder Center found that "long commuters" - those who travel one hour and 15 minutes or longer - have more sleep disorders and other health problems than the general population. There is also a significant danger of multitasking while commuting. The Harvard Center for Risk Analysis found drivers using cell phones are responsible for 2,600 traffic deaths per year and 330,000 traffic injuries (motorists on the road make 40% of all cellular telephone calls).

[6] **Digital Media Disturbing Sleep:** Daniel Reid's *The Tao of Health, Sex and Longevity* details how television disturbs the ocular-endocrine system. A US study showed that rats exposed to invisible television rays (screen was blackened) for six hours per day became hyperactive and extremely

aggressive for about a week, then suddenly become totally lethargic and stopped breeding entirely. A Columbia University Study conducted in New York suggests that "watching late night television may put people in a state of heightened alertness and physiological arousal, preventing them from falling asleep with ease. In addition, being exposed to many hours of the bright light of the television screen may throw people off their sleep-wake cycle, while too little physical activity may cause people to become restless and struggle with sleep."

A Rhode Island study published in journal of American Academy of Pediatrics suggests children's sleep is disturbed by watching TV before bedtime — causing them to become "over-stimulated, disturbed or frightened by the content of programs…particularly those containing violence." The "might" in this makes it pretty darn weak.

[7] **Sleep Medication**: 30 million people in the USA take sleep medications (*American Academy of Sleep Medicine*), an estimated 50% jump since 2000. With an ode to the "over x billion served" signs adorning McDonald's franchises, Sanofi-Aventis, maker of Ambien, boasts an aggregate total of 12 billion nights of patient use worldwide. $2 billion was spent on the drug worldwide in 2004. According to *LiveScience*, global sales for sleeping pills are estimated at $5 billion annually.

Daniel Kripke, UC San Diego psychiatry professor and author of *The Dark Side of Sleeping Pills*, conducted a revealing six-year sleep study with over one million adults. Kripke reported that the health risk of taking sleeping pills daily was not much different that the risk of smoking a pack of cigarettes a day! A study by researchers at Beth Israel Deaconess Medical Center and Harvard Medical School found that treating insomnia with habit and attitude modification was more effective – both immediately and over the long-term – than using Ambien. The sleep success techniques Kripke recommends include: don't go to bed until you're sleepy, get up at the same time each morning, avoid excessive stimulation or worry before bed, avoid caffeine for six hours before bed, avoid alcohol before bed, and spend adequate time outdoors.

[8] **Teenage Sleep**: A 2007 Mayo Clinic article suggests that teenagers require about nine hours of sleep to maintain optimal daytime alertness, but few actually get that much sleep due to jobs, homework, friends, digital media and other distractions (the National Sleep Foundation reports that 25% of teens report sleeping 6.5 hours per night or less). "Puberty changes a teen's internal clock, delaying the time he or she starts feeling sleepy until 11pm or later ("before adolescence, circadian rhythms direct most children to naturally fall asleep around 8 or 9 p.m"). "Staying up late to study or socialize can disrupt a teen's internal clock even more.

The article also notes that sleeping in or forcing an early bedtime are not adequate solutions, since they are not aligned with the teen's unique circadian rhythm. The Mayo Clinic staff suggests that you darken rooms at desired bedtime and expose teens to bright light in the morning, discourage naps longer than 30 minutes, discourage caffeine use and establish a consistent, quiet relaxing routine before bed – free of digital media.

[9] **Artificial sweeteners**: an on-line review mentioned by Dr John Briffa indicates that "100 per cent of industry funded studies proclaim aspartame to be benign; more than 90 per cent of independent studies and reports in the scientific literature say otherwise." Numerous studies suggest that intense artificial sweeteners increase appetite for sweet foods, promote overeating, and may even lead to weight gain. One study with rats from Purdue University concluded that "consuming a food sweetened with no-calorie saccharin can lead to greater body-weight gain and adiposity than would consuming the same food sweetened with higher calorie sugar." However, there are some other studies that refute the concept entirely. Perhapshe most relevant evidence is how obesity rates continue to climb even with the advent and increased used of artificial sweeteners in the modern diet.

[10] **Cardiovascular exercise heart rates**: My position that Chronic Cardio is harmful and that low level aerobic work is beneficial is based on personal experience over three decades as an elite athlete, personal trainer to clients of all ability levels and coach to elite professional triathletes. The extensive work of legendary coach Arthur Lydiard is a major influence as well. Lydiard, who pioneered the concept of overdistance endurance training for track and field athletes, developed numerous Olympic gold medalists and world record holders in his home country of New Zealand and for various other national teams. Elite athlete/authors like former professional triathletes Mark Allen (*Total Triathlete*) and Brad Kearns (*Breakthrough Triathlon Training*), former Olympic marathon runner and popular author and speaker Jeff Galloway, Joe Friel's popular series of "Training Bibles" for various endurance sports all echo these fundamental principles of endurance training:

• Building a base of comfortable aerobic activity is critical for success
• High intensity exercise should be strictly limited as a small percentage of total exercise volume and conducted only when a sufficient aerobic base is present

Conversely, the American College of Sports Medicine recommends exercise intensities of 55-90% of maximum heart rate, a ridiculously disparate range that stimulates vastly different metabolic responses in the body. Sadly, this information is widely circulated by health clubs, personal trainers, group exercise programs, books and magazines to the detriment of the average fitness enthusiasts. Exceeding 75% of maximum heart rate regularly (particularly for a non-elite athlete) will greatly inhibit the development of a strong aerobic base and invite increased risk of injury and burnout. Your cardio exercise range should be 55-75% of maximum heart rate, with occasional high intensity sessions where heart rate approaches maximum during short sprints.

[11] **Statin Side Effects**: Columbia University Study published in The Archives of Neurology suggests that even short term statin use depletes CoQ10 levels, a possible explanation for common statin side effects of exercise intolerance, muscle pain, and other indicators of muscle dysfunction.

The Conventional Wisdom connection between cholesterol levels and disease risk (and thus the popularity of cholesterol-reducing statins) is increasingly being called into question. Seventeen studies on lowering dietary cholesterol were assessed in a 2005 *Annals of Internal Medicine* article. Overall, the studies led to an average 10 per cent decrease in cholesterol levels, but there was no decrease in overall risk of death.

A long-term study published in the New England Journal of Medicine (in 1986, 1987 and 1991) showed that people who are taking multiple cardiac medications have 40 percent higher risk of mortality after four years than those who take nothing. Several other large studies (10,000 men in Europe, published in the European Heart Journal, 1986; 61,000 men in Europe, conducted by the World Health Organization and published in Lancet; 12,000 men in America, published in the Journal of the American Medical Association; a study in Finland published in the Journal of the American Medical Association, 1991) reported the same conclusion – medication either increased mortality or didn't increase survival time.

[12] **Walking To School**: CDC indicates that the percent of children who live within a mile of school and who walk or bike to school as their primary means of transportation has declined almost 25% over the past thirty years (from 87% to 63%) and that children who walk or bike from any distance has declined 26% (from 42% to 16%).

[13] **Poor compliance** with doctor prescribed exercise programs - is a major reason for the widespread condition of lower back pain, poor recovery from surgery and prolonged elevated risk factors for heart disease and cancer.

A 1998 *Journal of the American Medical Association* article noted that even when it comes to taking medication, the average compliance rate is only 50%. An article from *AlignMap – Beyond Patient Compliance*, further suggests that "noncompliance is underreported, typically hidden, and rarely detected by clinicians", and "research studies consistently reveal high levels of inadequate adherence to treatment recommendations throughout the healthcare spectrum, including cases of life-threatening illnesses. The indisputable conclusions are that medical noncompliance is, by any measure and from any perspective, pervasive, and that healthcare's failure to successfully address such a problem comes at the cost of diminished outcomes, unnecessary expense, and avoidable patient morbidity and mortality."

One Canadian study of heart attack victims published in the Canadian Medical Association Journal indicated a 43% noncompliance rate with rehabilitation and treatment recommendations. A Texas study of bariatric surgery patients revealed a noncompliance rate of 41% (female) and 37% (male).

[14] **Caffeine**: The average American uses about 230 milligrams of caffeine per day according to the Mayo Clinic. Side effects of consuming too much caffeine vary by individual (based on body weight, levels of physical and psychological stress and other drug use – according to MayoClinic.com), but can include "increased heart rate and urination, anxiety, headaches, nausea and insomnia", according to the online medical encyclopedia provided by the U.S. National Library of Medicine and the National Institutes of Health. The Mayo Clinic calls caffeine the "most popular behavior-altering drug", with nine of out ten Americans consuming some type of caffeine regularly.

[15] **Family Finances:** A 2003 book by Elizabeth Warren and Amelia Warren Tyagi called *The Two Income Trap: Why Middle Class Mothers and Fathers are Going Broke*, details the financial challenges faced even by working families who enjoy income levels far higher (even adjusting for today's dollars) than previous generations. While many point to the "*Affluenza*" mentality (The widespread cultural ill of excessive consumption habits detailed in John De Graaf's book of the same name) for the middle class's financial challenges, the authors make the convincing case that the larger, less optional expenses are the biggest culprit. Expenses for child care, car payments, college tuition and particularly suburban homes result in millions living in financial distress. Homes sold to families with children skyrocketed 79% in inflation adjusted dollars from 1983 to 1998. The two income couple (comprising some three quarters of all married couples) is a key component of the skyrocketing inflation of suburban home prices over the past 25 years. Hence a vicious circle emerges: home prices rise because many two-income couples can afford them…because they have two incomes! This sounds like "keeping up with the Joneses" times fifty million.

The *New York Times*, in 2003, revealed that a "typical household" (two income earners and one or two children – a demographic responsible for half the nation's personal consumption expenditures) making $60,000-$80,000 per year spends 70 to 75 percent of their take home pay on essentials such as home costs, groceries, vehicles and fuel, education and health care. The authors of *The Two Income Trap* point out that the figure for these expenses was only 54 percent in the early 1970's. Furthermore, the remaining 25% of disposable income, typically categorized as "discretionary", is further eaten up by expenses that might be better defined as "essential" due to social pressures and norms: cell phones, cable or satellite TV, Internet service, high definition TV sets, digital entertainment like iPods. Arguably the category could extend to fashion, cosmetics and popular diversions such as movies and vacations.

[16] **Childhood Obesity:** The CDC reports that nine million kids ages 6-19 are overweight or obese, and that 33% eat fast food every day, (American Academy of Pediatrics). The prevalence of children (ages 6 to 11) who are overweight has increased from about 4% in the 1960s to almost 19% in 2004. (Dr Richard Troiano and Dr Cynthia Ogden).

[17] **Children Recreation**: Dr. Sandra Hofferth and colleagues report that the way children spend their discretionary time has changed - less time is spent in unstructured activities (e.g., free play) and more time is spent in structured activities (e.g., sports and youth programs). Other changes of interest include a doubling of computer use.

[18] **Massive Multiplayer Online Role-Playing Games:** The popularity has skyrocketed from zero in 1998 (due to poor graphics quality, slow Internet connections, and a consequent lack of interest.) to an estimated 30-60 million active users in 2007, according to a Giga Omni Media article. Some consider this a vast underestimate, due to millions of Chinese playing in Internet cafés for four cents per hour but not registering as paid monthly subscribers. World of Warcraft (8.5 million users), Hobbo Hotel (7.5 million) and Runescape (5 million) are the leading games. Pre-teen games Club Penguin (4 million) and Webkinz (3.8 million) are also extremely popular. A survey published on Adpoll.com indicated that 45% of kids play for ten or more hours per week.

[19] **ADHD Prescriptions**: Diagnosis rates of Attention Deficit Hyperactivity Disorder (ADHD) have skyrocketed 500 percent since 1991, according to the Drug Enforcement Administration. An estimated 7 million schoolchildren are being treated with stimulants for ADHD, including ten percent of all ten-year-old American boys, according to an article published in the Journal of the American Medical Association.

A 1998 study by researchers Adrian Angold and E. Jane Costello found that the majority of children and adolescents who receive stimulants for ADHD do not fully meet the criteria for ADHD. The efforts of neurologist Dr. Fred Baughman, ADHD diagnosis critic, led to admissions from the FDA, DEA, Novartis (manufacturers of Ritalin), and top ADHD researchers around the country that "*no objective validation of the diagnosis of ADHD exists.*" A Maryland Department of Education study found that white, suburban elementary school children are using medication for ADHD at more than twice the rate of African American students.

[20] **Life Expectancy of Today's Child:** A 2005 report published in the New England Journal of Medicine suggests that the prevalence of obesity is shortening average lifespan by a greater rate than accidents, homicides and suicides combined. Children today will lose some two to five years of life expectancy due to the prevalence, and earlier onset of, obesity-related diseases like Type 2 diabetes, heart disease, kidney failure, and cancer. Dr. David S. Ludwig, director of the obesity program at Children's Hospital in Boston, said in the report, "Obesity is such that this generation of children could be the first basically in the history of the United States to live less healthful and shorter lives than their parents. There is an unprecedented increase in prevalence of obesity at younger and younger ages without much obvious public health impact. But when they start developing heart attack, stroke, kidney failures, amputations, blindness, and ultimately death at younger ages, then that could be a huge effect on life expectancy."

[21] **American Television:** A.C. Neilsen reports that the average American watches 28 hours of TV per week and that 66% of households have three or more televisions at home (A.C. Nielsen Co.). Dr Donald Roberts and colleagues and Victoria Rideout and colleagues with the Kaiser Family Foundation report that children between the ages of 8 and 18 years spend an average of nearly 6.5 hours a day with electronic media.

CHAPTER 3

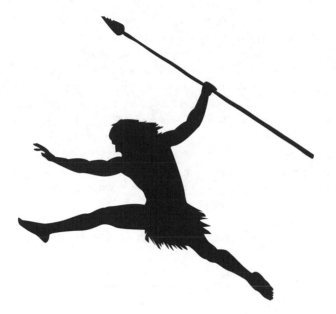

Primal Blueprint
Eating Philosophy

"Do These Genes Make Me Look Fat?"

In This Chapter

I present the philosophy, rationale, and benefits of *Primal Blueprint* eating, emphasizing the importance of moderating insulin production by limiting intake of processed carbohydrates—not only sugars but also all cultivated grains (yep, even whole grains). This simple dietary modification—perhaps the single most critical takeaway action item from the *Primal Blueprint*—will allow you to avoid the immediate unpleasant physical effects of high-carb eating, succeed with long-term weight-loss goals, and prevent many common lifestyle-related health problems and diseases.

You will learn why the Conventional Wisdom story about cholesterol as a direct heart disease risk factor is deeply flawed. The true culprit that triggers the development of atherosclerosis is Metabolic Syndrome, a serious condition that afflicts one in five Americans and is attributed to the typical modern diet and sedentary culture. I detail the dietary steps you can take to virtually eliminate your risk of heart disease. Chief among them is the ingestion of optimal amounts of omega-3s, which play an important role in controlling inflammation and preventing disease.

I detail how each macronutrient (protein, carbohydrate, fat, and the "fourth fuel" of ketones) affects your eating strategy, energy levels, and overall health. The Carbohydrate Curve reveals how various levels of average daily carb intake impact your health and weight management success. The concept of "eating well" means more than just making healthy food choices; it encompasses eating sensibly and intuitively, in a relaxed environment conducive to maximum appreciation of food, and avoiding regimented, restrictive diets that lead to negativity, guilt, and rebellion. Finally, I offer tips on how to succeed in converting to *Primal Blueprint* eating without causing additional stress or disappointment so common with unrealistic diet programs.

Obesity is really widespread
                    - Joseph O. Kern II

Primal Blueprint* eating offers many health benefits, which served Grok and his ancestors well for over two million years. The most important goal of eating like Grok is to regulate insulin production, which leads to success with losing unwanted fat, maintaining an ideal body composition for the rest of your life, and virtually eliminating the major disease risk factors that eventually kill more than half of all Americans. Here are some other major benefits of the *Primal Blueprint* eating style:

Enhanced Cellular Function: The ample levels of high-quality fat, especially the well-known omega-3 fats, found in *Primal Blueprint* foods provide optimum structural components for cell membranes and encourage your body to convert stored fat efficiently into energy. Yes, eating fat—healthy fat—will help you lose weight, as well as regulate your daily energy levels.

Improved Immune and Antioxidant Function: *Primal Blueprint* foods are higher in antioxidants and do not present the immune problems of grains and dairy. In contrast, diets with moderate to high levels of processed carbohydrates and simple sugars have been found to suppress immune function.

Lean Muscle Development and Maintenance: The high-quality protein found in *Primal Blueprint* foods will help you build or maintain lean muscle mass, achieve ideal bone density, and be better able to handle your body's day-to-day repair and renewal requirements. When you control insulin production and eat optimal amounts of protein, you become more *insulin sensitive*. This means the receptor sites in your muscle cells can assimilate amino acids and glucose efficiently, which is the key to muscle building and recovery. This touted benefit is dependent upon following a sensible *Primal Blueprint–*style exercise program that regularly burns stored glycogen and fat and promotes muscle growth.

Natural Weight Management: Plants and animals are much more nutritionally dense than processed carbohydrate foods, which constitute a large percentage of calories in the typical modern diet. Eat like Grok and you'll meet your nutritional needs in fewer calories. Secondly, the ample levels of protein and fat you will be eating have been shown by food scientists to provide deeper and longer lasting satisfaction levels—what they call *satiety*—than you get from a high-carb diet. Finally, when you consume fewer carbohydrates and, as a result, produce less insulin, your hunger and cravings (caused by insulin removing glucose from the bloodstream after high-carb meals or snacks) will subside and you'll intuitively moderate your caloric intake, simply by following your more regulated "natural" appetite.

Optimal Fat Metabolism: When you reduce your consumption of grains, sugars, and other simple carbohydrates in favor of plants and animals, your levels of insulin and its counterregulatory hormone, glucagon, will be in an ideal balance, enabling you to utilize fatty acids (from both food intake and stored fat) as your preferred fuel source.

Reduced Disease Risk Factors: Reducing intake of grains, sugars, other simple carbs, and processed foods, especially "bad fats" (trans and partially hydrogenated), will reduce your production of hormonelike messengers that instruct genes to make harmful pro-inflammatory protein agents. These agents increase your risk for arthritis, diabetes, cancer, heart disease, and many other inflammation-related health problems.

If you want to make an apple pie from scratch, you must first create the universe.
—**Carl Sagan**
American author and astronomer

Stable Energy Levels: *Primal Blueprint* foods help regulate daily energy levels, even if you skip meals, by optimizing insulin/glucagon balance so you can rely on your abundant fat stores for energy. Between-meal hunger subsides, while energy levels remain balanced. In contrast, excess insulin production from a high-carb diet depletes blood glucose levels, leading to fatigue and cravings for quick carbohydrate energy—and the need to eat every few hours.

A Separate Shelf for the Blueprint

You may be familiar with the decades-old best-selling Atkins diet program, named after Dr. Robert Atkins, the original proponent of "low-carb" dieting. Over the years, numerous similar programs (e.g., *South Beach Diet*) have battled for shelf space supremacy with everything from traditional low-fat programs favored by Conventional Wisdom to countless others and have varied from mostly credible to completely ridiculous. Followers of Atkins, South Beach, and other low-carb diets will indeed lose fat by strictly limiting carbohydrates and thus insulin production. However, a blanket, obsessive "ultra-low-carb" strategy can be unhealthy over an extended time period because it limits your intake of some of the most nutritional foods known to humans—vegetables and fruits.

While the *Primal Blueprint* also advocates eliminating the extremely harmful processed carbohydrates and sugars from your diet, vegetables and fruits are a central component of the *Primal Blueprint* eating strategy. Vegetables and fruits (which consist mainly of carbohydrate) are nutrient-dense yet calorically sparse, so that even generous portions of these foods will usually prompt minimal insulin production. One of the on-line *Primal Blueprint* appendices at MarksDailyApple.com compares and contrasts the *Primal Blueprint* with popular diets such as *Atkins,* low fat (e.g., Ornish, MacDougall, Pritikin), metabolic and blood typing, the *Paleo Diet, South Beach,* vegetarian, and the *Zone.*

Of all these mentioned, the *Paleo Diet* is probably most similar to the *Primal Blueprint.* However, I refrain from even calling the *Primal Blueprint* a "diet," due to its comprehensive nature. The Primal Blueprint is a lifestyle—with some important but extremely flexible eating guidelines. I prefer to keep the eating laws in context with the other eight *Primal Blueprint* lifestyle laws for best results.

It's All About Insulin (Well, at Least 80 Percent of "It")

The *Primal Blueprint* eating philosophy might seem a little unusual at first for those trying to do the right thing by Conventional Wisdom. After all, here's a plan that suggests that most fats are not bad at all. In fact, pundits might describe the *Primal Blueprint* as a high-fat, moderate protein, fairly low-carb diet—particularly in comparison to the exceedingly high-carb diet that has been recommended for years by the USDA Food Pyramid, American Heart Association, and American Medical Association.

We now know that these and other experts' outdated and never proven suggestion to essentially eat 300 or more grams of carbohydrates each day has contributed greatly to the destruction of human health. It's not unusual for an average American to consume 500 or 600 grams of insulin-generating, fat-storing carbohydrates daily. Keep in mind that Grok and his clan probably worked hard to gather an average daily intake of only 80 to 100 grams of carbs, most of which came from fibrous natural vegetables and fruits. By averaging between 100 and 150 daily grams (certain extremely active folks may adjust this upward, which I'll discuss later) of vegetable- or fruit-sourced carbs, you can achieve optimally low levels of insulin, enjoy stable energy levels, and easily reduce excess body fat and keep it off. If you want to accelerate your fat loss for a period of time, lowering your average carb intake to 50 to 100 grams or less per day will allow you to easily drop an average of one to two pounds of body fat per week. We will discuss this strategy in detail in Chapter 8.

Sitting down again? Here's another zinger that will blow your mind and set you straight from all the confusion and conflicting information about what the secret to weight loss and long-term body composition success really is....

Eighty percent of your ability to reduce excess body fat is determined by how you eat, with the other 20 percent depending on proper exercise, other healthy lifestyle habits, and genetic factors.

It's as simple as this: if you have excess body fat, it's directly reflective of the amount of insulin you produce from your diet combined with your familial genetic predisposition to store fat. In plain-speak, if you eat like crap and have bad (genetic) luck, you'll get fat and sick and you'll probably die early. On the other hand, bad diet and good luck (having the "skinny gene") might allow you to avoid a plump figure but also might result in a physique that I call "skinny fat"—having minimal subcutaneous fat, minimal lean body mass, and poor muscle definition but still having dangerous amounts of visceral fat surrounding the organs.

Furthermore, skinny fat folks can and do get heart disease, hypoglycemia, arthritis, sarcopenia (loss of muscle mass), chronic fatigue, compromised immune function, and a host of other adverse health consequences heavily attributed to diet. A slender type 2 diabetic can experience an even greater risk for serious disease, because he or she is less able to activate the so-called thrifty genes that efficiently store excess dietary glucose in fat cells (sort of a "toxic waist site" where it's relatively harmless in comparison with glucose that floats around in the bloodstream causing intense cellular damage). While the outward visibility and overall impact severity of poor lifestyle habits vary widely due to luck of the draw, we all share an evolutionary genetic predisposition to suffer chronic disease when we eat foods that are misaligned with our genes.

On the positive side, your ability to reduce excess body fat and maintain desirable body composition is directly reflective of your ability to moderate insulin production with healthy dietary habits and, to a lesser extent, your willingness to follow a sensible exercise program that combines extensive low-level cardio; frequent short, intense strength-training sessions; and occasional all-out sprints. Even if you have struggled with excess body fat for your entire life, you can quickly and dramatically alter your destiny by following the simple laws of the *Primal Blueprint.*

I'm not talking about achieving "success" with a short-term crash program. The *Primal Blueprint* is based on eating as much as you want, whenever you want, from a long list of delicious foods—and simply avoiding eating from a different list. When I say you will notice results quickly and dramatically, I'm referring primarily to the immediate increase and stabilization of energy levels, less hunger and mood swings related to "bonking" (running low on blood glucose), improved immune function, and a reduction in the symptoms of allergies, arthritis, and other inflammatory conditions.

Regarding weight loss, we must recognize that our minds are so messed up on this topic that it's hard even to have a sensible conversation about it. The stories of losing massive amounts of weight in a short time are so commonplace that we seem to expect nothing less when we pursue weight-loss goals. First, the *Primal Blueprint* is really about improving body composition, not about weight loss. For most, a reduction in body fat percentage and an increase or maintenance of muscle or lean body mass.

Clearly, altering your body composition by just a few net pounds by losing fat weight and gaining a little muscle weight produces more impressive appearance changes than someone who drops 20 quick pounds on a crash diet that depletes muscle mass and water. Lean body mass (muscle, skeleton, and all the rest of you that is not fat) is also directly correlated with "organ reserve"—the highly desirable ability of all your vital organs to function optimally beyond basal level (e.g., elevating your heart rate during exercise). We'll discuss this critical longevity component further in Chapter 6.

When you trigger your genes to stop storing body fat and start burning it, as well as to build or maintain muscle mass, you can sensibly and realistically lose a pound or two of body fat per week. You can even do this with minimal exercise, but the rate of fat loss (and the gaining, sculpting, or toning of lean muscle) can be accelerated significantly when you choose the right exercise regimen. Mostly, your success depends on how aggressive you are in keeping dietary insulin levels moderated, thereby extracting more of your caloric needs from fat stores.

Not a day goes by without a friend, client, or MarksDailyApple.com commenter relating to me how he or she notices improvements within days of switching to the *Primal Blueprint* eating style. As I will detail in this chapter, you have the chance to alter your biochemistry at each meal—to stimulate an efficient fat-burning metabolism and consistent energy levels or to do the opposite with poor food (and exercise) choices. The momentum you build with good choices will make it easier to discard old habits in favor of both instant gratification (from filling meals and stable energy levels) and positive long-term health and metabolic consequences.

No, Really—It's All About Insulin

The insulin story is perhaps the most health-critical concept in the book, so I want you to fully understand it on both a practical and a biochemical level. Like so many things in life, a moderate amount of insulin is good and a lot can be bad—very bad. By now you understand insulin's role as a storage hormone and that eating more carbs results in more insulin production. Insulin delivers nutrients to all cells, but for our purposes, we'll focus on insulin's role delivering nutrients to liver, muscle, and fat cells. When the system works as designed by evolution, cell receptors use insulin as a key to unlock pores within the membrane of each cell. With the cell door open, nutrients can then be stored inside the cell. It's an elegant way for cells to gather the nutrients they need and also to eliminate excess glucose from the bloodstream (remember, excess glucose is highly toxic) and store it as fuel for a later date.

Unfortunately, when we produce too much insulin over time, as happens when our modern diet is high processed carbohydrates, several things go wrong. First, muscle and liver cells aren't able to store a whole lot of glycogen (the stored form of glucose), so it's easy to exceed storage capacity with a typical moderate-to-high–carb modern diet. The average person can only store about 400 grams of glycogen in liver and muscle tissue (even a highly trained athlete can only store perhaps 600 grams). When your liver and muscles become filled with glycogen, any glucose remaining in the bloodstream that isn't used in "real time" by your brain or muscles (such as during an intense workout) gets converted into triglycerides in the liver and sent to fat cells for storage.

When blood insulin levels are high, those same fat cells store not only the excess glucose but the fat you ate at your last meal. Moreover, high insulin signals the fat cells to hold on to the fat and not release it for energy. If the pattern of high insulin-generating meals continues, fat cells swell up and we gain weight. Eventually, especially among people who don't exercise much, muscle and liver cells start to become *insulin resistant*—their receptors become desensitized to insulin's storage signals (the aforementioned insulin key doesn't unlock the cell membrane to allow nutrients in). Inactive folks generally have plenty of muscle and liver glycogen stored at all times. Because they are unpracticed at burning and inefficient at restocking energy from dietary nutrients, insulin takes ingested carbohydrates and fats on an express train, passing right through the liver, to their ultimate destination in fat cells.

Continuing this process can lead to severe obesity. Eventually, even fat cells become resistant to further storage, because we only have a fixed amount of fat cells. At that point, the body's last line of defense against glucose (the complete gorging of a finite number of fat cells) has maxed out. Consequently, all hell breaks loose in terms of blood glucose toxicity and insulin damage—leading to even greater risk for diabetes, heart attack, blindness, the need for limb amputation, and other disasters.

Unless you are exercising incessantly to burn stored glycogen and fat, the more insulin your pancreas produces, the more resistant your muscle and liver cells can get. This happens because the genes responsible for these receptor sites turn themselves off or "down-regulate" in response to—and defense against—the excessive insulin in your bloodstream. This is all part of the body's quest for homeostasis and balance and your genetic response to environmental signals. It is now becoming clearer how the shocking statistic of the average American gaining one and a half pounds of fat a year for 30 years is achieved. Conversely, when insulin levels are moderated (as happens with low carbohydrate eating and/or frequent exercise), your liver and muscle cell receptor sites become *insulin sensitive*—more effective at absorbing ingested nutrients transported by insulin. Furthermore, moderated insulin levels signal genes to make more receptor sites.

An insulin-resistant liver exacerbates the situation. The "No Vacancy" sign hanging on the liver (glucose is turned away due to insulin resistance) tricks some cells in your liver into believing they are starved for glucose. In response, genes in other liver cells get the signal to commence gluconeogenesis and dump more glucose into the bloodstream- despite the fact that there's already plenty in the bloodstream (talk about a communication breakdown!). Of course, your resistant muscle cells are deaf to insulin signaling as well, so the new, extra glucose your liver just made is also diverted to the eager fat cells – unless they too are resistant. Here is a quick summary of some of the unpleasant consequences of becoming insulin resistant:

Fat cells can't release their stored energy into the bloodstream, where the fatty acids could be used as fuel, because insulin keeps the fat locked inside.

Fat cells get bigger (and fatter), so you gain weight.

More glucose stays in your bloodstream longer, causing damaging AGEs (advanced glycation end products), chemical reactions that occur when blood-borne glucose molecules bind randomly with important proteins, rendering them useless. This can result in increased inflammation and risk of heart disease as well as the circulation problems and neuropathies (nerve damage) that characterize type 2 diabetes.

Pancreatic beta cells, continually sensing high levels of glucose in the bloodstream, keep working harder and harder to pump out more and more insulin. Eventually, the beta cells can become exhausted and stop working entirely—similar to the plight of insulin-dependent type 1 diabetics. All of this can happen as a result of eating too many carbohydrates for too long and/or not exercising enough to maintain insulin sensitivity.

But wait, there's more! As bad as all that glucose remaining in the bloodstream is, chronically high levels of insulin are almost worse. Insulin is very pro-inflammatory and can wreak havoc throughout the body. Scientists know that within any species, those that produce the least amount of insulin over a lifetime generally live the longest and remain healthiest (except type 1 diabetics, who might die but for supplemental insulin injections).

Excessive insulin is also now believed to be a central catalyst in the development of atherosclerosis. Insulin promotes platelet adhesiveness (sticky platelets clot more readily) and the conversion of macrophages (a type of white blood cell) into foam cells, which are the cells that fill with cholesterol and accumulate in arterial walls. Eventually, a cholesterol and fat-filled "tumor" blocks circulation in the artery, a situation further aggravated by increased platelet adhesiveness and thickness of the blood. In addition, insulin reduces blood levels of nitric oxide (a compound that relaxes the endothelium, the lining of your arteries), causing your artery walls to become more rigid. This drives up blood pressure and increases the sheer force of blood against the arterial wall, further exacerbating the atherosclerotic condition. I will further detail the chain of events causing atherosclerosis, and what you can do to prevent it, in the cholesterol section later in this chapter.

Once you understand the process, it's instructive to take a step back and realize how important exercise is to creating insulin sensitivity (along with low-insulin eating, of course). If you frequently empty your liver and muscle cells of glycogen with brief, intense workouts (you burn a little bit of glucose during the long, slow stuff, too), you become adept at not only burning calories but replenishing: accepting nutrients transported by insulin into your liver and muscle instead of just having them go straight to fat. If you are sedentary and eating a moderate or high-carbohydrate diet, there is no selection pressure (to borrow an apropos term from our evolution discussions) to be insulin sensitive. My foolproof prevention plan—or, dare I say, cure (you read my disclaimer legalese, right?)—for those with type 2 diabetes, obesity, and heart disease, no matter how overwhelming their genetic predisposition is to these conditions, is to exercise according to the *Primal Blueprint* laws and moderate insulin production with your diet.

It's interesting to note that levels of growth hormone and other important health-enhancing hormones are also adversely affected by insulin resistance. The pituitary gland makes growth hormone, which is then sent to the liver to signal the production of insulin-like growth factors (IGFs). Many of our cells have surface receptors for IGFs. Because of its similar structure, insulin binds to IGF receptors and prevents growth hormone-stimulated IGFs from doing their job. The thyroid gland produces a hormone called T4, which is converted in the liver to T3, the primary hormone that controls energy metabolism. When your liver becomes insulin resistant, conversion of T4 to T3 declines drastically. This leads to a decrease in metabolic rate, increased fat storage, and diminished energy levels and brain function.

High insulin levels over long periods of time also hamper sex hormone synthesis, causing levels of testosterone, DHEA, and other sex hormones to decline steeply as we age. Hormone levels naturally decline over time, but this flagship premise of the multi-billion-dollar antiaging industry is greatly exacerbated by insulin resistance as opposed to the mere passing of the seasons. Remember, if Grok was lucky, he could enjoy dramatically better health and physical fitness into his 70s than most of today's baby boomers. Sex hormones are supposed to be transported through the bloodstream by globulin (a blood protein) to act upon target organs and tissues. When excessive insulin is present, these hormones stay bound to globulin instead of getting dropped off at the target cells (e.g., the adrenal glands, sex organs, and brain are all strongly impacted by sex hormones) and doing their thing. Even an expensive antiaging hormone regimen cannot override this undesirable sex hormone-binding-to-globulin condition caused by excessive insulin.

Clearly, the ideal strategy is to assimilate your dietary nutrients using only the insulin you need to restock muscle and liver glycogen stores, rebuild muscle and other tissue with amino acids, and, finally, transport fatty acids to assist with a variety of essential metabolic functions (including energy storage). By maintaining an optimal balance between insulin and glucagon, you become like an ATM machine, always open for deposits and withdrawals based on your daily energy needs. Clearly, insulin is absolutely essential to life. It's just that chronic overproduction of insulin (also known as hyperinsulinemia) turns a good thing into a bad thing. It's as simple as this: when you eat the *Primal Blueprint*-style foods that fit your genes, you'll be able to fit into your jeans!

But a Little Bit Won't Hurt, Right?

If these clinical details about the long-term damage from a high insulin-producing diet are not sufficient to get you to change your breakfast order today, consider the short-term unpleasant effects of high-carbohydrate (and particularly high-sugar), insulin-producing meals and snacks (on otherwise healthy, nondiabetic folks). In short (sing along now), it's "high-low, high-low, toward insulin resistance you go!"

Ingesting a high-carbohydrate food or meal (sugary foods and beverages, desserts, processed grains, etc.) generates an immediate increase in blood glucose levels, which has the short-term effect of elevating your mood, energy level, and alertness (remember, your brain prefers glucose as fuel). In a matter of minutes, however, your pancreas (in a valiant effort to reduce the amount of toxic glucose in your bloodstream and store it someplace useful) is prompted to secrete a large amount of insulin. Depending on the type and amount of carbs you consumed and your degree of insulin sensitivity, this insulin rush can eventually cause your blood glucose levels to decline so much that your glucose-dependent brain is now low on fuel. As a result, you may soon feel sluggish, foggy, and cranky and have trouble focusing. While this explains the familiar post-lunch afternoon blues, extensive data also suggest a strong link between attention deficit/hyperactivity disorder (ADHD) and processed carbohydrate consumption/insulin production.

The ingestion of lots of carbohydrates, followed by the secretion of lots of insulin causing low blood glucose levels is perceived as a stressful event by the hypothalamic-pituitary-adrenal (HPA) axis. This homeostasis-monitoring part of your endocrine system triggers the fight-or-flight response, causing your adrenal glands to release epinephrine (commonly called "adrenaline") and cortisol into your bloodstream. Cortisol breaks down precious muscle tissue into amino acids, some of which are sent to the liver and converted into glucose through gluconeogenesis. The ensuing liver-generated blood glucose rush gives you the boost your brain thinks you need—at the expense of your muscle tissue! Depending on your individual sensitivity to glucose and insulin, the stress response to this seesaw process may now make you feel amped, jittery, edgy, and hyper, and you may have a racing heartbeat.

After some time passes and the stress response subsides, you can experience a post-stressful-event-combined-with-sugar-crash condition affectionately known as burnout. This physical, mental, and emotional lull prompts a strong craving for another quick high from sugar, and the cycle repeats. Over time, your continued abuse of the stress response system can overwork your pancreas and adrenal glands, paving the way for health problems like chronic fatigue, inflammation, and weight gain.

Besides the unsettling energy swings and added stress, sugar also seriously hampers immune function. We know that excessive and/or prolonged production of cortisol is a potent immune suppressor (the fight-or-flight mechanism diverts resources to provide an immediate energy boost). Research also shows that sugar itself can impair the function of immunity-related phagocytes (immune system cells that remove bacteria or viruses from the bloodstream) for at least five hours after ingestion. This impairment happens through a process known as competitive inhibition, when excess glucose prevents the all-important antioxidant vitamin C from being transported inside certain immune cells. Because both molecules use the same mechanism and entry point to gain access to the inside of the immune cells, the presence of excessive glucose can overwhelm the transporter site and block vitamin C from entering. With your guard summarily down, oxidative stress on your body increases as free radicals are allowed to run wild. Furthermore, your blood thickens as a response to these immune stressors, which is why heart attacks (in people predisposed to them) tend to occur after a meal.

Over time, the continued abuse of the insulin system leads to the serious health problems detailed previously in this chapter. Note that the chain of events described here happens routinely in a normal, healthy person who overdoes carbohydrate or sugar intake. Experiencing these high-low, high-low cycles from sugar ingestion is no fun, but it does mean you still have some sensitivity to the negative effects of sugar ingestion and insulin production. If you *don't* experience significant noticeable symptoms from eating lots of carbohydrates (particularly sugar), you are likely well on your way, or have already developed, the extremely problematic condition of insulin resistance. The analogy of a smoker feeling minimal to no immediate ill effects from his or her habit is relevant here. I'd argue that a vast majority of the population is somewhere on this continuum, far outside of the healthy ideal of a diet that moderates carb intake and insulin production in line with our genetic requirements for health.

Naturally, grain or sugar products will jack up blood glucose levels quickly and produce a greater insulin response than consuming a similar amount of calories from vegetables and fruits or combining a few carbs with slower burning protein or fat calories. While it's obviously preferable to mute the immediate insulin spike, your diet's total insulin load is still a serious concern. If you are routinely eating 150 to 300 grams (or more) of carbs per day, you will likely gain weight insidiously (unless you exercise like crazy) and still increase your risk of developing other associated health problems, including the "oxidation and inflammation" syndrome that is the major culprit behind heart disease, which I'll detail in the next section, about cholesterol.

It's Not About Cholesterol...Really, It's Not!

Big Pharma and your helpful friends at the FDA, the AMA, and other reputed health agencies have done a great job of vilifying cholesterol and saturated fat as the major causes of atherosclerosis and heart disease via the well-accepted lipid hypothesis of heart disease. You know their story by now. Your arteries are like pipes. Cholesterol is the fatty, sticky gunk that clogs them up if you eat too many high-cholesterol animal products (meat, eggs) or saturated fats in general. According to Conventional Wisdom, you should eat a low-fat, low-cholesterol, high complex-carbohydrate diet. If your diet or genetic "bad luck" results in a total cholesterol level over 200, you simply take cholesterol-lowering statin medicines to safely reduce your risk.

In recent years, many elements of Conventional Wisdom about cholesterol have been called into question. While there is significant dispute and uncertainty on the issue among respected experts, there is compelling evidence that freely dispensing powerful statin medications to reduce all forms of cholesterol offers only minimal protection from heart disease and stroke. Furthermore, it's almost universally agreed that lifestyle modifications (such as losing weight, reducing intake of processed carbs and fats, consuming omega-3 oils, exercising, and managing stress levels) can do a much better job than statins in eliminating the major heart disease risk factors.

Because I highly respect the valiant battle medical professionals are fighting with today's heart disease pandemic (after all, they often have little or nothing to do with patients until they show up on the appointment calendar with clogged pipes), I'd like to assert here that this is not a "Mark versus your doctor" battle of the egos. Rather, I believe this is an unbiased interpretation of cutting-edge data that extends beyond the narrow and dated "eating fat drives cholesterol drives heart disease" paradigm that most of us, including physicians, are familiar with.

> *Using total cholesterol level—or even your LDL cholesterol value—as a heart disease risk factor is like saying, 'Going to the beach is dangerous.' It's irrelevant in the absence of further context, such as Metabolic Syndrome and other accomplices to heart disease.*

This discussion will give you a deeper understanding of exactly what causes heart disease (*hint*: it's inflammation and oxidation, driven primarily by poor food choices, excessive insulin production and all forms of stress in excess, including overexercising) and help you do a better job minimizing heart disease risk than just following the party line of "Don't eat cholesterol—and take drugs if your numbers are high." If you are already familiar with the basics of blood chemistry and a firm believer in the concept that cholesterol is *not* an efficient marker for heart disease, you may want to skip ahead to the sidebar "How to Sneeze at Heart Disease." Otherwise, fasten your seat belt and hang on for the ride; it could save your life.

Among the most notable research refuting the cholesterol story is the highly respected Framingham Heart Study. The study (which I reference often at Marks-DailyApple.com) has followed the dietary habits of 15,000 participants (residents of Framingham, Massachusetts) over three generations. It is widely regarded as the longest (it began in 1948 and is still going strong!), most comprehensive epidemiological (study of health and illness factors on a population) assessment in medical history. It has led to the publication of more than 1,200 research articles in leading journals. Study director Dr. William Castelli summarized the issue unequivocally when he said, "Serum cholesterol is not a strong risk factor for coronary heart disease." Among the study's highlights are these:

- **There is no correlation** between dietary cholesterol intake and blood cholesterol levels.
- **Framingham residents who ate the most** cholesterol, saturated fat, and total calories actually **weighed the least** and were the most physically active.

Luckily for us, over the past decade, hundreds of bright, clear-thinking researchers have reexamined this data, conducted new research, and written extensively on how and why the Conventional Wisdom lipid hypothesis of heart disease is deeply flawed. (Google the term *cholesterol skeptics* and you'll discover an organized group called the International Network of Cholesterol Skeptics, populated by dozens of leading M.D.'s and Ph.D.'s in the field from across the globe.) Their research now shows that atherosclerosis is caused mainly by the excessive oxidation (and the ensuing inflammation) of a certain type of cholesterol that constitutes a small fraction of the mostly good stuff flowing through your bloodstream.

Ironically, in many cases, it appears that this oxidation might be made worse by consuming the very (cholesterol-free) polyunsaturated fats in vegetable and grain oils that the medical establishment led us to believe were healthier than animal fats! The millions who use statin drugs daily incur a significant expense and endure disappointing side effects. For nearly all users, there is little or no demonstrable reduction in heart disease risk.

Cholester-ALL—More Than Just a Number

Cholesterol is a little waxy lipid (fat) molecule that happens to be one of the most important substances in the human body. Every cell membrane has cholesterol as a critical structural and functional component. Brain cells need cholesterol to make synapses (connections) with other brain cells. Cholesterol is the precursor molecule for important hormones such as testosterone, estrogen, DHEA, cortisol, and pregnenolone. Cholesterol is needed for making the bile acids that allow us to digest and absorb fats. Cholesterol is made into all-important vitamin D in the presence of sunlight. Bottom line is that you can't live without cholesterol, which is why your liver actually makes up to 1,400 milligrams a day regardless of how much food-borne cholesterol you consume—or how much you avoid it like the plague—in your diet.

Because cholesterol is fat-soluble (it does not dissolve in water—think balsamic vinegar remaining intact in a dish of olive oil) but must travel to and from cells in the watery environment of the bloodstream, it needs to be carried by special spherical particles called lipoproteins (the name means "part protein and part lipid"). There are several varieties of lipoproteins with different transporting functions—chylomicrons, LDLs, IDLs, HDLs, and VLDLs (as well as subfractions of those)—but the three we are concerned with here are VLDLs, LDLs, and HDLs (very low-density, low-density, and high-density lipoproteins, respectively). Each of these lipoproteins carries a certain percentage of cholesterol, triglycerides, and other minor fats. Your blood test values for triglycerides and HDL, LDL, and VLDL cholesterol represent the combined total in your bloodstream of what all the lipoproteins are transporting.

VLDLs, the largest of these cholesterol complexes, are manufactured in the liver in the presence of high levels of triglycerides (triglycerides are also made in the liver—from excess carbohydrates and fats). Hence, VLDLs comprise 80 percent triglyceride (and a little cholesterol). After leaving their birthplace in the liver, these lipoproteins deliver their cargo to fat and muscle cells for energy. Once these VLDLs have deposited their triglyceride load inside a fat or muscle cell, their size decreases substantially and they become LDLs. At this point, they bear mostly cholesterol and a little bit of remaining triglyceride. In a healthy person, most of these LDL molecules are called "large fluffy" or "buoyant" LDLs. As such, they are generally harmless, even at relatively high levels, as they go about their assigned task of delivering cholesterol to the cells that need it.

The real trouble starts when triglycerides are unusually high in the bloodstream. This condition can occur routinely when you eat a high-carb diet (even if it's a low-fat diet), because, as you learned in the "It's All About Insulin" section, excessive insulin production drives the conversion of ingested carbohydrate into fat (triglycerides). Obviously, the condition can also occur when you eat a moderate-carb, high-fat diet, because insulin will see to it that both excess carbs and fat get circulated in the bloodstream and stored in fat cells.

> *Low-fat eating requires you to consume excessive carbs, by default, to obtain your daily energy requirements*

Dr. Dean Ornish and other proponents of low-fat eating will tell you that reducing fat intake reduces cholesterol and triglyceride levels. This is absolutely true, as confirmed by numerous best-selling books as well as newspaper and magazine feature stories touting quick and dramatic results (lowered cholesterol and triglyceride levels) from fat-restrictive diets. But one reason is this: your liver makes cholesterol as a raw material for the bile salts that help you digest fat, so if you aren't eating fat, your genes will be given the signal to down-regulate cholesterol production.

However, low-fat eating requires you to consume excessive carbs, by default, to obtain your daily energy requirements. This leads to excessive insulin production and, as you recall, kick-starts the cycle that eventually leads to heart disease. Any way you slice it, consuming too many carbs leads to high triglycerides (not to mention the other risk factors detailed in the sidebar "How to Sneeze at Heart Disease").

With high triglycerides in your blood, VLDL production skyrockets to handle the extra load. This can cause some of the VLDL particles to become altered into a more sinister form of LDL that has been shown to be a major factor in atherosclerosis and heart disease. These "small, dense LDLs" (why can't all medical nomenclature be this easy?) are thought to initiate the majority of atherosclerosis problems when they become stuck in the spaces between cells lining the artery and then become oxidized. This oxidative damage causes inflammation and begins a process of destruction that I will detail shortly. Research has shown that people with Metabolic Syndrome or type 2 diabetes all have elevated levels of both triglycerides and these small, dense LDL particles. Of course, these same people have substantially increased risks for heart disease and stroke.

The remaining cholesterol complex with which you might be familiar is the high-density lipoprotein (HDL), which takes cholesterol back to the liver for recycling. HDLs also clean up any damaged or oxidized cholesterol that might cause problems later—including removing the small, dense LDL particles and oxidized cholesterol that have become stuck in the artery wall. These tiny but powerful HDL cholesterol complexes are often called the "good cholesterol" or "nature's garbage trucks." Medical researchers generally agree that the more HDL you have, the lower your risk for heart disease. As you might have imagined, people with Metabolic Syndrome and type 2 diabetes also typically have low levels of beneficial HDL. Exercise is one of the cheapest, easiest, and most effective ways to raise HDL.

Murder Mystery Dinner—Oxidation and Small, Dense LDL Are Guilty!

As mentioned earlier, because lipoproteins have a lipid surface, they are subject to oxidation. Like oils left open in your kitchen, they can go rancid when they come in contact with oxygen. When this happens they—and the cholesterol inside—can become damaged. Of course, oxidation happens all the time throughout the body, and we have evolved some effective antioxidant enzyme systems (namely catalase, superoxide dismutase, and glutathione) to prevent too much of this damage from getting out of control. Furthermore, consuming ample levels of high-antioxidant foods (fruits, vegetables, nuts and seeds, dark chocolate, red wine, as will be detailed in Chapter 4) and antioxidant supplements (such as vitamin E, CoQ10, beta-carotene, and lycopene) can help mitigate some of the damage. It's also extremely convenient that HDLs can remove some of the damaged cholesterol and take it back to the liver for recycling.

Your cholesterol processing system clearly has evolved to expect a certain range and quality of dietary fat, protein, carbohydrate, and antioxidants, as well as a certain level of exercise (to help promote insulin sensitivity in the muscles and maintain high levels of HDL) to provide appropriate gene signals and avoid artery disease. And because HDL particles are very small, they can get into the spaces between arterial wall cells and clean up the oxidized cholesterol. That's why Big Pharma has tried—so far unsuccessfully—to create an effective drug to raise HDL and address existing atherosclerosis (some physicians prescribe the combination of prescription fibrates and over-the-counter niacin to raise HDL, but this treatment can be problematic and is not widely used).

The system has served humans and most all other mammals well for millions of years—until recently, when processed carbohydrates and partially hydrogenated fats entered the picture. As a result of unique gene signaling from consuming too much of these unnatural foods, small, dense LDLs are created and can become trapped in the spaces between endothelial cells lining the artery (sometimes called a gap junction). Even if they are not oxidized to begin with, once trapped, they can oxidize in place because they are sitting there continually exposed to oxygen passing by attached to hemoglobin in the red blood cells. Either way, this oxidation eventually causes injury and inflammation to the arterial wall, prompting the body's immune system to send macrophages (scavenging white blood cells) to gobble up the oxidized LDLs at the site where the first particles were trapped.

The immune system tries hard to do its job, but the macrophages are overwhelmed by absorbing so much oxidized LDL. Their gorging on oxidized LDLs signals specific genes to transform the macrophages into foam cells that attach to the arterial lining, laying the foundation for future trouble. The resulting lesion prompts more macrophages to come to the rescue. They try to gobble up more and more oxidized LDLs floating by, increasing the severity of the lesion over time. This is the familiar saga of plaque accumulation on the arterial wall. The plaque grows and eventually compromises the inner diameter of the artery. If allowed to continue, it can eventually occlude blood flow or break off as a clot, preventing blood—and oxygen—from reaching a vital organ (resulting in your classic heart attack or stroke).

The oxidation of these small, dense LDLs most likely happens for a variety of reasons that have to do with modern dietary habits more than anything else: a high intake of unstable polyunsaturated fats from vegetable oils in the diet (PUFAs incorporated into the lipid layer are much more prone to oxidation than are saturated fats); a reduced intake of natural antioxidants in the diet, which would otherwise mitigate oxidation; the presence of fewer HDL particles to remove oxidized lipids (low HDL cholesterol readings may be partly caused by high-carb diets); and the fact that small, dense LDL particles do not bind as easily to the normal LDL receptors on muscle and fat cells. Unable to release their cholesterol load and with typically fewer HDL particles to gobble them up, these small, dense LDL particles linger longer in the oxygen-rich bloodstream until they oxidize. By the way, the reason atherosclerosis happens in the arteries and not the veins is because venous blood has very little oxygen.

Note that the oxidation and inflammation process described has little or nothing to do with your total cholesterol or even your total LDL cholesterol levels. In most cases, atherosclerosis is a result of the oxidation of a small fraction of the total amount of LDL in your blood—the small, dense LDL particles. If you have little or none of these in your blood, your risk for heart disease drops dramatically. Also, if your HDL is high, it's very unlikely that you'll encounter a problem, because HDL does a great job of scavenging the oxidized cholesterol from LDL in the bloodstream.

Unfortunately for some of us, poor diet, lack of exercise, stress, certain drug therapies, and, yes, family genetic history can all contribute to the increased production of the dangerous small, dense LDL particles. Your doctor can test for them if you ask, but most common blood tests don't yet distinguish between the benign "fluffy" forms of LDL, sometimes called pattern A, and the small, dense particles, called pattern B. A comprehensive lipid blood panel will typically provide values for total cholesterol, HDL, LDL, VLDL, and triglycerides.

A physician will generally dispense medication if your total LDL levels exceed a certain figure (this varies by doctor and individual patient profile), knowing it will respond to the statins with a quick overall reduction. Statins will indeed lower all forms of LDL (including both the good stuff and the bad stuff), but it's a much more sensible—and safe—option to simply alter dietary and exercise habits and minimize insulin production, thereby preventing excess accumulation of triglycerides in the blood and allowing the cholesterol system to work as intended. In fact, the combination of low carbs and good fats in a *Primal Blueprint* eating plan, along with *Primal Blueprint* exercise habits, will generally raise HDL, lower both triglycerides and small, dense LDL, and allow you, regardless of your genetic predisposition, to essentially have no participation in this heart disease saga whatsoever. The choice is yours.

> *HDL does a great job of scavenging the oxidized cholesterol from LDL in the bloodstream… if your HDL is high, it's much less likely you'll encounter a [heart disease] problem.*

Statin Stats Stink!

Isn't it ironic, then, to discover that statins and other cholesterol-lowering meds do not have any ability to influence LDL particle size and can only lower total LDL by reducing both the good and the bad versions? The fact that some people taking statins experience a dramatic reduction in total cholesterol or in LDL means very little in the context of the true oxidation and inflammation nature of heart disease. To be clear, statins do slightly reduce the risk of additional heart attacks among men under the age of 65 who have had a prior heart attack. However, many doctors now believe that these benefits are independent of their "cholesterol-lowering" properties and instead come from an anti-inflammatory effect that addresses the more proximate cause of heart disease. A cheaper and more effective anti-inflammatory effect can be achieved by eating foods high in omega-3, taking fish oil supplements, or popping a small dose of aspirin daily.

By simply adopting the *Primal Blueprint* laws, you can enjoy superior results without the perilous side effects and huge expense of drug therapy. In the case of statins, known side effects include muscle pain, weakness and numbness, chronic fatigue, tendon problems, cognitive problems, impotence, and blood glucose elevations. These side effects are believed to be due in large part to statins' interference with the normal production of a critical micronutrient known as coenzyme Q10 (CoQ10). CoQ10 is essential to healthy mitochondrial function and defending our cells against free radical damage. Statin therapy is believed to lower CoQ10 levels by up to 50 percent. Ironically, CoQ10 plays a particularly important role in the healthy function of the cardiovascular system, and heart attack patients show depressed levels of CoQ10! Some researchers suggest that statins' depletion of CoQ10 may nullify any potential benefits of statin therapy.

So why are millions being misguided to take dangerous, powerful drugs when lifestyle intervention is more effective and less expensive and has no side effects? Perhaps we like to search for easy answers with quick results, and statins produce a graphic and quick decline in blood cholesterol levels. Like other elements of Conventional Wisdom, there are billions of dollars invested and powerful market forces pushing us in the direction of swallowing drugs and their side effects, while the full story is lost amidst the hype of "lower your numbers quick!"

> *By simply adopting the Primal Blueprint laws, you can enjoy superior results without the perilous side effects and huge expense of drug therapy.*

If you are currently taking statins or other medications, I realize that asking you to reject Conventional Wisdom and the specific recommendations of your trusted physician can put you in a very uncomfortable position. I strongly urge you to engage in lifestyle modification (after all, there are no side effects or potential compromises to your drug regimen when you improve your diet), while concurrently addressing the possibility with your doctor of gradually reducing your dependence on medication.

How to Sneeze at Heart Disease

The catchall term *Metabolic Syndrome* is used to describe an assortment of heart disease risk factors widely attributed to today's prevailing poor dietary and exercise habits. The highly respected Cleveland Clinic states that "the exact cause of Metabolic Syndrome is not known...[but] many features are associated with insulin resistance." When you have three or more of the following five markers, you are diagnosed as having metabolic syndrome.

Elevated fasting blood glucose: 100 mg/dl or greater
Blood pressure: 130/85 mm Hg or greater
Waistline measurement: 40 inches or more for men and 35 inches or more for women
HDL: less than 40 mg/dl for men and less than 50 mg/dl for women
Triglycerides: 150 mg/dl or greater

The U.S. government and other sources report that some 47 million Americans have Metabolic Syndrome—about one in five Americans. It's a chronic condition that develops and worsens over time (with no immediate discernable physical symptoms) unless you take dramatic steps to alter your lifestyle. The Cleveland Clinic and *Journal of the American Medical Association* report that more than 40 percent of Americans in their 60s and 70s have the condition. Dr. Richard Feinman, one of the most often-published and highly regarded researchers in the fields of nutrition and metabolism, has suggested that "Metabolic Syndrome may be defined by the response to carbohydrate restriction" (restrict carbs and immediately improve your five markers).

Supplemental Blood Tests

A routine physical exam and blood panel will give you an indication of your Metabolic Syndrome status. Many experts recommend a few additional blood tests to assess overall health and risk factors, including:

C-Reactive Protein: High sensitivity–C-reactive protein (hs-CRP) is produced by your liver as part of an immune system response to injury or infection. In the absence of other acute infections, high levels of hs-CRP in your blood are associated with an increased risk of heart attack, stroke, and sudden cardiac death. Because atherosclerosis is primarily a disease of inflammation, some researchers contend that hs-CRP is a strong predictor of your heart disease risk.

Lp2A: Another key inflammation marker associated with small, dense LDL particles.

A1c (estimated average glucose): A1c measures how much glucose is attached to a hemoglobin molecule, a reliable marker for the dangers of elevated blood glucose levels over an extended time period (i.e., a dietary "batting average" versus a single trip to the "plate" for a sugar rush home run).

Fasting Blood Insulin Levels: High levels are indicative of prediabetic conditions.

Vitamin D: indicates adequate exposure to sunlight, a critical health component we'll discus in Chapter 7.

continued

Put Inflammation at Ease with Omega-3s

A major feature of *Primal Blueprint* eating is that it provides high levels of healthy saturated and unsaturated fats. While Conventional Wisdom generally positions saturated fats as something to diligently restrict, they are an excellent energy source and offer a variety of nutrients critical to health. Consuming ample amounts of saturated fat helps prevent oxidative damage to your cells (saturated fat is an integral part of cell membranes). While your eyes might bug out at this statement, it's virtually irrefutable and proven by many respected long term studies:

Eat (healthy) fat and help prevent cancer and heart disease. Avoid fat and increase your risk of cancer, heart disease, and even obesity.

Fortunately, omega-3 polyunsaturated fatty acids don't have an image problem and are universally regarded as healthy. Adequate omega-3 consumption supports healthy cardiovascular, brain, skin, and immune function. By turning on genes that improve blood circulation, reduce inflammation, and support healthy cholesterol and triglyceride levels, omega-3s help reduce the risk of high blood pressure, blood clots that cause heart attacks, arthritis, autoimmune disorders, and cognitive problems such as depression, Alzheimer's, and even ADHD. The important role of omega-3s in supporting cognitive function is made even more evident by the fact that half the brain consists of fat, including concentrated levels of the omega-3 docosahexanoic acid, DHA.

The benefits of high omega-3 intake and optimum fatty acid balance are strikingly evident from data on cultures that consume substantial amounts of fat but have markedly reduced heart disease rates compared to Westerners, such as the *traditional* Japanese diet (i.e., for those who frequent sushi bars instead of the 3,598 McDonald's in Japan) centered around fish and vegetables.

Another form of polyunsaturated fats called omega-6s plays a vital role in our health as well, but their extreme prevalence in the Western diet—from vegetable oils, animal fats, bakery items (donuts, cookies), and processed snacks (the highly offensive trans and partially hydrogenated fats are classified as omega-6)—leads to a dangerous imbalance of excessive omega-6 and deficient omega-3. The ideal omega-6 to omega-3 balance is 1:1 or 2:1, ratios that Grok likely met with ease. Even 4:1 is okay today, but the typical modern eater has a ratio of 20:1 or worse! It's also interesting to note that imbalanced fatty acid intake can exacerbate the insulin resistance problem discussed earlier. Omega-6 fats (particularly arachidonic acid) suppress expression of the major insulin receptor gene governing insulin sensitivity (GLUT4), while omega-3 fats increase expression of GLUT4.

Once again, your genes are only doing what they are told to do by the signals you give them. The imbalance of fatty acids in the typical modern diet triggers a genetically programmed inflammation response throughout the body. Under normal circumstances, inflammation is your body's highly desirable first line of defense against pain, injury, and infection. Inflammation detects and destroys toxic material in damaged tissue before it can spread to the rest of the body. Consider examples like a bee sting, taking a fastball to the eye, or turning an ankle on a hiking trail—the reddened skin, black eye, and ballooned ankle help your body quarantine the damage from the trauma to the inflamed areas, instead of letting toxins run wild through the bloodstream. Unfortunately, an out-of-control body-wide inflammatory response (also known as systemic inflammation)—resulting from stress and imbalanced dietary and/or exercise habits—confuses your body into thinking it's under assault from destructive, infectious foreign agents or that a major trauma has just occurred. That's when the disease process begins.

The extreme stress of my Chronic Cardio training regimen and my highly inflammatory grain-based diet led to excessive and prolonged inflammation throughout my body. What I should have been seeking was a more desirable temporary state of moderate inflammation (pumped muscles, elevated heart rate, oxygenated lungs, etc.—factors that enhance peak performance), from a *Primal Blueprint*–aligned training regimen and plenty of recovery time and good food choices for my body to return to homeostasis. My undesirable "overtraining" inflammatory response compromised the optimal function and recovery of my muscles, joints, and immune system. Interestingly, after extreme endurance events like a marathon or ironman race, blood levels of CPK (creatine phosphokinase; it leaks into the bloodstream when muscle, heart, or brain tissue is traumatized) can be elevated for weeks afterward. In fact, if you presented in the ER with such levels and didn't explain that you had recently run a marathon, the doctor might think you were suffering from a heart attack! In my case, when I adjusted my diet and training habits, virtually all my inflammatory symptoms vanished.

We know that most forms of systemic inflammation have a strong dietary component and can usually be resolved with a few dietary modifications. Nevertheless, Conventional Wisdom within the medical community has recommended fighting our widespread inflammation-related health problems with corticosteroids, COX-2 inhibitors such as Vioxx and Celebrex, and other nonsteroidal anti-inflammatories (asthma meds work on a similar chemical pathway). I have a nonscientific name for this approach: *digging a hole to install a ladder to wash the basement windows.* As you might imagine, because these medications interfere with normal hormone pathways and gene expression, they almost never address the underlying cause of inflammation. They simply mask the pain in the short term—if they mask it at all. Dietary modification (and exercise modification if you are overdoing it) is almost always a superior method of treatment and protection against pain and serious diseases triggered by systemic inflammation.

> *I have a nonscientific name for this approach: **digging a hole to install a ladder to wash the basement windows.***

The *Primal Blueprint* eating style, with its emphasis on high omega-3 foods (such as organically grown animal meats, eggs, fish, nuts and seeds) and its aversion to processed foods, provides an ideal dietary fatty acid balance without you really having to worry about it. When you combine healthy eating with the other *Primal Blueprint* laws, you can naturally avoid the systemic inflammation that is now believed to be the root cause of the major health problems affecting modern humans.

Context In, Calories Out—
Understanding the Macro Nutrients

While you likely have a basic understanding of what carbohydrate, protein, and fat do in the body, it's important to examine the role of each nutrient further in the context of how they support the *Primal Blueprint*. This is particularly true in light of the massive misinformation, distortion, and confusion presented by opposing camps on this issue. For decades, we've been bombarded with messages, ranging from hairsplitting debates on what percentage of total dietary calories should come from carbs, protein, and fat (I'm never concerned where my own percentages fall, because I know they will land in the optimal range when I choose the right foods) to campy marketing glitz served up by the diet celebrity of the month.

Most popular daily diets (and fitness programs) follow the "calories in, calories out" Conventional Wisdom to pursue weight loss, failing to understand the importance of context when making this otherwise literally true statement. Your body uses macronutrients for a variety of different functions, some of which are structural and some of which are simply to provide energy (as calories)—immediately or well into the future. The food you eat can be stored as glycogen and/or body fat or used to build muscle. But just as easily, you can burn off that body fat, deplete glycogen and even tear down muscle for fuel. It's all based on signals you provide in what you eat, how much you eat, when you eat, what you're doing before or after you eat—even what you're thinking when you eat. Yet because your body always seeks to achieve homeostasis (balance), the notion of you trying to zero in on a precise day-to-day or meal-to-meal eating plan is generally fruitless, not to mention practically impossible and incredibly frustrating.

To figure your true structural and functional fuel needs (and, hence, to achieve your body composition goals), it's far more effective to look at a much larger span of time, like a few weeks, and aim for an "average" consumption. This approach will allow for the occasional party splurge, a preplanned (or incidental) calorie-restriction period, an over-the-top workout, or even a week of laziness—without any disastrous long-term effect.

With a big-picture approach, we can appreciate the three macronutrients as more than just typical sources of caloric energy where protein and carbs provide four calories per gram and fat has nine calories per gram. For example, the first 10, 20, or 30 grams of protein you consume daily go toward muscle and other cell repair and growth, not energy. Do we therefore discount those first 30 grams when we count calories? It depends on the context. If you don't exercise much and you eat copiously as a habit, maybe most of the protein you eat will indeed count toward your energy budget (because your structural protein turnover rate is much lower when you don't exercise). On the other hand, if you run yourself ragged, are under a great deal of stress (lots of catabolic hormones are tearing you down), and generally don't consume much protein, most of that high-protein meal might go toward repair and will be unlikely to be called upon as fuel. Simply saying that protein provides four calories per gram for energy needs is like saying that the two-by-four studs that support the walls of your house will burn nicely if you run out of firewood. They will in that emergency situation, but you'll normally choose to burn other fuel first!

Fats aren't just for fuel either. They are integral parts of all cell membranes and hormones and serve as critical protective cushioning for delicate organs. At what point do the fats we consume stop becoming structural raw material and start becoming calorically dense fuel? It depends again on the context. If there's a ton of carbohydrates accompanying the fat on a daily basis, you can bet that dietary fat will be stored as adipose tissue sooner rather than later, because the insulin prompted by the carbs ingested will also deliver those other nutrients right to your fat cells. That's nine calories per gram in the tank to use in the future (or never, considering that introductory stat about Americans adding one and a half pounds of body fat every year).

On the other hand, if you are eating insulin-balancing *Primal Blueprint* meals, fat consumed at a meal might be used quickly to provide fuel for normal metabolic processes at rest or during very low-intensity exercise, or for structural uses and never get stored. If your carb intake drops below 100 grams a day, you can dip into a mild state of ketosis, a fat-burning mode that creates what many now refer to as the metabolic advantage. In this context, fats are fueling most of the body's energy demands either directly as fatty acids or as fat-metabolism by-products called ketones, which I will discuss at length shortly. The following sections define the macronutrients in the context of the *Primal Blueprint* and help you determine how much of each you really need.

Protein

Most nutrition researchers are in agreement that protein is essential for building and repairing body tissues and for overall healthy function. Intake recommendations among doctors and nutritionists vary, with most falling in the range of 0.5 to one gram of protein per pound of lean body mass per day (I favor an average of 0.7 to 1.0). There were days when Grok and his family probably obtained two or three times that amount, so if you happen to overdo your protein significantly on any given day or aren't the type to obsess about such things, you'll almost certainly be well within safe guidelines.

To calculate or estimate lean body mass, you must first determine your total weight and percentage of body fat. You can do this using any of numerous methods ranging from costly and highly accurate water tank tests to the easier fat scales, skinfold calipers, or online calculators using certain body measurements. Most good gyms can help you with this, or you can just estimate roughly for these purposes, knowing that the average moderately fit male and female carry about 15 percent and 22 percent, respectively.

Multiply your total weight by your percent body fat to attain your "fat" weight, and then subtract that figure from your total body weight to obtain your lean body mass. For example, a 155-pound woman with 25 percent body fat has a lean body mass of 116 pounds (155–39=116).

At a minimum you need 0.5 gram of protein per pound of lean mass per day to maintain your "structure" and healthy body composition. If you are even moderately active, you need closer to 0.7 gram, and if you work out regularly (or under a fair amount of stress), you need as much as one gram of protein per pound of lean mass. That's at a minimum, but it's on a daily average. So, our 155-pound moderately active woman with 116 pounds of lean mass needs an average of 82 grams of protein per day (116 x 0.7). If she gets 60 or 70 some days and 110 on others, she'll still be in a healthy average range. She could even fast a day or two occasionally and, provided she has been regularly eating low carb and doesn't overexercise on fasting days, easily preserve her muscle using the body's tendency to retain protein stores in the short term. On the other hand, if she exceeds the 110 grams, it's also no problem if she's eating low carb because the excess protein will convert to glucose, which will reduce her effective carbohydrate needs (see next section). At four calories per gram, her daily average of 82 grams is only 328 calories per day in protein.

Again, I'm not concerned with you counting or even meeting this requirement every single day. You'll find yourself intuitively arriving at a comfortable number or range of protein grams within a week of *Primal Blueprint*–style eating. You will discover that it's quite easy to eat one gram of protein per pound of lean body mass without a lot of planning and pretty difficult to eat much more than two grams per pound without forcing yourself to. You simply aren't as hungry when you regularly eat a low-carb diet. While Grok often ate more than two grams per pound, he was far more active all day long. Grok never knew when the next meal was coming, so he had to stock up in times of feast in order to be prepared for the times of famine. We have a little more leeway today!

If you have ample stored glycogen in your muscle tissues and liver (not a problem for most people unless you are engaged in high-volume, high-stress endurance training or severely restricting your carbs a la the Atkins diet) and your body is getting the rest of its energy efficiently from fats, it's likely that the protein you consume will go first toward the repair or building of cells or enzymes. Proponents of the "a calorie is a calorie" Conventional Wisdom will pipe in here that excess calories are always converted or stored as fat, regardless of their original ingested state. This is true, of course (remember, the *Primal Blueprint* doesn't like to piss off scientists!), and when we eat a high-carb, high-insulin diet, those excess calories indeed are stored as fat. But we must then ask what excess fat calories do when there is not a lot of insulin in the bloodstream (given that they cannot easily be stored as fat without insulin giving them a ride). No problem; the body will respond by raising metabolic rate (to burn more calories at rest) and by increasing the production of ketones, which may be burned or excreted (more on this shortly).

In summary, if you are the type to enjoy and observe details in your macronutrient intake, I suggest you strive to obtain your protein requirements first, in the activity level–influenced range discussed previously. Focus on quality sources of protein such as the organic animal products that will be detailed in the next chapter.

Carbohydrates

If you've forgotten everything you ever learned in biology, just remember this and own it: *carbohydrate controls insulin; insulin controls fat storage.* Carbohydrates are not used as structural components in the body; instead, they are used only as a form of fuel, whether burned immediately while passing by different organs and muscles or stored for later use. All forms of carbohydrates you eat, whether simple or complex, are eventually converted into glucose, which the brain, red blood cells, and nerve cells generally prefer as a primary fuel. For reference, a little less than one teaspoon of glucose dissolved in the entire blood pool in your body (about five quarts in the case of a 160-pound male) represents a normal level of blood glucose.

In most healthy people, glucose that is not burned immediately (exercising muscles prefer glucose, if it is available, but don't absolutely require it unless they are working at high intensity for long periods) will first be stored as glycogen in muscle and liver cells. When these sites are full, glucose is converted into fatty acids and stored in fat cells. It's insulin's job to take glucose out of the bloodstream and put it somewhere fast.

Unless you burn an extreme amount of energy every day (competing endurance athlete, etc.), there is no physiological reason for you to consume high levels of carbohydrate. In fact, carbohydrates are not required in the human diet for survival the way fat and protein are. The body has several backup mechanisms for generating glucose from dietary fat and protein, as well as from proteins stripped from muscle tissue (all done via gluconeogenesis). Some researchers have estimated that the body manufactures up to 200 grams of glucose every day from the fat and protein in our diet or in our muscles. Entire civilizations have lived for thousands of years on 50 or fewer grams of dietary carbohydrate a day.

That said, the *Primal Blueprint* is not designed to be a ketogenic (extremely low-carb) diet, because this strategy would restrict your intake of the most nutrient-dense foods on the planet—vegetables and fruits. I don't even characterize the *Primal Blueprint* as a "low-carb" diet, as much as it is an "eliminate bad carbs" diet. I don't advocate portion control or even diligently counting your macronutrient intake beyond a few days of journaling now and then to establish benchmarks and reference points (visit

FitDay.com or TheDailyPlate.com to calculate your macronutrient amounts from a food diary if you are trying to lose weight). It's really easy to stay in the optimum range of 100 to 150 grams per day even when you eat a ton of colorful vegetables and liberal servings of fruit—as long as you stay Primal and consume no grains. For example, a huge salad, two cups of Brussels sprouts, a banana, an apple, a cup of blueberries, and a cup of cherries totals only 139 grams of carbs.

Note: Perhaps you are familiar with the concept of "net carbs" when measuring macronutrient intake. This is a calculation that subtracts fiber, because fiber is usually not digested and moderates the blood glucose impact of a carbohydrate food. For the sake of simplicity (and to assert the *Primal Blueprint* philosophy that you don't need many carbs, nor any additional fiber from grain foods), all the calculations and zones in this book are represented by *gross* total carbohydrate grams.

The effects on the body of various levels of carb intake (detailed next in "The Carbohydrate Curve") are a critical component of the *Primal Blueprint*, so I should mention a few caveats and exceptions to the guidelines that follow. Obviously, a light, moderately active female has different energy requirements from those of a heavy, active male. The 50-gram/200-calorie variation within each range on the curve attempts to account for the majority of these individual disparities. Also, if you are insistent upon doing Chronic Cardio, you must increase carb intake to account for regular depletion of stored liver and muscle glycogen and an elevated metabolic rate. You can experiment with consuming perhaps 100 additional grams of carbs per day for every extra hour of training and notice how your body responds. However, I'd prefer that you simply adjust your training program to conform to *Primal Blueprint* guidelines and thus reduce your need for dietary carbohydrate.

Hard-core *Primal Blueprint* enthusiasts who have the time and energy to compile many hours of low-level cardio and a steady dose of intense strength training and sprinting and who enjoy abundant servings of fruits and vegetables, trace amounts of carbs from nuts, seeds, and other Primal foods (e.g., even an almond is 14 percent carbohydrate), and the occasional indulgence will quite possibly exceed the 100 to 150 grams per day optimum zone. If you are eating and exercising Primally, feeling energized throughout the day, and effortlessly maintaining ideal body composition, it's a safe bet that the *Primal Blueprint* is working—even if your carb intake at times exceeds the ideal zone described here.

> *It's really easy to stay in the optimum range of 100 to 150 grams per day even when you eat a ton of colorful vegetables and liberal servings of fruit—as long as you stay Primal and consume no grains.*

The Carbohydrate Curve—What'll It Be?
The "Sweet Spot" or the "Danger Zone"?

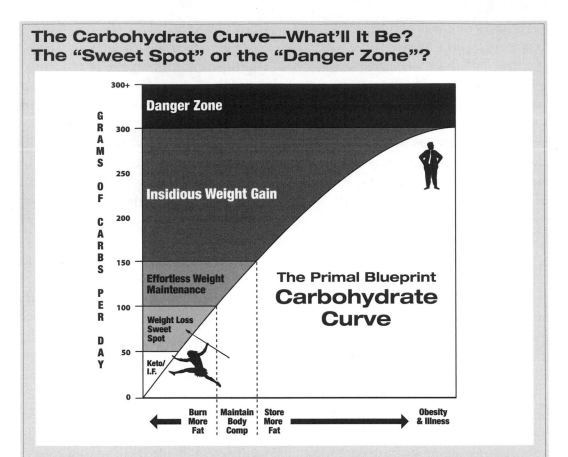

Carbohydrate intake is often the decisive factor in weight loss success and prevention of widespread health problems like Metabolic Syndrome, obesity and type 2 diabetes. These average daily intake levels assume that you are also getting sufficient protein and healthy fats, and are doing some amount of Primal exercise. The ranges in each zone account for individual metabolic differences.

- **0-50** grams per day: *Ketosis and I.F. (Intermittent Fasting)* zone. Excellent catalyst for rapid fat loss through I.F. Not recommended for prolonged periods (except in medically supervised programs for obese or Type 2 diabetics) due to unnecessary deprivation of plant foods.
- **50-100** grams per day: *Sweet Spot for Weight Loss.* Steadily drop excess body fat by minimizing insulin production. Enables 1-2 pounds per week of fat loss with satisfying, minimally restrictive meals.
- **100-150** grams per day: *Primal Maintenance* zone. Once you've arrived at your goal or ideal body composition, you can maintain it quite easily here while enjoying abundant vegetables, fruits and other Primal foods.
- **150-300** grams a day: *Insidious Weight Gain* zone. Most health conscious eaters and unsuccessful dieters end up here, due to frequent intake of sugar and grain products (breads, pastas, cereals, rice, potatoes - even whole grains). Despite trying to "do the right thing" (minimize fat, cut calories), people can still gain an average of 1.5 pounds of fat every year for decades.
- **300+ grams** a day: *Danger Zone* of average American diet. All but the most extreme exercisers will tend to produce excessive insulin and store excessive fat over the years at this intake level. Increases risk for obesity, Metabolic Syndrome and type 2 diabetes.

Here are more details about how carbohydrates impact the human body and the degree to which we need them, or don't need them, in our diet. Carb intake level is the decisive factor in your weight-loss success or failure, and excessive carb consumption is arguably the most destructive behavior disparity between ourselves and what our genes crave to support health, longevity, and peak performance. Eliminating grains and sugars from your diet could be the number one most beneficial thing you ever do for your health!

0 to 50 grams per day *Ketosis and Accelerated Fat Burning*

Acceptable for occasional one- to two-day Intermittent Fasting efforts toward aggressive weight loss (or longer term, for medically supervised weight-loss programs for the obese and/or type 2 diabetics), provided adequate protein, fat, and supplements are consumed. Excellent catalyst for quick, relatively comfortable weight loss and not at all dangerous. (Grok relied heavily on fat metabolism and ketosis to account for the difficulty in obtaining appreciable amounts of carbs in daily life.) Not recommended as a long-term practice for most people due to resultant deprivation of high-nutrient-value vegetables and fruits.

50 to 100 grams per day *Primal Sweet Spot for Effortless Weight Loss*

Minimizes insulin production and accelerates fat metabolism. By meeting average daily protein requirements (in grams per pound of lean mass, as detailed previously), eating nutritious vegetables and fruits, and staying satisfied with delicious high-fat foods (meat, fish, eggs, nuts, seeds), you can lose one to two pounds of body fat per week in the "sweet spot." Delicious menu options that land in the sweet spot are detailed in Chapter 8.

100 to 150 grams per day *Primal Blueprint Maintenance Range*

Allows for genetically optimal fat burning, muscle development, and effortless weight maintenance. Rationale supported by humans eating and evolving in this range or below for millions of years. Dietary emphasis of vegetables, fruits, nuts, seeds, and animal foods, with grains and processed sugars eliminated.

A prior history of heavy carb intake may result in a brief period of discomfort during the transition to *Primal Blueprint* eating. Adequate consumption of satisfying foods (high-water-content fruits and vegetables, high-fat snacks like nuts and seeds, and meals emphasizing animal foods) helps protect against feeling deprived or depleted.

150 to 300 grams per day *Steady, Insidious Weight Gain*

Continuous insulin-stimulating effects prevent efficient fat metabolism and contribute to widespread health conditions. The de facto recommendation of many popular diets and health authorities—including the USDA Food Pyramid!—is 150 to 300 grams per day, despite clear danger of developing Metabolic Syndrome. Chronic exercisers and active growing youth may eat at this level for an extended period without gaining fat, but eventually fat storage and/or metabolic problems are highly probable.

This "insidious" zone is easy to drift into, even by health-conscious eaters, when grains are a dietary centerpiece, sweetened beverages or snacks leak into the picture here and there, and obligatory fruits and vegetables are added to the total. Recall that Wendy Korg's trip to Jamba Juice for a healthy afternoon snack resulted in 187 grams of carbs ingested at one sitting. Starting your day off with a bowl of muesli cereal, a slice of whole wheat toast, and a glass of fresh orange juice might seem as healthy as can be—but the numbers start racking up (that's 97 grams right there!), and the disastrous insulin-sugar crash-stress response cycle is set in motion. Despite trying to do the right thing and cut fat and calories, many frustrated people still gain a pound or two of fat per year for decades as a result of the carb intake in the insidious range.

> *Despite trying to do the right thing and cut fat and calories, many frustrated people still gain a pound or two of fat per year for decades as a result of carb intake in the insidious range.*

300 or more grams per day *Danger Zone!*

The zone of the average American's diet, and in excess of official USDA dietary guidelines (which suggest you eat 45 percent to 65 percent of calories from carbs), thanks to stuff like soda tipping the scales over. Extended time in the danger zone results in almost certain weight gain and Metabolic Syndrome. The danger zone is the primary catalyst for the obesity and type 2 diabetes epidemics, as well as numerous other significant health problems. Immediate and dramatic reduction of grains and other processed carbs is critical.

Fat

I've already discussed how the common admonition to keep dietary fats low is truly unfounded in most credible research. As far as I'm concerned, fat is your friend. Consuming healthy fats from animal and plant sources supports optimal function of all the systems in your body. Furthermore, ingesting fat helps you feel full and satisfied in a way that carbohydrates cannot. Because fat has little or no impact on blood glucose levels and insulin production and takes far longer to metabolize than carbohydrates, you will feel a deep and long-lasting satisfaction from consuming ample amounts of fat in your diet.

I understand that this is a controversial topic that will be met with some opposition. Please take it upon yourself to gain a clear understanding of the issue, learn to distinguish healthy fats from unhealthy, and sort out misleading Conventional Wisdom that frowns upon food staples that drove human evolution. The highly respected Nurses' Health Study, tracking dietary habits of 127,000 nurses over two decades (the largest epidemiological study of women in history, it has led to the publication of 265 scientific papers in leading journals), showed no statistically significant association between total fat intake (or cholesterol intake) and heart disease. Many other studies have attempted to establish a firm connection, yet none have demonstrated that a high-fat diet by itself causes heart disease. So how can it be that low-fat eating became the Conventional Wisdom? I believe that the otherwise well-meaning, well-educated folks in the low-fat camp are influenced by a few factors that lead them to the party line conclusion that a high-fat diet is unhealthy.

1. Failure to distinguish between good fats and bad fats. The skyrocketing rates of obesity, heart disease, and cancer that have ensued over the past half-century from consuming high-fat processed foods have unfairly implicated all fats as dangerous. As I discussed earlier and will cover further in the next chapter, the typical modern diet is grossly imbalanced between omega-6 fats and omega-3 fats. We ingest way too much of the former (from processed foods, partially hydrogenated vegetable oils, and grain-fed animal products) and way too little of the latter (from organic meats, eggs, and fish, and certain nuts, seeds, and omega-3 oils).

Furthermore, we consume excessive amounts of the highly toxic partially hydrogenated fats and trans-fats (they are not quite the same but are closely related and both evil). These "Franken-fats" are created by heating and chemically treating vegetable and seed oils to render them solid, effectively extending shelf life and improving the flavor of processed foods. They are easily oxidized to form free radical chain reactions that damage cell membranes and body tissue, and compromise immune function. Because your brain, nervous system, and vascular system are primarily composed of membranes, any dysfunction in these critical areas can be devastating. Research confirms that consumption of trans-fatty acids and partially hydrogenated fats may promote inflammation, aging, and cancer. The *New England Journal of Medicine* reviewed numerous studies and reported a strong link between processed fat consumption and heart disease.

2. Carbs making fat "look bad." Fat is calorically dense at nine calories per gram. If you consume excessive carbs (150 to 300 grams or more per day), produce a high level of insulin, and eat any appreciable amount of fat along with your high-carb diet, yes, your fat intake will contribute directly to making you fat. You know the saying "Which came first, the chicken or the egg?" Well, in this case, it's neither the chicken nor the egg making you fat—it's the carbs! High levels of insulin direct both carbs and fat (and protein) into your fat cells. Limit your carbs and fat will make you healthy, help moderate your appetite and total caloric intake, and greatly enhance the satisfaction level of your diet.

> *Which came first, the chicken or the egg? In this case, neither. It's the carbs that make you fat!*

3. Propaganda and flawed science manipulated into Conventional Wisdom. The machinations of public policy bureaucracy often leave rational thinking in the dust in favor of protecting and promoting corporate interests and the reputations of politicians. While I am all in favor of capitalism, it's unsettling how much decision-making power is controlled by corporations that spend billions of marketing dollars molding and shaping Conventional Dietary Wisdom in the direction of profits, with little regard for health.

The story of how saturated fat came to be vilified should mention the work of American scientist Ancel Keys. Keys was an eloquent and dynamic early promoter of the link between saturated fat intake, cholesterol levels, and heart disease—a driving force in the origination and promotion of the lipid hypothesis of heart disease mentioned earlier. Keys received notoriety in the 1960s for his efforts to transition the public away from saturated fats to replacements like polyunsaturated oils or low-fat eating in general. It has taken decades, at a dawdling pace, to recognize the folly of his health suggestions. For example, Keys didn't even connect obesity to heart disease risk, and the foundation of his work was compromised when he was criticized for hand-picking examples (comparisons of fat intake and heart disease rates among different cultures) that supported his hypotheses. In fairness, Keys later did some great work helping to popularize the Mediterranean diet (highlighted by the liberal intake of healthy fats), even spending his last few decades living in a small town in Italy and studying the residents' dietary habits.

On a bureaucratic level, the U.S. government has time and again shown a penchant for doggedly defending the status quo and vigorously squashing voices opposing Conventional Wisdom. A sordid example of the influence of power and money on the development of public policy is found in the FDA's so-called imitation policy, passed in 1973 (without Congressional approval, thanks to some clever legal maneuvering). The legislation relieved food manufacturers from having to use that pesky "imitation" designation on labels of foods created with artificial ingredients (coffee creamers, imitation egg mixes, processed cheeses, whip cream, and hundreds more), as long as manufacturers added synthetic vitamins to their concoctions to approximate the benefits of similar whole foods.

Mary Enig, Ph.D., a renowned nutritionist, lipid biochemistry expert, and author of *Know Your Fats*, from the University of Maryland, has spent a career battling Conventional Wisdom's position take on fat intake and heart disease. In the 1970s she was a central figure in challenging the corruption and misinformation dispensed by the USDA and the U.S. Senate's McGovern Committee (headed by former presidential candidate George McGovern). Influenced by highly questionable, lobbyist-tainted testimony, the committee published its report (many believe McGovern was hoodwinked by subordinates to buy into flawed conclusions) directing Americans to replace saturated fat with PUFAs and to limit fat intake in general (which was then disastrously replaced with excessive carbohydrates).

Ensuing government-funded research was essentially mandated to fall in line with the committee recommendations, and the notion that fats are bad took hold and flourished into Conventional Wisdom for decades (and is still going strong!). The discussion of the food propaganda topic is compelling enough to fill entire books (check out *Fast Food Nation*, *Food Politics*, *Appetite for Profit*, and *Good Calories, Bad Calories* for fascinating and detailed examinations of how Conventional Wisdom has led us astray), so we'll wrap here by asserting the point that it's clearly unwise to blindly trust Conventional Wisdom when it comes to fat and to dietary habits in general.

Ketones—The Fourth Fuel

By now you know that we evolved to burn primarily fats and a little glucose. We can also burn protein, when certain amino acids enter the energy pathways through a part of the glucose cycle (as happens when we run out of glucose or glycogen during a long workout or during starvation). Protein can also be converted to glucose in the liver. While most cells in our body can easily burn both fats and glucose, there are a few select cells that function only on glucose (some brain cells, red blood cells, and kidney cells, for example). Without glucose, those cells would cease to function and we would not last very long. The minimum daily glucose requirement to keep those systems running has been estimated at between 150 and 200 grams per day, but recent research shows that after a little adaptation, some of these cells can operate effectively on a fuel known as ketones, further reducing the overall glucose requirement.

Ketosis was crucial to our evolution. As we have already discussed here, our ancestors didn't always have access to a handy-dandy daily supply of glucose-containing carbohydrates like we do today. In fact, they may have gone weeks or months without appreciable carbs, so they had to evolve a system whereby the liver could take protein either from the muscles or directly from the diet and convert it into glucose through gluconeogenesis. This system worked to keep Grok alive during short periods of starvation or longer periods when meat (protein and fats) was plentiful but plants (carbs) were not. Today we can tap into this same system and prompt our genes to speed up the process of fat loss when we cut carbs while still consuming adequate dietary protein. In this scenario, we never have to sacrifice muscle in pursuit of fat loss (the unfortunate M.O. for traditional calorie-restriction weight loss) if we eat according to the *Primal Blueprint*. And the best part of all this is that gluconeogenesis tends to "waste" fat in the process.

Manufacturing glucose from protein requires its own source of energy, so liver cells happen to use fats (fatty acids, really) to fuel this conversion. When liver cells are involved in gluconeogenesis, they are unable to completely burn off those fats to the final end products of carbon dioxide and water. Consequently, they produce an energy-rich by-product known as a ketone (also called a ketone body). Ketones are very safe, desirable, energy-efficient forms of fuel in and of themselves. They are quite literally the fourth fuel. A 2004 article in the *Journal of the International Society of Sports Nutrition* referred to numerous studies suggesting that a low-carbohydrate intake and the resulting mild ketosis may offer many benefits, including reduction of body fat, minimized damage from insulin resistance and free radicals (from metabolizing a high-carbohydrate diet), and a reduction of LDL cholesterol.

Many cells actually prefer ketones to glucose, given the choice between the two. Cardiac muscle, skeletal muscle, and even certain brain cells thrive on the four and a half calories per gram delivered by ketones. After a little adaptation, the brain can do very well getting 75 percent of its energy from ketones. The fact that we can so easily convert to this alternative energy source plan may be the best proof that Grok didn't always have access to lots of carbs.

So what exactly is ketosis? Ketones can't be stored conveniently the way fats (and excess glucose) can be stored in fat cells or the way glucose can be stored as glycogen. Ketones simply circulate in the bloodstream where they are available to be picked up by any cells that want and need the energy they provide. *Ketosis* is the scientific name for a relative condition in the body where ketones start to accumulate in the bloodstream to a point beyond which they can all be picked up for energy. There is nothing wrong with being in ketosis. It is a natural, normal part of human energy production and metabolism. You have probably been in mild ketosis any time you have fasted or skipped a couple meals in a row.

Ketones happen to be somewhat acidic, and because the body works hard to maintain a slightly alkaline (nonacidic) state, unused ketones are excreted in urine, stool, or even breath (some describe the smell of ketone breath as that of overly ripe apples or acetone). People who are trying to stay in a mild state of ketosis often use "ketostix" to measure the amount of ketones in their urine. For them, more is better because each gram of ketones excreted means extra fat has been burned.

Some people—including some misinformed doctors—maintain an unnecessarily dim view of ketones and ketosis. I believe these criticisms arise because the diets in question allow for only 20 grams or less of carbs per day, a level that does not allow for the plentiful intake of nutrient-rich vegetables. While we are not meant to run primarily on carbohydrate energy, we do depend heavily on the nutrients offered by low-carb vegetables and most fruits. Other people may be mistaking ketosis for ketoacidosis, a much different (and deadly) condition that affects insulin-dependent diabetics and alcoholics.

In the normal *Primal Blueprint* maintenance program, we rarely even get to a state of ketosis. (But we still burn lots more fat and produce more ketones than high-carb people.) Because 100 carb grams a day seems to be the cutoff point above which ketosis is reduced, the recommended range of 100 to 150 grams per day of vegetable- and fruit-based carbs is plenty to fuel those glucose-/glycogen-dependent systems while the majority of our energy comes from fat.

On the *Primal Blueprint* accelerated fat-loss program (detailed in Chapter 8), we will look to achieve what I call the weight loss "sweet spot"—a level of mild ketosis—by dropping carbs into the range of 50 to 100 grams per day. For Primal weight loss efforts, we ensure that protein needed for gluconeogenesis comes from our diet (not our muscles) and that we have plenty of fat to meet our daily fuel requirements. Primal diehards who average very low-carb intake over extended periods (50 to 100 grams or less per day) will likely benefit from having an occasional higher-carb day (maybe 250 to 300 grams of nonsugar carbs) to fine-tune insulin sensitivity.

> *My doctor told me to stop having intimate dinners for four. Unless there are three other people.*
> —*Orson Welles*

By understanding how the metabolic processes work for protein, fat, carbohydrate, and ketones and knowing that you can control these processes through your diet and exercise habits, you needn't agonize over day-to-day calorie counting. As long as you are generally eating a *Primal Blueprint*–style plan and providing the right context of calories, your body will ease into a healthy, fit, long-term comfort zone effortlessly.

Eating Well

The *Primal Blueprint* is about enjoying a healthy, happy, balanced lifestyle. As Dr. Andrew Weil said in describing the title of his book *Eating Well for Optimum Health*, "eating well" refers not only to choosing natural, nutritious foods but also to enjoying the experience as one of the great pleasures of life. It's likely that Grok appreciated food much more than we do today, because he had to work so hard for his meals and was never assured of success. Throughout history, food has represented a centerpiece of cultural celebration—let's not kill the momentum now!

The "Oh, Positive!" Diet

If you wish to succeed with healthy dietary habits, it's important that you discard any negative emotions you have toward eating and embrace each meal as an opportunity to enjoy yourself. I strongly recommend that you give yourself permission to eat as much as you want (from the broad list of *Primal Blueprint*-approved foods), whenever you want, for the rest of your life. While this suggestion might scare the heck out of you, releasing yourself from restriction and deprivation enables you to become more connected with your physical nutritional needs rather than being driven by emotional triggers. Take notice of that point in every meal where you have attained satisfaction and feel comfortable stopping—not the point at which you are full, but the point at which you are no longer hungry for the next bite—knowing that you can eat again whenever you like. If you wish to enjoy a indulgent treat, do so with full attention and awareness to the pleasure that every single savored bite gives you. Reject feelings of anxiety, guilt, or rebellion connected to your food choices and replace them with the idea that you deserve to eat the most delicious, nutritious foods possible.

When it comes to specific meal choices, I prefer to let my taste buds guide me to the most enjoyable and nourishing foods within the broad guidelines of the *Primal Blueprint*. Forget the scientifically unproven admonitions to eat certain food-type combinations at certain times or align your food choices with your racial heritage, body shape, or blood type (I can't remember if my blood is O positive or O negative, but when I eat my Primal Salad most afternoons, my brain always thinks, "Oh, positive!").

Humans have evolved on widely differing diets from settlements all over the globe. While there are certain genetic predispositions to grain or dairy allergies, for example, *Primal Blueprint* foods satisfy and nourish everyone, regardless of where the last five or 500 generations in your bloodline lived or what they ate. In the Q&A section, I'll comment further how to reconcile the evolutionary-based *Primal Blueprint* diet with concepts like the metabolic-type eating recommendations that have become popular in recent years (hint: one is a gimmick and one is aligned with the fundamental basis from which all human biology originates—evolution).

Essentially, my goal is for you to become a modern forager with a keen sense of what you need to do (or not do) to thrive day in and day out. When you understand this basic concept, the resulting sense of personal power you will gain is tremendous. When you eat *Primal Blueprint* style, there is no city you can't travel to, no restaurant you can't negotiate with, no grocery store you can't shop in…no family holiday you can't endure!

Eating on Grok's Clock

Ever notice how some people freak out if they miss a meal or can't find exactly what they want on a menu? They become irritable and start complaining about being light-headed—as if their world might stop if they don't inhale some calories right away. Ironically, other than a lifetime of cultural socialization and a metabolism they've built to depend on sugar instead of fat, there is no reason skipping a meal should be a big deal. Our ancestors ate sporadically—with continually varied mealtimes and food choices. It's quite certain that they didn't always have enough, with the seasons and hunting success being major factors for their amount and diversity of food choices. Our genes thrive on intermittent scarcity and can even handle occasional excess. In fact, they expect it.

Our genetic ability to thrive on intermittent eating habits is an important concept to retain, because it unburdens us of having to eat every meal on a set schedule, to balance food groups (meat with starch, grains with protein, etc.), or to align our foods with time-of-day traditions (cereal for breakfast, sandwich for lunch, etc.). Skipping meals, fasting briefly, and simply freeing yourself from an obsessive need to eat three squares or six small meals a day when the clock strikes a particular hour might actually benefit your body by aligning more closely with your historic genetic experience to eat sporadically. Unburdened by the strict and ill-advised "rules" of Conventional Wisdom, eating becomes much simpler and more enjoyable. You might even discover that you experience even greater pleasure from food if you miss a meal here or there or alter your eating pattern from time to time.

On this topic, it's interesting to note that your need to consume calories on a regular schedule will diminish substantially when blood glucose levels are moderated and you start burning fat more efficiently through low-insulin *Primal Blueprint* dietary choices. In contrast, if you eat the typical Western diet of 300 to 500 grams of

> *Perhaps the single quickest and most exciting revelation for converts to the Primal Blueprint eating style is that by eliminating sugars and grains from your diet and emphasizing plant and animal foods, you will experience more consistent energy levels and a naturally diminished appetite.*

carbohydrate per day (instead of the 100 to 150 from complex sources as suggested by the *Primal Blueprint*), you are going to experience significant blood glucose fluctuations and corresponding cravings for quick-energy, high-carbohydrate foods. Perhaps the single quickest and most exciting revelation for converts to the *Primal Blueprint* eating style is that by eliminating sugars and grains from your diet and emphasizing plant and animal foods, you will experience more consistent energy levels and a naturally diminished appetite.

These benefits will be long lasting, but they might take a bit of time to realize. Every once in a while, people commenting on MarksDailyApple.com mention difficulties with energy level swings when participating in my online 30-day *Primal Blueprint* Challenge. When switching from a carbohydrate-based diet to a Primal eating style, keep in mind that it takes your body two to three weeks to "learn" how to burn fats better. During that time, your body expects sugar as fuel (which it's getting less of—perhaps for the first time in decades) but hasn't perfected yet how to get the most out of your fat reserves. Don't worry, it will. By limiting carbs (and, hence, lowering insulin) you are sending a new series of hormonal signals to your genes. In turn, they are down-regulating their sugar-burning systems and up-regulating their fat-burning machinery.

While you may experience a few episodes of light-headedness during the transition, rest assured that the shift will be complete in a few weeks and energy levels will dramatically improve. Meanwhile, grab a handful of nuts or a cold drumstick to munch on if you get hungry for a snack (I'll detail some of my favorite snack choices in Chapter 4). You should always satisfy your cravings with abundant amounts of approved foods instead of suffering through them with willpower and other flimsy, short-duration weapons. Don't worry, these primal food choices will deeply satisfy you without bringing about a sugar crash later, as will happen when you reach for a bagel. This is due to the high caloric density and slow burn rate of foods high in fat and protein (such as meat, nuts, and seeds) and the high water and fiber content (which moderate the blood glucose impact) of fruits and vegetables.

Because modern life is all about schedules, we often find it convenient and enjoyable to eat regular meals. I'm simply suggesting you pay more attention to your hunger levels than the clock. For example, I eat breakfast nearly every day, but in a wide range of food choices and total calories—based on my appetite, activity level, and the day's schedule. Often I will have my huge Primal Omelet with four to five eggs; chopped mushrooms, peppers, onions, and tomatoes; cheese; avocado; turkey meat; and salsa. On other days I will grab a few pieces of fresh fruit and some nuts or make a protein smoothie to have on the go. Some days I simply skip breakfast altogether, with no accompanying guilt, hunger pangs, or low blood glucose. As long as you are eating Primally most of the time, fluctuating habits work fine, and definitely help with weight control.

When you can be flexible with your food choices and eating schedules, your diet becomes more psychologically pleasing and less stressful to follow. However, the key is to make informed choices that minimize your exposure to toxic foods and, when you indulge or get off track, allow your body to return quickly to balance. If you enjoy a decadent dessert or a weekend away from healthy food options, simply eat a few low-insulin meals in a row and return to regulated energy levels and optimal metabolic function. Even a short walk after a big meal and rich dessert can mitigate the insulin response by diverting some of the glucose from your bloodstream into working muscles.

Dealing With the (Maybe Radical) Change to Primal Blueprint Eating

If you argue that life will never be the same without your bowl of Raisin Bran or a heaping plate of pasta and garlic bread, see if these suggestions can ease your transition:

"80% Rule": If you are someone who has a difficult time transitioning to a new habit, call to mind the spirit of the 80% Rule and do your best. Take it step by step and relieve yourself of pressure so you can adapt more comfortably. Be sure that your indulgences are sensible, as I detail in the next chapter. Over time, you will naturally and comfortably become more compliant, particularly with the restriction and elimination of grains and processed carbohydrates from your diet.

Build Momentum: As you continue to make progress eating the way you were designed to eat, you will notice a heightened sensitivity to how food affects your body, both positively and negatively. During my years as an athlete, I thought my recurrent digestive bloating and postmeal fatigue were due to my hard training regimen or simply the end of a long day—not from a subclinical allergic reaction to excessive processed carbohydrates and/or dairy products. Can you relate to that hyper, racing heart sensation that comes after consuming a sugary dessert? It's probably something that we've been aware of since childhood—a little annoying but no big deal, right?

It was only when I started to really clean up my already quite healthy diet a decade ago that my sensitivity went to the next level. What a pleasure it was to leave the dinner table feeling totally satisfied, yet alert and energetic—and not having to unbuckle the belt a notch or two! Passing on dessert took a little getting used to, but I noticed that the minimal sacrifice of instant gratification paled in comparison to not having to deal with sugar highs and sugar crashes. Plus, as you cut out those simple carbs, you begin to lose the craving for them. Hence, you escape the vicious cycle that befalls even those with tremendous willpower trying to do the right thing but eating the wrong stuff.

Five Favorite Meals Strategy: Pick your five favorite *Primal Blueprint*–approved meals and rotate them for the first two weeks of your transition to *Primal Blueprint* eating. Maybe it's broiled salmon and steamed broccoli. Lamb chops with grilled zucchini and summer squash. Rotisserie chicken (with the skin—preferably organic) and a large steamed vegetable. As much colorful, creative salad as you want. Liberal snacking on *Primal Blueprint*–approved snacks. Yes, you are removing the baked potato, corn on the cob, Cheerios, baguettes, and other beige staples from the picture, but the discomfort of a habit change can be greatly assuaged when you can look forward to as much as you want of your favorite Primal foods during the crucial transition period to the *Primal Blueprint* eating style.

Never Struggle, Suffer, or Go Hungry: Surround yourself with *Primal Blueprint*–approved foods and enjoy them as much and as often as you like. Always have a Primal snack nearby to help you through the transition period. That said, respect the Primal philosophy and pay close attention to your hunger levels, eliminating emotional triggers that negatively influence healthy eating. The key is to stop eating not when you are full—by then you've had too much—but when you are no longer hungry.

Substitute: Consider whether you can switch out *Primal Blueprint* meals for some of your old favorites. I used to be a big blueberry pancakes and granola guy, but whatever deprivation I might have felt at first in eliminating the "stack" from my life was more than made up for by a dozen bites of a delicious, deluxe high-fat omelet. Consider the overall impact of your current favorite foods on your body and if they are all truly worth it. A fine Italian meal of pasta with gelato for dessert will please most any palette, but if you feel bloated, gassy, and sleepy in the hours afterward, a better strategy might be to consider some of the many other delicious, *Primal Blueprint*–approved items on the menu (or off it, from a polite request) at the same restaurant.

One Small Scoop for Mankind

When you eat *Primal Blueprint* style, the consequences of your food choices become crystal clear. Eat right and you have discernibly more energy and health. Stick with it and your body composition goals happen effortlessly. Slide a little bit and you might get halfway to your goal (or less, owing to the vicious cycle of insulin-driven sugar crashes and cravings), have a little less energy, and maybe catch an extra cold or two due to compromised immune function.

Every once in a while, I'll have a lapse in judgment and indulge in something like a small scoop of gourmet ice cream. It tastes delicious for the four minutes it takes to eat it (but not quite on a par with a bowl of fresh blueberries and raspberries with homemade whipped cream), but invariably I experience bloating and gas in the ensuing hour as well as a bit of a sugar crash. Because these lapses are out of my normal habit pattern, I am highly sensitive to the consequences of choices like these.

Understand that I enjoy the taste of ice cream as much as anyone, but I will assert my position that after eating Primally for some time, even the occasional treat that's not *Primal Blueprint* approved—for me—is *just not worth it*. I don't mean to come off as a food nazi here. I assure you that I'm tempted frequently and in the future will certainly indulge in a non-Primal manner again (and again after that…hopefully we're talking *years* now!). I'm merely trying to illustrate how, once you're sensitized to the negative effects of unhealthy choices, it gets easier to turn down what used to seem impossible to resist. This is especially true when you clearly understand the consequences of each and every food choice that you make, whether they are aligned with your primal genes or whether they are not.

When you use defense mechanisms like "Everything in moderation," "You only live once," and the like, you disguise the fact that over years and decades, those little ice cream outings can add up literally to hundreds of pounds of ingested substances that are toxic to your body. Furthermore, as unhealthy food choices ingrain themselves (pun intended) into your daily life, I believe you become desensitized to the negative effects they have on your health. This concept is illustrated by heavy tobacco or caffeine users who are able to function somewhat normally (that's not saying much) with volumes of chemicals in their bloodstream that would floor the casual user.

The complete lack of regimentation or caloric deprivation in the *Primal Blueprint* eating style (I refuse to use the word *diet* because it implies regimentation) is the secret to its long-term success. You don't have to force yourself to go hungry or to feel deprived or negative about eating. Simply make sensible choices by welcoming the abundant selection of delicious foods whenever you want and transition out of habitually consuming foods that may taste great for a brief moment but make your body feel bad or create long-term metabolic stress.

> *Once you're sensitized to the negative effects of unhealthy choices, it gets easier to turn down what used to seem impossible to resist.*

Chapter Summary

1. Primal Blueprint Foods: Eating lots of vegetables, fruits, nuts, seeds, and animal foods, and avoiding processed foods, creates a more calorically efficient, nutrient-dense diet. These *Primal Blueprint* foods have driven human evolution for two million years. Benefits of *Primal Blueprint* eating include enhanced cellular function, improved immune and antioxidant function, optimal development and repair of muscle tissue, enhanced fat metabolism and weight management, a reduction in disease risk factors, and a stabilization of daily appetite and energy levels. While the *Primal Blueprint* advocates restriction of processed carbs like some popular diet programs, it does not restrict most nutritious natural carbs and, furthermore, takes a comprehensive lifestyle approach rather than being a mere diet.

2. It's All About Insulin (Well, at Least 80 Percent of It): Eighty percent of your ability to achieve body composition goals is determined by your diet—essentially, your ability to moderate insulin production so you can access and burn stored body fat for energy, while preserving or building muscle. Insulin is an important hormone that transports nutrients into cells for storage. When the delicate insulin balance is abused by habitually consuming too many carbs, cells become insulin resistant; more fat is stored and it becomes increasingly difficult to burn. This sets the stage for the development of serious conditions like Metabolic Syndrome, type 2 diabetes, and heart disease. Synthesis of testosterone and human growth hormone are hindered by excessive insulin production, creating an artificially accelerated aging process. There are also serious immediate drawbacks to consuming high-carb snacks or meals. The sugar high–insulin release–stress response cycle causes problems with fatigue, mental focus, mood swings, and jitters, resulting in the familiar condition of burnout. The regulation of insulin production is perhaps the most important takeaway message of the *Primal Blueprint* for preventing obesity and many modern health problems.

3. Cholesterol: Cholesterol is critical to healthy cell structure and numerous metabolic functions. Conventional Wisdom's lipid hypothesis of heart disease is a flawed and narrow perspective on the actual chain of events and risk factors that contribute to heart disease (a premise supported in recent years by the Framingham Heart Study and many other respected studies and experts). In many cases, only one specific lipoprotein, small, dense LDL, is most related to heart disease and usually only causes problems when triglycerides are high and systemic inflammation is present (typically a consequence of excessive insulin production, a poor omega-6 to omega-3 ratio, and poor exercise habits—either sedentary or too stressful). Furthermore, sufficient levels of HDL—generated by healthy eating and exercise habits—can often mitigate the damage caused by small, dense LDL. The primary function of statin drugs—lowering cholesterol levels—does not directly address these risk factors. Statin's purported anti-inflammatory benefits can be easily achieved through diet, exercise, and supplementation—it's cheaper and without side effects!

4. Omega-3s: *Primal Blueprint* eating provides higher levels of the highly touted omega-3 polyunsaturated fatty acids, which support healthy cardiovascular, brain, skin, and immune function, primarily by keeping the inflammation response under control. The ratio of omega-6 to omega-3 intake is dangerously out of balance in the modern diet, due to excessive consumption of processed foods and oils.

5. Macronutrients: Understand the context of calories to see a bigger picture than the overly simplistic "calories in, calories out" concept of weight loss. Obtain between 0.7 and one gram of protein per pound of lean body weight per day (observing the adjustment factors detailed). Limit carbohydrate intake to an average of 100 to 150 grams per day (or 50 to 100 grams per day if you seek accelerated fat loss), something that will happen automatically when you enjoy plenty of vegetables and fruits and avoid grains, sugars, and other processed carbs. The Carbohydrate Curve summarizes how various levels of carbs impact your health and weight management success.

With protein intake in optimum range and carb intake strictly controlled, fat becomes your main caloric energy variable. This allows you to enjoy deeply satisfying high-fat foods whenever you are hungry (knowing they will more likely be burned as energy than make you fat—if you moderate insulin production). Although fat has been maligned by Conventional Wisdom for years, it's largely due to mistakenly attributing the negative effects of processed fats (and high carb diets) to fat intake in general. Ketones (a by-product of gluconeogenesis in the liver) are known as the fourth fuel because they provide an efficient energy source when carbohydrate intake is low. Occasional mild ketosis during weight-loss efforts is a safe strategy to burn off excess body fat more rapidly.

6. Eating Well: Eating well means enjoying one of the great pleasures of life without deprivation, restriction, stress-related bad habits, or other negativity. Choose the foods that you enjoy most from the broad list of *Primal Blueprint* choices and don't obsess about calories, nutrient ratios, regimented mealtimes, or food combinations. Eat until you feel satisfied instead of habitually stuffing yourself. Realize that our genes evolved to easily handle sporadic eating habits without energy lulls or metabolic slowdowns.

7. Transitioning to the Primal Blueprint: Discover desirable substitutes (rotate them over and over if desired) to avoid feelings of deprivation from discarding old meal choices. Ensure you have plenty of *Primal Blueprint* foods available for snacks and meals so you don't suffer or feel depleted. Follow the 80% Rule by striving for total compliance (realizing this should get you to 80 percent) and not stressing about perfection. Notice your heightened sensitivity to how foods affect your body and leverage that instant gratification to stay on the path of high-energy, effortless weight management and optimal gene expression with *Primal Blueprint* foods.

CHAPTER 4

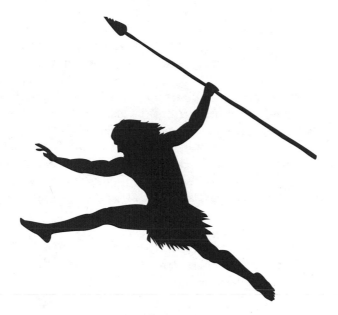

Law #1:
Eat Lots of Plants
and Animals

(Insects Optional)

In This Chapter

I detail the health benefits of eating *Primal Blueprint* style and how to choose the best products in the food categories of vegetables, fruits, nuts, seeds, animal foods (meat, fish, fowl, and eggs), and herbs and spices. I pay particular attention to the benefits of choosing organic plants and animals and contrast the often offensive ingredients (hormones, pesticides, and antibiotics) and processing methods found with conventional foods and mass-produced animal products.

Organic, locally grown vegetables and fruits are the most nutritious and safest. They are teeming with antioxidants and micronutrients that support health and help prevent disease. Organic animal foods are healthy and nutritious and will help you reduce excess body fat and build lean muscle. Eggs are healthy and nutritious. They have been mistakenly maligned due to the flawed assumption that their high-cholesterol content is a heart disease risk factor. The budget increase for buying organic products pales in comparison to the importance of leading a healthy life and avoiding disease risk factors.

Nuts, seeds, and their derivative butters offer high levels of beneficial unsaturated and omega-3 fats, phytonutrients, fiber, antioxidants, and numerous vitamins and minerals, and they make for delicious and satisfying snack options. Herbs and spices offer tremendous micronutrient value and high antioxidant values. Spices enhance your enjoyment of meals, while herbal extracts can benefit numerous health conditions.

I detail foods that you can enjoy in moderation, including how to make the best choices among certain fruits, coffee, dairy products, fats and oils, starchy tuber vegetables, and wild rice. I refute Conventional Wisdom's notion that you should routinely drink extensive amounts of water and instead assert that, like Grok, we simply use our thirst to guide us to proper hydration. A few sensible indulgences like alcohol, dark chocolate, and high-fat treats should be chosen discriminately, but enjoyed guilt-free. Certain high-quality supplements (multivitamin/mineral/antioxidant formula, omega-3 oil, probiotics, and protein powder) can provide a strategic boost for our high-stress lifestyles and often nutrient-challenged food supply.

If we're not supposed to eat animals, how come they're made out of meat?

—Tom Snyder

I f you are trying to memorize the most important, life-changing sound bites from the *Primal Blueprint*, here's another one: plants (vegetables, fruits, nuts, seeds, and herbs and spices) and animals (meat, fish, fowl, and eggs) should represent the entire composition of your diet. While vegetables, fruits, and herbs and spices don't provide a ton of calories, they should represent your main source of healthy carbohydrates and micronutrients (vitamins, minerals, antioxidants, anti-inflammatory agents, and thousands of other phytonutrients). Nuts, seeds, and their derivative butters, and animal foods are calorically dense, stimulate minimal insulin production, offer the best forms of healthy protein and fat, and should represent the bulk of your caloric intake.

Brightly colored fruits and vegetables supply high levels of antioxidants that are critical to good health. The flavonoids, carotenoids, and myriad other important phytonutrients found in these foods can serve as a powerful first line of defense against oxidative damage from aging, stress, and inflammation. Moreover, antioxidants and other phytonutrients appear to contain cancer-fighting properties, support immune function, aid in digestion, and help preserve muscle mass, a critical longevity component for those of advanced age.

While leading a healthy, balanced lifestyle will activate the genes that make our built-in antioxidant systems (catalase, superoxide dismutase, and glutathione) fight hard against cellular and DNA breakdown, research suggests that we may require additional antioxidant support from foods and supplements. Of course, most processed foods and starchy carbohydrates are devoid of antioxidants, while vegetables, fruits, and nuts are the best sources of these natural antioxidants. It follows that if you want to be healthy and prevent disease (recall from Chapter 3 the discussion of oxidation as a central heart disease component; antioxidants protect against oxidative damage in the body), vegetables and fruits must take center stage in your diet. It is also apparent that modern food-processing methods, which include growing produce in soil bereft of important minerals and the widespread use of pesticides, may further hamper our efforts to get enough antioxidants. Consequently, many people may benefit from a prudent supplementation program.

> *Plants (vegetables, fruits, nuts, seeds, and herbs and spices) and animals (meat, fish, fowl, and eggs) should represent the entire composition of your diet.*

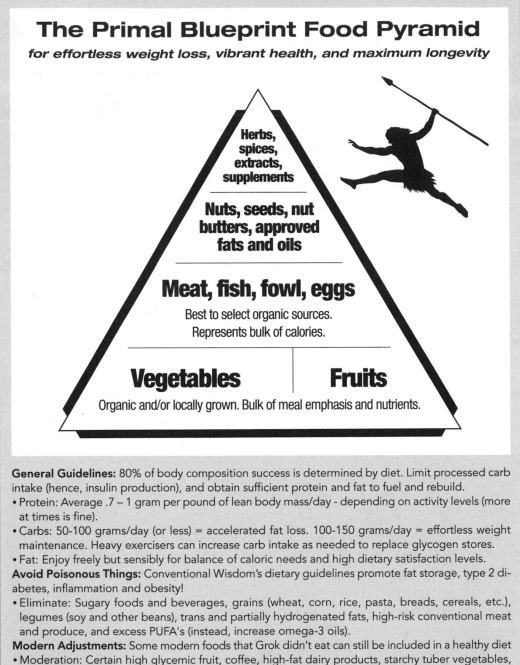

The Primal Blueprint Food Pyramid

for effortless weight loss, vibrant health, and maximum longevity

Herbs, spices, extracts, supplements

Nuts, seeds, nut butters, approved fats and oils

Meat, fish, fowl, eggs
Best to select organic sources.
Represents bulk of calories.

Vegetables | **Fruits**
Organic and/or locally grown. Bulk of meal emphasis and nutrients.

General Guidelines: 80% of body composition success is determined by diet. Limit processed carb intake (hence, insulin production), and obtain sufficient protein and fat to fuel and rebuild.
• Protein: Average .7 – 1 gram per pound of lean body mass/day - depending on activity levels (more at times is fine).
• Carbs: 50-100 grams/day (or less) = accelerated fat loss. 100-150 grams/day = effortless weight maintenance. Heavy exercisers can increase carb intake as needed to replace glycogen stores.
• Fat: Enjoy freely but sensibly for balance of caloric needs and high dietary satisfaction levels.

Avoid Poisonous Things: Conventional Wisdom's dietary guidelines promote fat storage, type 2 diabetes, inflammation and obesity!
• Eliminate: Sugary foods and beverages, grains (wheat, corn, rice, pasta, breads, cereals, etc.), legumes (soy and other beans), trans and partially hydrogenated fats, high-risk conventional meat and produce, and excess PUFA's (instead, increase omega-3 oils).

Modern Adjustments: Some modern foods that Grok didn't eat can still be included in a healthy diet
• Moderation: Certain high glycemic fruit, coffee, high-fat dairy products, starchy tuber vegetables, and wild rice.
• Supplements: Multivitamin/mineral formula, probiotics, omega-3 fish oil and protein powder.
• Herbs, spices and extracts: Offer many health benefits and enhance enjoyment of meals.
• Sensible indulgences: Dark chocolate, moderate alcohol, high-fat treats.

For a quick primer, red plants (pomegranates, cherries, watermelon, etc.) have been shown to help reduce the risk of prostate cancer as well as some tumors. Green fruit and vegetables (avocados, limes, green beans, zucchini, etc.) are high in carotenoids that have a powerful antiaging effect and are especially helpful for vision. Yellow and orange produce (bananas, papayas, carrots, butternut squash, pineapple) offer beta-carotene for immune support as well as bromelain, which has been shown to aid in digestion, joint health, and the reduction of inflammatory conditions. Cruciferous ("cross"-shaped, with a branch and leaves) vegetables, including broccoli, Brussels sprouts, kale, arugula, turnips, bok choy, horseradish, and cauliflower, have demonstrated specific anticancer, antiaging, and antimicrobial properties. Nuts and seeds provide high levels of beneficial monounsaturated and omega-3 fatty acids, fiber, phytonutrients, antioxidants (e.g., vitamin E and selenium), and a host of essential nutrients (e.g., manganese, magnesium, zinc, iron, chromium, phosphorous, and folate).

Plant foods also naturally promote a beneficial balance between acidity and alkalinity (also known as "base", or non-acidic) in your bloodstream. Almost all cells prefer a slightly alkaline environment to function properly, but many metabolic processes, including the normal production of cellular energy, result in the release of acidic waste products. The buildup of acidic waste is toxic to your body, so it works very hard at all times to preserve a slightly alkaline environment, measured by the familiar "pH" levels. While we have evolved several highly refined buffering systems to balance our pH, ingesting acid-producing foods makes it that much more difficult to achieve pH homeostasis.

As you might guess, consuming heavily processed foods, sugars, grains, deep-fried foods, alcohol, caffeine, cigarettes, carbonated drinks, artificial sweeteners, and many recreational and prescription drugs promotes an acidic imbalance in the body, a precursor of many health problems and diseases. In contrast, by emphasizing alkaline-forming foods—vegetables, fruits, nuts, and seeds—in your diet, you optimize your acid/base balance and improve metabolism to burn fat, build muscle, and reduce your susceptibility to environmental and dietary toxins. While they have tremendous health benefits, meat and dairy products also happen to be acid-producing, making it essential to balance the intake of these foods with sufficient vegetables and fruits that support alkalinity.

Vegetables

It is preferable to select locally grown, in-season, organic vegetables whenever possible. The shiny, buffed-up vegetables on display in our local supermarkets are typically cultivated in an objectionable manner—sprayed with pesticides, picked too early (and then artificially ripened by exposure to ethylene gas), jet-lagged from their distant origins (thumbs-down from a green perspective), and even genetically modified to grow bigger and more colorful, albeit at the cost of being less nutritious.

It may take some acclimation to center your diet around vegetables, as we are so accustomed to reaching for packaged, high-carbohydrate snacks as a first option. Don't follow the example of restaurants that serve skimpy vegetable portions seemingly just for decoration; serve yourself heaping portions that crowd everything else on your plate! Enjoy vegetables raw, steamed, baked, or grilled—even slathered in butter if you like. Cook or slice up extra portions for easy preparation or snacking the following day. Reject your attachment to cultural meal traditions centered on starches or grains and get wild and colorful with your meals! Have some steamed carrots and beets with your eggs for breakfast or kale, squash, and chicken for lunch. Try some of the many delicious vegetable-focused recipes at MarksDailyApple.com. Grab some stuff you've never tried before and ask your grocer about the best preparation methods.

> *It may take some acclimation to center your diet around vegetables, as we are so accustomed to reaching for packaged, high-carbohydrate snacks as a first option. Reject your attachment to cultural meal traditions centered on starches or grains and get wild and colorful with your meals!*

While virtually all vegetables offer excellent nutritional value, some offer particularly high levels of antioxidants. One of the best objective resources to determine the antioxidant power of any vegetable, fruit, herb, or other food is the USDA's ORAC (Oxygen Radical Absorbance Capacity) report. I like to aim for at least 10,000 ORAC units a day, which is easily obtained from a few servings of the top fruits and vegetables (the USDA recommends a much lower number, between 3,000 and 5,000 per day).

Here (in alphabetical order, not point value order; but don't worry—they're all gold medal winners) is a list of some of the highest antioxidant vegetables. Make a special effort to include these regularly in your meals: avocado, beets, broccoli, Brussels sprouts, carrots, cauliflower, eggplant, garlic, kale, onion, peas, red bell pepper, spinach, yellow squash

If, for reasons of budget or availability, you decide to eat nonorganic produce, note that there are varying levels of residue exposure risk depending on the item. Be particularly careful to avoid conventional sources of vegetables that have a large surface area (leafy greens, including spinach and lettuce, are treated with some of the most potent pesticides) or a skin that is consumed (bell peppers are perhaps the most pesticide-tainted vegetable; also avoid conventional celery, cucumbers, green beans, winter squash, and carrots). If you do find yourself purchasing these, be sure to soak and/or rinse them with soap or a "fruit and vegetable wash" solution, which you can find in any health food store. On the other hand, conventional broccoli (also a good source of omega-3s), asparagus, avocados, cabbage, onions, and other vegetables with an easily washable or non-edible skin have minimal pesticide exposure risk.

Fruits

Fruits are outstanding sources of fiber, vitamins, minerals, phenols, antioxidants, and other micronutrients. Generally speaking, the *Primal Blueprint* plan allows you to eat generous amounts of fruit (unlike many low-carb programs), with a few important caveats. For one, modern cultivation and chemical treatments have resulted in fruits that are large, brightly colored, uniformly shaped, and extra sweet, with much less micro-nutrition than the small, varied, highly fibrous, deep-colored, less sugary, and less insulin-stimulating fruits that Grok foraged for. As with Olympic gymnasts, higher presentation value means nothing if you receive poor scores in execution.

Choosing the Best Fruits

Three major categories that affect fruit quality are growing methods, nutritional value (glycemic and antioxidant levels), and risk of pesticide exposure. The "Fruit Power Rankings" chart in this section details which types of fruits to enjoy in abundance, which to eat in moderation, and which to strictly avoid. Regarding growing methods, organic fruit offers vastly superior nutritional value to conventionally grown fruits. Some experts estimate that organic fruits are 10 times richer in key micronutrients than their conventional counterparts! Organic fruits must manufacture high levels of antioxidants to defend themselves against pests—something conventional fruits don't have to worry about, thanks to their treatment with synthetic herbicides and pesticides. (Notice an analogy here? Think Grok and his lean, strong, fit body hustling for food every day versus today's channel-surfing couch potato enjoying delivered pizza).

Organic is not always the be-all and end-all, however. Organic fruits from distant lands are less tasty and nutritious because of their premature picking and long transit time to market. Thus, many experts advocate conventionally grown local fruit over organic fruits grown remotely. Even if local fruit is not certified organic, your local farmer likely uses less offensive growing methods than large commercial operations, and the optimum picking time means the fruit has matured to be bursting with great nutrition and taste. Those living in progressive areas with thriving farmers' markets and food co-ops might even encounter fruits designated as "wild." As the term conveys, these fruits are as good as it gets…if you can find them. If you are so inclined, you may want to visit seedsavers.org or seedsofchange.com to purchase seeds and plant your own wild-variety fruit trees, berry bushes, and vegetable plants.

> *Many experts advocate conventionally grown local fruits over organic fruits grown remotely.*

Be strict (particularly with children, due to their substantially higher risk of harm from pesticides) about avoiding conventionally grown fruits with a soft, edible skin that is difficult to wash, such as berries. You can be less strict on fruits with tough, inedible skins that peel; they offer a protective barrier against chemical ingestion. If you must eat conventional fruits, wash your fruit thoroughly with soap or a special solution. Avoid genetically modified fruit, a concept that elicits serious health and philosophical concerns and is about as far away from Grok as you can get. Genetically modified organisms (GMOs) have insufficient research to guarantee their health and safe ingestion, as I discuss at length on MarksDailyApple.com.

Most all fruits offer a host of nutritional benefits, but some (detailed on the chart) are relatively low in antioxidant values while having a high glycemic effect. You may have heard of the glycemic index (G.I.; how the food impacts blood glucose levels in comparison to the benchmark of pure glucose) and glycemic load (basically, the total sugar content of the food), and perhaps you have seen popular foods with a point score attached to them. While a high glycemic response is undesirable (because it triggers a big insulin response), I'm wary of placing a numerical judgment on foods without further context. For example, carrots have a high glycemic index score in a calorie-for-calorie comparison with other foods on the chart. However, one is more likely to drink a 20-ounce bottle of Coke than eat four and a half cups of carrots to get an equivalent 240 calories. When comparing fruits to fruits, however, it's obviously best to emphasize high-antioxidant, low-glycemic fruits over lower-antioxidant, higher-glycemic fruits.

In light of the popularity of juicing, it's important to note that whole fruits are vastly superior to juice – even the most nutritious, freshly squeezed glass. Juice is generally higher in sugar and lower in many other micronutrients than its produce sources, because juicing eliminates the nutrient-rich skin and fiber (which help moderate the glycemic impact of the food). Recall that Kelly Korg's 24-ounce Strawberry Surf Rider smoothie contained 71 grams of sugar! I strongly suggest drinking only moderate amounts of juice and sticking with freshly squeezed when you do. Bottled juices are heated for safety and stability, which reduces their nutrient content and compromises their great natural taste. Making your own juice is preferable to getting it from a juice bar, where your beverage can be quite pricey and comes with uncertain quality standards for produce selection.

All that said, a moderate serving of fresh juice (or even bottled juice) can hardly be described in critical terms, and it's a good choice for nutrients on days when you can't obtain adequate whole foods (such as when traveling). Furthermore, I'm not keen to get painted with the same brush as Atkins and other across-the-board "carbophobes." If your eyes are bouncing up and down the page sorting out which fruits are good and bad, relax! If you've junked grains and moved on to prioritizing your fruit choices, you're far ahead in the battle to eat whole, nutritious foods and avoid processed foods. I'm certainly not advocating sitting forlornly off to the side at the Fourth of July picnic, watching others eat the hot dogs, corn on the cob, and watermelon. By all means enjoy the watermelon guilt-free (just forget the former two and smuggle in your own smoked wild salmon for a main course!). Simply use a bit of restraint for fruits on the moderation list, particularly if you are pursuing ambitious fat-reduction goals.

Fruit Power Rankings

This is by no means a comprehensive list, but it should help you successfully navigate the grocery store (or, better yet, the farmers' market). Each list is in rank order of best to worst.

Growing Methods

Wild: Difficult to find, but the best choice due to their high-antioxidant production (think survival of the fittest), and lack of cultivation. Plant your own or scour the farmers' market!

Local organic: Superior choice for nutritional value, taste, and safety.

Local conventional: Superior to remote organic due to freshness and ideal picking time. Wash thoroughly with soap or vegetable solution.

Remote organic: Ranks below local conventional due to harmful effects of transportation and premature picking that compromise nutritional value.

Remote conventional: Strictly avoid due to diminished nutritional value and pesticide risk. (*Hint*: if it's out of season in your area, don't eat it!)

GMO fruit: Don't even think about it. Instead, ask yourself, "What would Grok do?" 'Nuff said.

continued

Fruit Power Rankings (continued)

Nutritional Value

Outstanding: High-antioxidant, low-glycemic fruits, including all berries and stone (pitted) fruits.

Great: Lower-antioxidant, higher-glycemic fruits, including apples, bananas, cherries, kiwi, and pomegranates.

Exercise some moderation: Low antioxidant, high glycemic fruits, including dates, dried fruits (all), grapes, mangoes, melons, nectarines, oranges, papayas, pineapples, and tangerines.

Pesticide Risk

Low risk: Fruit with tough, inedible skin, including bananas, avocados, melons, oranges, tangerines, mandarins, pineapples, kiwis, mangoes, and papayas.

High risk: Fruit with soft, edible skin, including apples, apricots, cherries, grapes, nectarines, peaches, pears, raisins, raspberries, strawberries, and tomatoes.

Mark's Top 10 Favorite Fruits

Naturally, everything on this list assumes an organic, locally grown variety. Consult the three previous sections to ensure your pesticide risk is minimized and you otherwise choose the best fruit possible—and avoid problematic fruits. These are in my personal rank order, but again, anything on this list is superior.

1. Blueberries, strawberries, raspberries, blackberries, and nearly all other berries
2. Cherries
3. Prunes
4. Apples
5. Peaches
6. Pears
7. Figs
8. Grapefruit
9. Kiwis
10. Apricots

Animal Foods

In Grok's time, the bulk of calories in the human diet (estimates range from 45 to 85 percent, depending on geography) came from eating a variety of animal life, including insects, grubs, amphibians, birds, their eggs, fish and shellfish, small mammals, and some larger mammals. In general, those living closer to the equator consumed more plants and less animal food,

> *My favorite animal is steak.*
> **—Fran Lebowitz**
> *American author and humorist*

while those at colder latitudes with fewer plant options consumed more meat. These meat sources provided significant amounts of protein and all types of essential fatty acids and vitamins. Grok often ate as much as 300 or 400 grams of protein and up to 200 or more grams of fat in a day during times of plenty—and yet maintained a svelte physique. Of course, he also ate very limited amounts of carbohydrates, produced moderate levels of insulin, and excelled at using stored fat as fuel. These macronutrient breakdowns allowed him to build or preserve muscle and provided ample fuel for both long treks and short bursts of speed.

Animal foods are healthy and nutritious and will help you reduce excess body fat, build lean muscle, and generally promote peak performance. While I highly respect those who have philosophical objections to consuming animal flesh, I want to dispel Conventional Wisdom that eating a diet high in animal foods leads to obesity and heart disease or that vegetarianism is somehow healthier. Like it or not, our bodies have evolved for two million years on animal foods, ever since meat eating became a survival factor and a trigger to population expansion on earth (our ability to migrate to the higher latitudes depended on us developing "meat-adaptive" genes).

The fact remains that no culture or society has ever survived for an extended period of time on a meatless diet. While it would seem to be much easier to live and evolve without having to run around and kill animals, the truth is that we need concentrated, nutrient-rich energy sources like meat to support accelerated brain development—our distinguishing feature that brought us to the top of the food chain. Remarkably, about 500 calories a day are required just to fuel the human brain (both primitive and modern). Anthropological evidence strongly suggests that it was protein and omega-3 fatty acids from animal foods that provided both the raw materials and energy necessary for the human brain to grow larger over the course of evolution. Our ability to hunt and catch animals and cook their meat (cooking makes meat easier to chew, swallow, and digest) was critical in our branching up and away from our mostly vegetarian ape cousins.

At this point in our discussion, it's important to acknowledge that over the past decade, some studies about red meat consumption have prompted alarming headlines that "excessive" consumption of red meat may be associated with a slightly increased risk for cancer and heart disease. In all such studies to date, however, there has been no distinction or separation between groups who consumed organic, hormone-free, 100% grass-fed or otherwise "clean" red meat versus the vast majority of participants who ate the standard hormone-laden, grain-fed, antibiotic-laced meats that I decry here. Nor has there been any necessary correlation with carbohydrate intake (remember that carbs *and* fats consumed together increase triglyceride production from both sources). Most of these studies (in which participants self-report their dietary intake) include in the general red meat category all manner of processed meats (hot dogs, breakfast sausage, chemically-treated jerkys, bacon, bologna, salami). These foods may contain preservatives that act as potential carcinogens. Furthermore, their nutrient value is diminished from the mechanical processing and addition of preservatives, artificial colors and often a significant level of simple sugars or artificial sweeteners. Of course, the *Primal Blueprint* suggests that you generally avoid these meats.

Authors of these studies also offer another possible explanation for the minimally increased risks: overcooking of meat. You may have heard that some forms of seared, burned, or overcooked meat may contain heat-altered chemical by-products called heterocyclic amines (or HCAs) which may be carcinogenic if consumed frequently over long periods of time. Since mankind has been cooking with fire for hundreds of thousands of years, it's apparent that we have developed a host of natural genetic adaptations to allow us to eat most properly cooked foods without problems. Furthermore, some studies indicate that consuming antioxidant-rich foods (such as fruits, vegetables, herbs and spices, and even red wine) along with cooked meats can essentially neutralize any HCAs during digestion. Of course, using appropriate cooking techniques, avoiding deep-fried or high-heat barbequed meats, and eating certain forms of meat raw (sushi, tartar, etc.), can help you eliminate your risk altogether.

While it's indisputable that our bodies thrive on the rich and unique nutrients provided by animal foods, it is possible—albeit pretty darn difficult—to be healthy and enjoy a nutritious diet without consuming meat. However, it will be a real challenge to obtain sufficient protein and fat—or simply enough calories—to fuel an active lifestyle while also avoiding grains and other processed carbohydrates. By choice or default, these foods constitute a high percentage of calories for vegetarians and vegans. If you consume moderate to high amounts of grains in an effort to make up for the absence of meat, you are probably going to encounter a host of possible health challenges, as I will detail in the next chapter.

Animal fats used in cooking (e.g., lard, tallow, chicken fat, and butter) have long been maligned by Conventional Wisdom in the movement toward polyunsaturated fatty acids (PUFAs) that has spanned the last few generations. However, saturated fats (solid at room temperature, unlike PUFAs) are the most beneficial fats with which to cook. They are not teeming with micronutrients, so you may wish to limit them somewhat in favor of more densely nutritious calorie sources (such as the meat or vegetables you might be cooking!). However, they are not at all bad for you, as we've been conditioned to believe. In contrast, PUFAs contain too much omega-6 and can contribute significantly to the oxidation and inflammation conditions detailed in Chapter 3. The sidebar "Mark's Primer on Fats and Oils" later in this chapter details my favorite fats and oils, as well as which ones to avoid.

Meat and Fowl

Many of the Conventional Wisdom health objections to eating animal foods can easily be countered by eating organic sources of meat, a suggestion that is, in my estimation, highly recommended due to the extremely poor quality of much of today's conventionally processed animal foods. Mass-produced ranch animals can contain hormones (to grow them bigger quickly and therefore increase profits), pesticides (ingested from their own inferior food sources; vegetarian advocates claim that 80 to 90 percent of your total dietary pesticide exposure comes from eating meat, although that's disputed by the EPA), and antibiotics (to prevent widespread illness resulting from consuming immune-suppressing feed and living in filthy, cramped, artificial conditions). These three stooges can really mess up your efforts to eat healthfully.

Furthermore, today's mass-harvested cattle, chickens, and other animals are fed a diet of fortified grains, which have a similar effect on their bodies as on humans! Purchase your meats at a chain grocer or big-box store, and there's a good chance you'll end up eating a malnourished, insulin-resistant, and quite possibly diseased animal whose meat is high in omega-6 fats—a far cry nutritionally from Grok's fresh, lean, wild kills. Finally, humane reasons compel many to avoid meat. The animals we typically dine on consume half of our crop harvest; their waste pollutes air, rivers, and streams; and many claim they are subjected to horrifying treatment at unsanitary production facilities (as detailed in such books as *Fast Food Nation*, *The Omnivore's Dilemma*, *Diet for a New America*, and even *Skinny Bitch*).

For these reasons, I strongly urge you to look for USDA-certified organic meat whenever possible. Clearly, there is a continuum here where you can find options that are various degrees away from ideal. While the ultimate meat would be a wild animal with lots of lean mass, little fat, and a nutritious, high omega-3 natural diet, there aren't many of them running around the continent these days. If organically raised meats are not available, suitable alternatives would be hormone-free, antibiotic-free meat or meat from animals that were "100% grass-fed" or "100% grass-finished" (as denoted on the label). While there is minimal regulation in this industry, you can educate yourself, obtain trusted sources of healthier meats, and alleviate nearly all of the objections mentioned previously. Fortunately, the popularity of organic eating is skyrocketing, so you should have good luck finding healthier animal products in your area. If not, you can utilize some of the excellent resources on the Internet, such as americangrassfedbeef.com and eatwild.com.

Besides being free of hormones, pesticides, and antibiotics, animals raised organically offer higher levels of healthy omega-3 and monounsaturated fats (two to six times more omega-3 than commercial beef). The main reason to avoid the very high-fat commercial meats is because these animals, just like humans, tend to store toxins (pesticide residues, hormones, and antibiotic metabolites) in their fat cells. If, for reasons of budget or availability, you find yourself eating a less-than-ideal source of meat, always choose the leanest possible cuts and trim the excess fat. This will significantly limit your potential exposure to these toxins.

A Little Meet and Greet for Your Meat

Following are brief descriptions of common labels on meat products to help you make informed purchasing decisions. Admittedly, navigating this topic is extremely difficult. All manner of impressive terms are commonly used to convince you that you are eating a product that is superior to the conventional, mass-produced animals that are the norm today. Many of the terms have no official designation or are not regulated in a meaningful manner. For further insights, *The Omnivore's Dilemma*, by Michael Pollan, is a highly regarded book that offers extensive commentary on the subject of eating meat in a healthy manner.

Certified Organic: This is the premier choice for meat. The USDA is making a serious effort to enforce a comprehensive national definition of the term certified organic. Those using the label are subject to regular inspection (by USDA-approved third parties) and record-keeping requirements. Certified organic meat comes from animals raised on grass or grain feed without antibiotics, hormones, genetic engineering, irradiation, sewage sludge, or artificial ingredients. Furthermore, certified organic animals are afforded "conditions which allow for exercise, freedom of movement, and reduction of stress appropriate to the species." Certified organic meat is likely rivaled in health quality by animals raised locally from a trusted source (who might not carry official designation due to being a small-sized operation or other economic reasons).

Certified: The USDA Food Safety and Inspection Service has evaluated the meat for class, grade, or other quality characteristics (e.g., Certified Angus Beef).

Chemical-Free: This vague term is not defined or recognized by the USDA and has virtually no significant meaning on a package.

Conventional (i.e. - absent any specialty designations): You are likely buying a mass-produced animal raised on feedlot grains with pesticide residues, growth hormones, and antibiotics and often treated inhumanely.

Country of Origin Labeled (COOL): This labeling program, regulated by the USDA, specifies where the animal was raised, slaughtered, and processed—sometimes including multiple locations. As with produce, local products are preferred.

Free-Range: Applies only to poultry, indicating the animals are given "access" to outdoors. However, free-range has no legal definition or third-party verification, and many growers cut corners to slap the impressive distinction on their labels. Furthermore, the term does not guarantee that the meat is free of hormones and antibiotics.

Fresh: This label implies that the meat has not been frozen (internal temperature dropping below 26 degrees Fahrenheit) prior to sale. It does not pertain to how the animal was raised, fed, or slaughtered, and it is not third-party verified.

Grass-Fed, Grass-Finished, Pasture-Raised, Pasture-Finished, etc.: These designations require that animals are afforded access to grass in their diet but do not guarantee that the animals' diets are free from grains, unless you see the "100%" qualifier before the description. Even then, there is no guarantee that the meat is free of hormones or antibiotics. Furthermore, "access" to pasture is loosely defined and can often refer to a large indoor facility (where animals have been conditioned to remain) with a door to a small outdoor area. The terms are not regulated or third-party verified and are certainly inferior designations to USDA certified organic.

Hormone/Antibiotic Free: This label carries no official meaning from the USDA. Growers must provide documentation to make this claim on their products, but they are not verified by a third party. It certainly suggests an improvement from conventional products, but USDA certified organic is far superior.

Humane Designations: Animal Welfare Approved, American Humane Certified, Certified Humane Raised & Handled, or Free Farmed are common terms. The first designation, from the Animal Welfare Institute, certifies that animals were treated humanely throughout all life stages. Their designation (and the others) has strict standards for outdoor access; diets free of hormones, pesticides, or antibiotics; and freedom from overcrowded conditions. Furthermore, the terms are third-party verified. This is probably a suitable choice in the absence of USDA-certified organic meat.

Kosher: Meats with this label have been prepared under rabbinical supervision and the corresponding guidelines mandated to be awarded the distinction. The guidelines relate more to slaughtering methods, segregation of implements and production facilities (meat cannot be mixed with dairy products, etc.), and other factors that may or may not be related to health quality.

Natural: To the USDA, this term merely means the meat is free of artificial flavors, colorings, and preservatives. It has no relevance to how the animal was raised, fed, or slaughtered, and it is not third-party verified.

Vegetarian Diet: This pertains to the animal's diet only and does not guarantee that the animal had access to pasture or humane treatment.

Fish

Fish offer a rich source of omega-3 fatty acids (particularly the important omega-3 fractions known as DHA and EPA, which are not present in most other foods), complete protein, B complex vitamins, selenium, vitamin D, vitamin E, zinc, iron, magnesium, phosphorous, antioxidants, and other nutrients. A 2006 study by the Harvard School of Public Health indicated that regular consumption of fish helps dramatically reduce the risk of heart disease and that the benefits (particularly the omega-3 content) outweigh the potential risks of ingesting toxins from polluted waters. Regular consumption of fish has been shown to exert a strong anti-inflammatory effect, reduce risk for heart disease, help protect against asthma in children, moderate chronic lung disease, reduce the risk of breast and other cancers by stunting tumor growth, and ease the symptoms of rheumatoid arthritis and certain bone and joint diseases. Nursing and pregnant women enjoy a host of benefits from fish consumption, including support for fetal and early childhood brain and retinal development and a lowered risk of premature birth.

While the benefits of eating fish are substantial, you should choose wisely to avoid fish possibly tainted with environmental toxins and steer clear of the increasingly popular farmed sources that are inferior to wild-caught fish. The risk of ingesting fish tainted by environmental contaminants (heavy metals such as mercury, polychlorinated biphenyls [PCBs], dioxins, and other toxins) can be countered by emphasizing fish caught in remote, pollution-free ocean waters. The healthiest sources of fish are small, oily fish, such as wild-caught Alaskan salmon, sardines, herring, anchovies, and mackerel. Domestic mahimahi, Pacific halibut, pollack, white sea bass, and shellfish (e.g., oysters, calamari, and American lobster) are also healthful and carry a lower risk of contaminants. The fish at the top of the marine food chain are the least desirable, due to their tendency to accumulate concentrated contaminants. Hence, you should avoid or limit your consumption of swordfish, ahi tuna, shark, and Chilean sea bass, to name just a few.

The reason to avoid farmed fish is that they are generally raised under unsanitary conditions similar to those of ranch animals, and exposed to high levels of dangerous chemicals, such as dioxins, dieldrin, toxaphene, and other pesticides or toxic residue. These chemicals (from contaminated sediments in their fish meal) are easily absorbed into fat cells. Farmed fish are constantly exposed to their own waste and are often fed artificial dyes (to match color with wild varieties; e.g., wild salmon derive their pink color from the healthy carotene astaxanthin in their natural diet) and antibiotics to ward off the high risk of infection and disease from living in cramped farms. The waste from a large salmon farm is estimated to equal the sewage from a city of 10,000 people. A 2004 report in the popular journal *Science* warned that farmed salmon contained 10 times the amount of toxins of wild salmon and should be eaten rarely—once every five months—due to their high cancer risk. (Hey, *Science*—how about never?)

While wild salmon, trout, and catfish offer 19 to 27 percent of their total fat in omega-3s, the farmed varieties of these fish contain significantly less omega-3s, less protein, and much higher levels of omega-6 fats (obtained from their commercial feed, unlike the omega-3-rich algae that nourishes wild fish). Of additional concern is the estimated three million salmon that escape from their pens into the ocean each year, contaminating and genetically diluting nearby wild salmon (farmers' daughters sneaking out to fool around with wild boys from out of town—what else is new?). Use discretion and look for wild Alaskan salmon (distant from the escaped convicts of the major farms located in the North Atlantic, the North American continent, and Chile).

If you are wild about salmon and willing to endure the trade-off of a big carbon footprint and substantial expense to get a quality product, you can do your shopping online at such Web sites as wildpacificsalmon. com, seabeef.com, jdockseafood.com, or vitalchoice. com. The first site, wildpacificsalmon.com, offers a choice of a half-dozen different species, all caught in Alaska and shipped across the United States via FedEx next-day in vacuum-packed, cold-insulated containers. This site also features extensive details about the benefits of eating wild salmon and the dangers of eating farmed salmon.

> *Farmed fish should be avoided because they are raised in unsanitary, waste-infested waters; have dangerous chemical additives in their diets; and offer much lower levels of omega-3s than their wild counterparts.*

Eggs

Eggs can be freely enjoyed as an excellent source of healthy protein, fat, B complex vitamins, and folate. Be sure to obtain organic chicken eggs, which contain up to 20 times more omega-3s (obtained from green leaves in the chickens' natural diet) than factory-produced, grain-fed chicken eggs. The popular Conventional Wisdom "heart-healthy" concept of discarding the yolk to avoid cholesterol is misguided, as the yolk is one of the most nutrient-rich foods you can find—laden with omega-3s and the other aforementioned nutrients. In contrast, egg whites, besides being a good source of complete protein, have otherwise a rather low nutrient content. Furthermore, and contrary to Conventional Wisdom, there is no proof that egg consumption raises blood cholesterol or affects your risk for heart disease.

A Harvard Medical School study of 115,000 subjects over the span of eight to fourteen years demonstrated no correlation between egg consumption and heart disease or stroke. A 2008 study published in the *International Journal of Obesity* suggests that

> *Even the most vocal complainers about high-priced organic food might benefit from examining their discretionary purchases and moving healthy food up the priority list. Eliminating processed or packaged foods and bottled beverages and growing your own fruits and vegetables can reduce your budget and improve your dietary quality.*

eating two eggs for breakfast (not just the whites—the whole deal) is healthier than eating a bagel. Most quality grocers, health food stores, co-ops, and national chains (e.g., Trader Joe's and Whole Foods) stock abundant sources of organic eggs. If you have trouble finding organic eggs near you, visit localharvest.org and perform a zip code search.

Going Primal on a Dime

I understand that buying organic animal products can be cost-prohibitive. I will accept criticism that the distinctions I elaborate here could characterize the *Primal Blueprint* eating style as elitist in the eyes of some. I'll discuss this philosophical issue with great enthusiasm and detail in Chapter 9. For now, I'll proudly stand as an advocate for healthy living and getting your priorities straight, including budgeting for the best foods you can afford—even if this means your diet potentially (but not necessarily, if you do a little legwork) becomes more expensive and cumbersome for you than for the other families on your block. The fact is, to reprogram your genes for optimal health, you must make every effort to eat as cleanly as Grok did.

Even the most vocal complainers about high-priced organic food might benefit from examining their discretionary purchases and moving healthy food up the priority list. For example, if you sharply cut back or eliminate processed carbohydrates from your diet, you avoid the vast majority of the high-cost (and high-profit), low-nutritional-value products in the store. Shifting from bottled waters, juices, and all manner of sweetened beverages to a simple water-filtration system in your home can save money and improve dietary quality. Shifting from designer foods such as synthetic energy bars and meal replacements (Kelly Korg spends about 70 bucks a month on her twice-daily Slim-Fast shakes) to such basics as trail mix, jerky, or farm-fresh eggs can also reduce your budget while improving dietary quality.

Consider growing your own fruits and vegetables in your backyard garden or rent a patch in a community garden if your urban environment is short on soil. Part-time employees at many food stores enjoy a purchase discount. Perhaps there is even a co-op or farmers' market in your area where you can trade time for food? One popular post on MarksDailyApple.com detailed the concept of "cowpooling"—chipping in with other families to purchase and divide up all or part of a butchered cow, typically raised locally and naturally. I've written numerous other posts detailing ways to make *Primal Blueprint* eating convenient and affordable.

A concerted effort to follow the simple tips listed here will likely get you very close to break-even with your "before" *Primal Blueprint* grocery expenses (pricey sweetened beverages, brand-name packaged snacks, and prepared meals) compared to your "after" expenses (fruits and vegetables from the farmers' market, organic meat options such as cowpooling, filtered water as your main beverage, healthy bulk items like nuts, seeds, and increasingly more fresh produce, as well as a little high-fat dairy, instead of processed, packaged foods). You have the right and also the obligation—to yourself and your loved ones—to pursue the absolute highest dietary quality possible. Yes, it may require more time, energy, and even expense, but the payoff here is arguably greater than from any other lifestyle change you ponder (new TV, new car, new clothes, vacation, etc.). And not to sound trite, but an investment in your health today pays dividends far greater and far longer than you might ever see in your 401(k).

Now that I've climbed down off my soapbox, let's admit that real-world concerns may have you falling short here and there of the ideal spelled out in these pages. It's important to default back to the big-picture view that the *Primal Blueprint* is a way of life, not a boot camp. If you are agonizing over which fruit stimulates less insulin or you find yourself eating commercial hamburger at the company picnic yet are diligent enough to toss the buns in the garbage before you dig in, congratulations are in order for the momentum and awareness you have already created. When it comes to health and fitness, there is always a higher standard to strive for, but the *Primal Blueprint* allows for enough deviation from "ideal" never to compromise your enjoyment of today. Every step you take toward living Primally puts you that much closer to your health and fitness goals-and that much more adept and righting course when the inevitable deviations happen.

> *Forget love—I'd rather fall in chocolate!*
> *—Sandra J. Dykes*

Nuts and Seeds and Their Derivative Butters

Nuts and seeds and their derivative butter products are filling and nutritious and may be consumed liberally in place of high-carbohydrate snacks. Nuts and seeds are concentrated foods that represent an energy source (some might call it a "life force") for future generations of their plant—packed with protein, fatty acids, enzymes, antioxidants, and abundant vitamins and minerals. Their incredible nutrient density may result in you consuming fewer calories to satisfy your hunger and energy needs in comparison with cycling through the ups and downs of carb snacking throughout the day. You can conveniently carry and eat nuts and seeds anytime, anywhere. They stimulate minimal insulin production and will keep you satisfied for hours until your next meal.

Numerous respected studies (Iowa Women's Health Study of 40,000 women, Harvard School of Public Health's Nurses' Health Study of 127,000 women, and Physicians' Health Study of 22,000 men are among the most prominent) suggest that regular consumption of nuts significantly reduces the risk of heart disease and diabetes. Walnuts are known for their high omega-3 levels. Other highly nutritious choices that have earned the FDA's "heart healthy" distinction include almonds, hazelnuts, pecans, pine nuts, pistachios, flaxseeds, pumpkin seeds, and sunflower seeds. I'd add chia seeds and macadamia nuts to that list. Conversely, the ever-popular peanuts (technically a legume, not a nut) are among the most allergenic foods and also may contain dangerous molds that produce aflatoxin, a potent carcinogen. Definitely skip the Skippy and replace peanuts and peanut butter with less objectionable alternatives. Obviously, avoid nuts that have been processed with sugary or oily coatings or other offensive ingredients.

You can mix and match nuts and seeds with a little dried fruit to create nutritious trail mix snacks. The national chain Trader Joe's has an abundant selection of affordable, creative, delicious trail mixes, as do many local health food stores. Moderate your intake of the fancy bags that throw in a lot of dried fruit or chocolate, as the sugar and other carb count can creep up accordingly. Use a mini food processor to grind nuts and sprinkle onto salads, over baked vegetables, or even into omelets. Whole nuts (in the shell) will last up to a year without spoiling. Shelled nuts have less shelf life, and sliced nuts less again. Store excess in the refrigerator (or freezer if longer than six months) to prolong freshness. If your nuts have a rancid, oily smell or any discoloration, fleckings, or signs of mold, discard them. While there are some concerns about pesticide exposure from consuming nuts, they are minimal in comparison to concerns about animal products, fruits, and vegetables. Furthermore, because less than 1 percent of U.S. tree nut farmland is certified organic, finding organic nuts is problematic.

Nut and seed butters offer a versatile and great-tasting way to spread your intake of nuts and seeds over different meals and snacks. Take care to choose cold-processed butters that are simply ground up (at low temperatures and free of added ingredients—except salt, which is fine), and refrigerate them at all times. Many health proponents claim raw nuts, seeds, and butters have superior nutritional value to those that have been roasted, so by all means choose raw products if you can find them. Almond butter is believed by many to be the best butter choice. Almonds have the highest protein content of any nut (20 percent of total calories) and are high in antioxidants, phytonutrients, vitamins, minerals, and plant sterols that support health and lower disease risk.

Mark's Favorite Primal Snacks

Beef Jerky: How Primal can you get? Branch out and try buffalo, turkey, and venison, too. Be sure to choose a quality product without all the unhealthy additives as found in the typical jerky displayed in gas stations and liquor stores. Search the Web or your local health food store for natural products with only a few light seasonings listed on the label.

Celery: Enjoy with cream cheese or almond butter. Celery offers that satisfying texture and is a great vehicle to carry these and other low-carb toppings.

Cottage Cheese: Enjoy with nuts, berries, balsamic vinegar, or other creative toppings. While I don't like dairy as a centerpiece of the diet, using a cottage cheese base to top with the nutritious options mentioned (and more) is a sensible snack from time to time.

Dark Chocolate: Any lingering sweet tooth issues relating to your transition to Primal eating can be assuaged with a couple of squares of dark chocolate (with a 70 percent or greater cocoa content).

Dried Fruit: Snack on these in moderation. Apricots, blueberries, and coconut are good choices.

Fish: Canned tuna or sardines (yes, packed in oil) can easily replace a full meal for nutrient intake and satiety. Peel off the roll top and all you need is a plastic spoon to dine in style!

Fresh Berries: Raspberries, blueberries, blackberries, strawberries—all are Grok-like, nutritious, and very satisfying. Add some heavy cream to liven up the berries a little bit.

Hard-Boiled Eggs: Sprinkle some salt and seasoning in a ziplock bag and then roll the peeled egg around in the bag for a tasty snack. You don't have to go Cool Hand Luke crazy with several per day, but once in a while these make a nice change of pace from the usual carb-centric snacks.

Nuts and Seeds: Walnuts offer the best Primal health value; almonds, macadamias, pecans, and nut butters (except peanut) are great, too. Pumpkin, sunflower, and sesame seeds are also tasty and filling.

Olives: These delicious, nutrient-dense handy snacks are a great source of monounsaturated fatty acids and a central reason for the compliments lavished on the Mediterranean diet.

Trail Mix: Make sure your mix emphasizes nuts and seeds. A little dried fruit or even some dark chocolate chips are okay, but avoid the exotic offerings that have high-carb additions, such as yogurt-covered raisins, M&M's, and the like. Stay away from peanuts; they are technically legumes and can be highly allergenic.

Web Site: MarksDailyApple.com has hundreds of postings for snack and recipe ideas, including some creative make-your-own Primal snacks. We also have dozens of our ever-popular "top 10 lists" for everything you can think of relating to meat, vegetables, fruits, seasonal favorites, recipes, foods to avoid, and healthy dietary habits.

Herbs and Spices

No discussion of healthy eating would be complete without the inclusion of herbs and spices. Although these tasty additions provide minimal calories, they are packed with significant amounts of important micronutrients. Extensive evidence suggests that herbs and spices support cardiovascular and metabolic health, may help prevent cancer and other diseases, and improve mental health and cognition. Some of the highest antioxidant values (from ORAC scores) among all foods can be found in herbs and spices. Certain marinades and herbal preparations are so powerful in their antioxidant capacity that they have been shown to mitigate or eliminate potential issues that may arise from overcooking meat.

Herbs are generally green plants or plant parts used to add flavor to foods. Herbal extracts have been used for thousands of years in Eastern medicine and continue to enjoy widespread popularity today, for their powerful immune and health-supporting properties. Spices, on the other hand, are typically dried seeds, fruits, and plant parts. Spices are used to enhance flavor, add color, or help prevent bacterial growth on food.

Grok surely partook of the many varieties of plants he encountered. Throughout history, herbs and spices have played a large role in the human diet and even in culture as a whole. During the Middle Ages, spices were a currency with substantial economic value. Their popularity to enhance flavor and preserve food was a catalyst for the fervent exploration of the globe by Marco Polo, Columbus, Magellan, and others.

The specific health properties of individual herbs and spices could fill an entire book. A couple of headliners that are easy to integrate into everyday meals include curcumin (offers potent anti-inflammatory effects and high antioxidant value) and cinnamon (regulates blood sugar and demonstrates high antibacterial, anti-inflammatory, and antioxidant values). Visit MarksDailyApple.com for extensive coverage of numerous herb and spice benefits.

Foods to Enjoy in Moderation

While they may not be exactly what our ancestors ate, moderate consumption of the following foods can add some nutritional benefit to your diet without negative consequences, provided they are not overemphasized. If you are pursuing ambitious fat-reduction goals, you will probably want to eliminate some of these from the picture.

Certain Fruits

As previously mentioned, you may wish to exert a little restraint when eating fruits that carry relatively high glycemic values and low antioxidant values. These include melons, mangoes, papayas, pineapples, nectarines and dates, bananas, oranges, tangerines, plums, grapes, pomegranates, and all dried fruits.

Coffee

Coffee is fine in moderation, as long as you avoid using caffeine as a crutch to raise energy levels. Proper diet and exercise should enable you to wake up feeling refreshed and energized and avoid afternoon blues caused primarily by high-carbohydrate eating habits. Make an effort to drink organic coffee, as many big coffee-producing countries don't regulate chemical and pesticide use with their conventional brands.

Research is mixed on the effects of caffeine on the body. Some studies suggest that caffeine can actually reduce risk of heart disease and cancer and enhance fat metabolism, particularly during exercise. Other studies are inconclusive, while still others suggest that caffeine is harmful to the cardiovascular system, does not enhance fat metabolism, and stresses the adrenal glands as an artificial central nervous system stimulant. It seems reasonable that it's unhealthy to habitually ingest a beverage that can keep you cranking at warp speed when what you really need is a nap! However, it appears that a cup or two a day won't hurt. I myself enjoy coffee, especially after adding heavy cream and a pinch of sugar (yes, a pinch won't hurt). It's a warm and comforting element to my morning routine, especially on those freezing cold winter mornings in Malibu....

Dairy Products

Certain dairy products can offer a decent source of nutrition for those who don't suffer from lactose intolerance or casein sensitivities. My friend and health expert Scott Kustes (at modernforager.com) recommends eschewing normally processed or pasteurized dairy products entirely and ranks the best options in this order:

1. **No dairy** at all (gotta love this guy's style!)
2. **Raw, fermented** dairy (yogurt, kefir)
3. **Raw, high-fat** dairy (butter, cream)
4. **Raw milk and cheese**
5. **Organic, hormone- and antibiotic-free** dairy

Raw dairy products retain more nutritional value due to their minimal processing. Fermented dairy products may help you avoid the immune system issues and allergenic reactions that many have toward the lactose and casein in cow's milk. They also offer a good source of probiotics (healthy bacteria for your intestines). High-fat dairy products have low levels of the objectionable casein protein, which I will discuss shortly. And how can you not love an eating style that lets you have butter and heavy cream? As a last allowable choice, organic products protect you from the dangers of the hormones, pesticides, and antibiotics prevalent in commercial dairy products.

> *Milk doesn't really "do a body good." Objections include lactose, casein, hormones, pesticides, antibiotics, and high-temperature processing methods, while the calcium benefits are overstated.*

Cheese does have broad appeal and can play a minor role in a healthy diet. Play it snooty and go for the high-quality, aged stuff—not the weirdo processed stuff reminiscent of school lunches. Aged cheese is a fermented food, so it contains little to no lactose (for those with intolerance concerns). Cheese offers high-quality fats and proteins, as well as many other essential nutrients, with a satisfaction level that's just as important as the aforementioned health benefits. For a change of pace, try some raw, nonpasteurized cheese that is loaded with good nutrition.

Having offered possible options of what might constitute acceptable dairy, let's now look at why milk in and of itself doesn't really "do a body good." Lactose is a carbohydrate in milk that is difficult to digest for many who stop producing lactase (the enzyme that helps digest lactose) after age three or four. This is in alignment with our genetically programmed transition away from breast-feeding in early childhood (breast milk contains significant lactose). The incidence of lactose intolerance varies widely by ancestral heritage—something that is believed to be a rare example of genetic change through selection pressure in the manner of evolution (I'll discuss this topic at length in the Q&A appendix at MarksDailyApple.com). People from cultures with long histories as herders (and, hence, high dairy consumption)—like the Swedes and Dutch—are very tolerant. Other ethnic groups—like those of African or Asian descent—have high rates of lactose intolerance. If you carefully examine your dietary habits, you may discover incidences of bloating, gas, cramping, or diarrhea in conjunction with consuming milk products—all indications that you have some level of lactose intolerance and should avoid all dairy that is not fermented.

Casein is a protein that has autoimmune-stimulating properties and can initiate very serious allergic reactions. Casein is believed to contribute to or exacerbate conditions like celiac disease, Crohn's disease, irritable bowel syndrome, asthma, and possibly autism. Success has been reported treating these conditions naturally with a wheat- and dairy-free diet. *Paleo Diet* author Loren Cordain mentions how a substance known as epidural growth factor (EGF) in milk and other dairy products can increase cancer risk and tumor progression and also suggests that milk and other dairy products worsen acne cases. These negatives do not even address the consequences of consuming the hormones, pesticides, and antibiotics contained in conventional milk and dairy products (which was discussed at length in the context of conventional animal meats). Fortunately, the dangers and objections of the commonly used recombinant bovine growth hormone (rBGH; a treatment given to cows to increase their milk production) are well publicized, leading some forward-thinking nations to ban its use and sophisticated consumers to steer clear of milk made with rBGH.

Milk's modern processing methods also present health objections. Milk that is homogenized and pasteurized is certainly free of dangerous bacteria, but it is also devoid of beneficial bacteria, vitamins, and enzymes due to the heating process. Even if you don't have any acute symptoms, it's sensible to conclude that milk consumption should be limited to mother's milk in the first couple years of life.

For those who recoil at the suggestion to limit intake of milk, let's examine further why some of the Conventional Wisdom about dairy is flawed. Yes, most dairy is an excellent source of calcium, but we don't need nearly as much calcium as we have been led to believe. The United States and other Western nations with high dairy intake nevertheless have high rates of osteoporosis, suggesting that calcium is not the be-all and end-all for bone health. Experts are in agreement that magnesium, vitamin D, vitamin K, potassium, and other agents are also extremely important. Furthermore, just like with omega-3 and omega-6 fatty acids, these agents need to be obtained in proper balance to provide optimal bone health benefits, an area where the average Western diet falls short. Today, we generally consume too much calcium, largely from heavy use of dairy products. This hampers our ability to absorb magnesium because they compete on the same absorption pathways.

To make matters worse, many of us don't consume enough magnesium (found in leafy greens, nuts, seeds, and fish) nor synthesize enough vitamin D (from sun exposure, as I will detail in Chapter 7). Many experts believe that vitamin D intake might be more critical than calcium to bone health. Furthermore, chronic stress may play a huge role in osteoporosis, because the stress hormone cortisol inhibits calcium uptake by bones (rendering ingested calcium less effective). How about that? Taking a break from your busy day to bag some rays in your lounge chair might be better for your bones than drinking a glass of milk and swallowing a bunch of calcium pills!

Since we've discussed the importance of promoting an alkaline environment in the body, it should be noted that dairy foods are acid forming—a reality that actually hampers calcium absorption. For your calcium needs, you will better off consuming easily assimilated, high-calcium, alkaline-forming foods, such as leafy greens, nuts, oranges, broccoli, and sweet potatoes, or calcium-rich fish, including wild salmon and sardines. All told, it would be preferable to push dairy aside in favor of the *Primal Blueprint* stalwarts of vegetables, fruits, nuts, seeds, and meat. That said, when you look at the spectrum of foods from best to worst, the previous list of allowable dairy is still a preferred choice over grains, if you depart from the *Primal Blueprint* now and then.

Fats and Oils

Many oils offer significant health benefits, but they are generally high in calories with minimal vitamin and mineral values. Obviously, Grok didn't press oils in his day, but his omega-3 intake was quite high from animal and plant sources. Today, we need all the help we can get toward optimum essential fatty acid balance. Many oils offer a way to boost your intake of omega-3s and other healthy monounsaturated and saturated fats, but moderation is advised in this food category. Nuts and avocados offer similar health benefits to oils but carry much greater nutritional value. It's important to choose your oils wisely and strive to balance omega-6 and omega-3 intake. Stay with nut oils as they offer a healthy alternative to the decidedly less healthy polyunsaturated oils from vegetables, grains, and other sources.

Olive oil, the most monounsaturated oil, offers proven cardiovascular benefits (raises HDL and lowers LDL cholesterol) and has powerful anti-inflammatory and antioxidant properties. It's very good for cooking at low heat, but be careful because excessive time at high temperatures can compromise the health benefits of any oil. As you probably know, various processing methods dramatically affect the health quality of olive oil, with extra virgin designated as the purest form. As with fruit, you should strive for oil produced locally or at least domestically (instead of the vast majority of products shipped from Greece or Italy) for maximum freshness. The additional distinction "first cold press only" suggests that the olives have been pressed only once and bottled immediately, instead of being repeatedly pressed for maximum crop yield (this is the most common method, particularly with the large bottle–low price imports). You'll notice the difference with a single taste of a locally grown, first cold-pressed extra virgin olive oil in comparison with a much blander, duller-tasting extra virgin import. The aroma and taste are incredibly powerful—the high level of tocopherols (a potent antioxidant) may actually sting the back of your throat! In my estimation, nothing beats a Primal salad with generous drizzling of olive oil.

High omega-3 oils are a great dietary addition. These oils are extremely delicate and easily suffer damage from exposure to heat, light, and oxygen. Thus, you'll find them in health food stores refrigerated in small black containers (recognize that all bottled oils are damaged by heat, light, oxygen, and time). It's best to store your oils in the refrigerator and use them quickly—usually within six weeks of opening. Every time oils are exposed to air, they oxidize a bit. If you detect a slightly rancid smell in any oil or if it's been on the shelf for more than six months, discard the product immediately.

High polyunsaturated oils (corn, safflower, sunflower, cottonseed, and all partially hydrogenated oils) should be avoided, because they also oxidize easily. Canola oil, while enjoying mainstream popularity due to its high monounsaturated content, is inferior to olive oil because it's a heavily refined, genetically engineered product only recently cultivated (in contrast to olive oil's reign of thousands of years). Canola oil is derived from the rapeseed plant, which is thought to be toxic to humans and animals (particularly harmful to respiratory function). Most canola oil is put through a deodorizing process that converts some of its natural omega-3s into harmful trans fats.

Coconut oil offers numerous health benefits but has received a bad rap because it's the most saturated of all oils (at 92 percent, it's nearly solid at room temperature; this is the distinction between a saturated and an unsaturated fat). Of course, you know by now that saturated fat offers many health benefits. Coconut oil has been found to help normalize blood lipids and protect against damage to the liver by alcohol and other toxins, and it has anti-inflammatory and immune-supporting properties. Coconut oil is less sensitive to heat than unsaturated oils, making it the best choice for cooking. Butter and unprocessed palm oil are also great choices for cooking.

Mark's Primer on Fats and Oils

Approved Fats and Oils (in alphabetical order)

This list contains a variety of saturated and unsaturated types. The saturated fats listed here (animal fats, butter, coconut oil, and palm oil) are great choices for cooking because they are temperature stable (they won't oxidize under high heat). Review the list carefully, stockpile your fridge, and be sure to stick to the best intended use for each.

Animal Fats: Chicken, duck, or goose fat; lard (aka pork fat), beef, or lamb tallow; and other animal fats are excellent for cooking because their saturated composition makes them temperature stable.

Butter: An excellent choice for cooking or enhancing taste of steamed vegetables. A good source of vitamins A and E as well as selenium.

Coconut Oil: Temperature stability and numerous health and immune-supporting benefits make it the premier choice for cooking. Find an organic brand and try it in the Primal Energy Bar recipe at MarksDailyApple.com!

Dark Roasted Sesame Oil: This oil's intense flavor makes it a great choice for wok vegetables, meat, or salads.

High Omega-3 Oils: These delicate oils come in small dark containers and require refrigeration and quick use. They are a great addition to salads or protein shakes for an omega-3 boost. Recent research suggests that it may be more difficult to assimilate omega-3 benefits from flaxseed oil than other types. Choose borage, cod-liver, krill, salmon, hemp seed, or hi-oleic sunflower or safflower seed oils (not to be confused with their unhealthy polyunsaturated derivatives) as alternatives.

Marine Oils: Typically delivered in capsule or soft-gel supplement form, these fish or krill oils are an excellent source of omega-3s.

Olive Oil: Choose extra virgin, first cold press, locally grown, and savor the flavor! Best not to cook with olive oil due to temperature fragility.

Palm Oil: The unprocessed variety (not to be confused with widely used partially hydrogenated palm oil) is great for cooking.

continued

Mark's Primer on Fats and Oils (continued)

Oils and Fats to Strictly Avoid (in alphabetical order)

Many of these oils are considered polyunsaturated fatty acids (PUFAs), which have a variety of serious health objections. The concerns stem from PUFAs' long-chain fatty acids, which are unstable, quickly go rancid, and are easily oxidized in your body. Consequently, PUFAs have a pro-inflammatory effect and disturb homeostasis in many other ways. The endocrine system is especially vulnerable to the effects of PUFA ingestion, leading to symptoms like a slowed metabolism, low energy levels, and sluggish thyroid function. Heavy consumption of PUFAs in the modern diet is blamed as a leading contributor to obesity, diabetes, heart disease, cancer, immune problems, arthritis, and other inflammatory conditions. Strictly avoid PUFAs, trans and partially hydrogenated fats, and the other fats and oils detailed as follows:

Canola Oil (PUFA): Heavily refined and genetically engineered. Contains trans fats.

Cottonseed Oil (PUFA): Heavily processed oil popular in packaged and frozen foods, often in partially hydrogenated form.

Corn Oil (PUFA): Derived from a grain! High omega-6, low omega-3 value.

High-Temperature Processing: Avoid all oils heated to high temperatures in the course of frying or deep frying food.

Margarine: Contains objectionable ingredients and processed with chemical additives at high temperatures. While most margarines today have the "trans-fat free" distinction proudly adorning the label, the PUFAs that some margarines contain still potentially raise LDL, lower HDL, and suppress immune function and insulin sensitivity. Research strongly suggests an increased risk of cancer and heart disease from margarine use.

Partially Hydrogenated Oils: High-temperature, chemically altering processing methods makes these toxic to your DNA. Extreme health hazard!

Safflower and Sunflower Oils (PUFAs): Some of the most popular PUFAs.

Soybean Oil (PUFA): High omega-6, low omega-3 values. There is evidence that some forms may disturb thyroid function.

Trans Fats: Similar, but not identical, to partially hydrogenated oils. Also an extreme health hazard!

Vegetable Shortening: Similar to lard in appearance but chemically produced to create a trans fat. The brand name Crisco is an acronym for "crystallized cottonseed oil." Bad stuff—stay away!

Starchy Tuber Vegetables

Potatoes, yams, and sweet potatoes are considered tubers (vegetables that grow underground and have a swollen stem). Grok probably found the occasional wild tuber in his travels and enjoyed its starchy contents, particularly after learning how to roast it. However, most potatoes in general are another domesticated, recently introduced product that happens to stimulate a high insulin response when eaten. Yams and sweet potatoes are nutritionally superior to the lighter colored potatoes (russets, reds, whites, new potatoes) and stimulate a lower insulin response. Starchy vegetables might be a particularly appealing choice for those who require more than 150 grams per day of carbs to replenish their frequently depleted muscle and liver glycogen stores. This would include the Chronic Cardio crowd and those with very active lifestyles and high metabolisms.

Water: Obey Your Thirst, It's *Not* Too Late

"Drink eight glasses of water a day to ensure good health." "By the time you're thirsty, it's too late." We've heard these adages our entire lives as part of Conventional Wisdom's 10 (or 20, or whatever) commandments to be healthy—right up there with "Drink milk to get your calcium," "Eat your grains for fiber," "Stay out of the sun," "Cut down on fat intake to lose weight," and other fables. While adequate hydration is paramount to good health, there is absolutely no scientific evidence to support the age-old rule of thumb that you should drink eight glasses of water per day.

Dr. Heinz Valtin, former chair of physiology at Dartmouth Medical School and one of the world's foremost experts on kidney function, after conducting research for 11 months with the assistance of a professional librarian, discovered no conclusive studies about drinking eight glasses of water per day. Valtin believes that the myth originated in the 1940s when the National Institute of Medicine first issued recommendations for dietary nutrient intake, including water. Their suggestion to consume about two liters of water per day (this equals about eight 8-ounce glasses) for optimum hydration contained the long-forgotten comment that "much of this can be gained from the solid food we eat."

Indeed, raw milk is 90 percent water, chicken 54 percent, ground beef 53 percent, pizza 50 percent, white bread 30 percent (but, of course, we wouldn't be eating any pizza or bread, right?), and so on. Caffeine and alcohol, which constitute a significant portion of total fluid intake for many adults, have long been thought of as diuretics that dehydrate you by increasing urine flow. While this is true when you drink in excess, your daily cup of coffee, bottle of beer, or glass or two of wine will actually contribute to hydration levels and not lead to any appreciable fluid loss.

When you experience such variables as hot weather and increased activity levels, your thirst mechanism works wonderfully to dictate how much you need to drink each day. This is a mechanism that has evolved over millennia to prevent dehydration, which is one of the quickest ways you can die. To date, there is no archaeological evidence that Grok wore a CamelBak during his active life (or even a leather bota bag, for that matter!), but he did just fine scooping water out of streams, licking the dew off of leaves, and maintaining adequate hydration incidentally through his diet.

Even when your water intake fluctuates significantly, your kidneys and endocrine system work very efficiently to promote optimum fluid levels in your bloodstream. When you experience even a slightly higher than normal concentration of your blood volume, an agent known as antidiuretic hormone goes to work increasing the absorption of more water from the kidneys and returning it to the bloodstream. According to Dr. Valtin and other experts, if your blood becomes concentrated by about 2 percent, your thirst mechanism will kick in and send a strong signal to consume additional fluids. It is only when your blood becomes concentrated by 5 percent that the symptoms of dehydration present themselves. Dr. Valtin further asserts that while dark urine indicates a need to drink perhaps a glass of water, there is no validity to the idea that your urine needs to be clear to indicate that you are adequately hydrated.

Even with a wide variation in water intake, our bodies will do a great job at maintaining normal blood concentration. And yes, there is such a thing as too much water. Hyponatremia is a serious and occasionally fatal condition where sodium levels become too diluted in the blood as a result of overconsumption of water. Some believe that drinking too much fluid near or during meals can result in poor digestion and excretion due to the dilution of stomach acids that are critical to the digestive process.

As an alternative to the bottled water industry–influenced mantra, "drink, drink, drink!" without regard to your thirst, I recommend consuming a sensible amount of fluid each day, using your thirst as a guide to maintain optimum hydration. Sometimes this might be eight glasses of water, sometimes much less than half that. Heavy exercise, hot temperatures, body weight, and the water content of the foods you eat are obviously all significant variables. When in doubt, obey your thirst! (finally, a marketing slogan with a ring of truth to it!).

Wild Rice

Even though wild rice is a high-protein, gluten-free, high-nutritional-value natural species grass, it is still technically a grain that has a relevant carbohydrate load. Nevertheless, it is an excellent substitute for white rice or brown rice.

Sensible Indulgences

One issue I have with our modern lifestyle is the emphasis on perfection. Newer, slimmer, bigger, better, faster—the message screams out to us from glossy magazines, slick television ads, and one pop-up Web banner after another. While I do believe fundamentally in pursuing your personal definition of peak performance, and I think we could generally be doing far better in terms of diet and exercise, I have a hard time with the constant barrage of images telling us that, in short, we suck.

This brings me to indulgences. I'm a pretty disciplined—okay, very disciplined—guy, but I stop short of attempting perfection. Sure, I could stress over those missed workouts when I'm vacationing with my wife and kids. I could forever kiss berries and cream, cheesecake, and chocolate good-bye. But why? Furthermore, when you choose wisely, many "indulgences"—such as those on the following list—may even support your health when you partake sensibly. With that in mind, here are a few items that Grok rarely or never enjoyed but which can be added to a Primal lifestyle with little or no downside.

Alcohol

If alcohol is something you enjoy and can consume moderately, go for it. Yes, these are calories devoid of nutritional value, so you don't want to go overboard, but some of the potential health benefits may be worth noting. Wine is a bit better for you than beer, but these are both beverages you can sensibly enjoy on a regular basis. Red wines are the best, owing to their high phenol content. Recent studies have shown so many health-enhancing benefits from the resveratrol in red wine that red wine extracts have become very popular as supplements.

On the flip side, studies have clearly shown that alcohol in excess of one or two glasses a day can increase the risk of cancer (as well as auto accidents, divorces, bar fights, and other tribulations), so let's be clear that I'm not leaving the door open for alcohol abusers. Furthermore, it's believed that alcohol is the first fuel to burn when ingested. That means even the most Primal eaters will put fat metabolism on hold while the alcohol calories are burned.

Dark Chocolate

Most of us know by now that dark chocolate is rich in antioxidants, brain-stimulating compounds, and that it offers impressive health benefits, such as reducing the instance of blood clots, lowering blood pressure, and helping prevent cancer. It's all in the antioxidants—specifically, compounds known as phenolic phytochemicals or flavonoids. Some studies have shown that cocoa contains considerably more flavonoids than acclaimed heavy hitters like green tea and red wine (but I'd add that red wine has resveratrol going for it as well). The ORAC values of cocoa powder and dark chocolate are higher than those of virtually any fruit or vegetable!

Chocolate is the most craved food in the world, thanks to it's rich supply of phenylethylamine, an agent that is believed to trigger a feeling similar to falling in love. Be sure to choose the absolute highest-quality chocolate you can find, because not all chocolates are created equal, from both a taste and a health perspective. The higher the cocoa content, the more you'll enjoy the aforementioned health benefits. This means milk chocolate is a distant also-ran to dark chocolate. Commercial bars like good old Hershey's have diminished cocoa content and such additives as sugars and milk solids, agents that dramatically compromise health benefits. I recommend choosing chocolate that is 70 percent cocoa or greater (anything with more than 50 percent cocoa content is classified as bittersweet chocolate). Unsweetened chocolate (aka chocolate liquor—100 percent cocoa) is the healthiest option, but you may not enjoy the taste.

Organic chocolate offers you the comfort of greater oversight along the growing, harvesting, and processing procedures—important due to the fact that conventional cocoa beans have a high pesticide concern and commonly often arrive from countries with questionable growing regulations and safety standards. Enjoy your chocolate guilt-free, with total awareness of a taste so rich that even a small portion can deepy satisfy you.

High-Fat Desserts

Dessert—the tradition of eating a high-calorie, high-sugar meal after you have just eaten your regular meal—is a bizarre concept that has become perverted by modern American society. (I was once asked in Texas, after eating a four-egg omelet for breakfast, whether I wanted some dessert!) We rarely have dessert in my house, and my kids never ask for it. Grok certainly had no choice in the matter, but you do. Avoiding dessert is probably one of the easiest ways to start going Primal.

Nevertheless, if you feel the urge to indulge, do yourself a favor and choose a high-fat, fresh-made, premium-quality treat instead of a store-bought product that comes with too much sugar and unpronounceable chemicals and preservatives and that falls well short of homemade in the taste category. My favorite choice for dessert is a bowl of fresh berries with a small dose of homemade whipped cream and mascarpone cheese. If you have a thing for cheesecake, have a small slice—not the 1,400-calorie insulin tidal wave–producing monsters offered by the Cheesecake Factory. Or maybe try some sliced apples with nut butter or fry some plantains in coconut oil with a pinch of sugar (there I go again!). Experiment with simple desserts that you can make with your kids. Then take a walk after your meal to burn off some of the glucose and moderate the insulin response. Wake up the next morning and eat a delicious low-insulin breakfast to get your body back into hormone and blood glucose balance.

Finally, a Word About Supplements

While there are many things we can do (or eat) today that very closely approximate what Grok did to trigger positive gene expression, there are also a number of obstacles that can thwart our attempts to be as Primal as possible. Artificial light prompts us to stay up too late and sleep too little. Electronic entertainment competes for our time when we should be out walking and basking in sunlight. We don't always have access to ideal foods. We use medicines to mask our symptoms instead of allowing our bodies natural symptoms to strive for homeostasis. You get my point. It's tough going "full Primal" today. Hence, I enjoy discovering modern adaptations that produce the same gene expression Grok experienced—but by using 21st-century technology or just plain old common sense. Given the lack of certain critical nutrients in even the healthiest diets (refer to the discussion on the drawbacks of conventional animal, vegetable, and fruit products), using premium-quality supplements is a great example of a "modern Primal" adaptation.

As you may know, I own and operate a supplement company called Primal Nutrition, which markets products of the nature I describe here. While I am not keen to blend my company's marketing efforts with my literary efforts to help you get Primal, the question arises often enough that a basic explanation of what and why is appropriate. I agree that the supplement industry does have its share of shady characters. Most of the products you see on store shelves are probably harmless, but some are also probably useless—with more smoke, mirrors, and hype than credible research backing them up. However, there are also some high-quality products that deliver proven benefits and that I wouldn't be without in my own regimen. Here I will discuss the most important supplement categories and also discuss the ways that you can ensure that the brands you choose are of the highest quality.

Multivitamin/Mineral/Antioxidant Booster

The flagship product of the supplement industry is designed to offer complete protection and nutritional balance to make up for any inadequacies in your daily diet. The popularity of this category makes it rife with poor-quality offerings, so be sure to review the product quality selection tips in the coming section. You'll want to choose a supplement with natural forms of all the vitamins.

The topic of free radicals and oxidative damage has been covered in depth at MarksDailyApple.com beyond the scope of this book. Suffice to say, we want to do everything we can to reduce oxidative damage to our cells (and particularly inside our mitochondria, the energy-producing component of our cells). Eating and exercising according to the *Primal Blueprint* (particularly avoiding excessive high-end cardio) and managing stress effectively with *Primal Blueprint* lifestyle laws are your first lines of defense. However, our powerful antioxidant systems can fall short when we face even the routine level of stress inherent in modern life. If you challenge your stress-management system by eating sugar, drinking alcohol, taking prescription (or nonprescription, ahem) drugs, skimping on sleep or sunshine, or arguing with your spouse about the particulars of the dreaded holiday trip to the in-laws, you can overwhelm your defenses and find yourself in sincere need of a boost.

Furthermore, many of the best sources of dietary antioxidants historically have all but disappeared or have been rendered impotent by today's aggressive factory farming techniques. Among industrial fruit growers, for example, obtaining the highest possible sugar content has replaced antioxidants as the focus. Even if you are eating really well, I believe we need a broad mix of different antioxidants on a daily basis, because different antioxidants work in different ways and in different parts of the cell. Furthermore, too much of any one single antioxidant (in the absence of others) has been shown to have potentially negative effects, as a few recent studies have demonstrated where subjects supplemented with only vitamin E to their detriment.

When you take a quality broad-spectrum antioxidant formula (containing hard-to-get nutrients like full-spectrum vitamin E [not just alpha-tocopherol], mixed carotenoids [not just beta-carotene], tocotrienols, n-acetyl-cysteine, alpha-lipoic acid, curcumin, resveratrol, milk thistle, CoQ10, and quercetin, to name a few), the agents can work synergistically to mitigate oxidative damage and then help each other recycle back to their potent antioxidant form after donating an electron to the antioxidant effort. For that reason, I take my high-potency Damage Control Master Formula multivitamin loaded with extra antioxidants every day.

Omega-3 Fish Oil

In Grok's day, virtually every animal he consumed was a decent source of vital omega-3 fatty acids. The fish he caught had eaten algae to produce omega-3 fatty acids rich in EPA and DHA (which helped build the larger human brain over the previous few hundred thousand years). The animals he hunted had grazed on plants that generated high levels of omega-3 in these meats. Even the vegetation Grok consumed provided higher levels of omega-3s than found in today's vegetables. In Grok's diet, the ratio of pro-inflammatory (bad) omega-6 to anti-inflammatory (good and healthful) omega-3 was close to 1:1. Unfortunately, most of us with a typical American diet today get way too much omega-6 and way too little omega-3, and that unhealthy ratio tends to keep many of us in a constant state of systemic inflammation.

Because omega-3 oils are found in fewer and fewer modern foods (fish being one of the few, but fresh wild fish also being impractical to eat regularly due to expense, availability, and objections over contaminants), the single easiest way to overcome this serious deficit and rebalance your omegas is to take highly purified omega-3 fish or krill oil supplements. The research on fish oils is extraordinarily positive, showing such benefits as decreased risk for heart disease and cancer, lowering of triglycerides, improvement in joint mobility, decreased insulin resistance, and improved brain function and mood. The drug companies are even starting to recognize the power of this "natural" medicine and have begun promoting prescription fish oil (at four times the price of a comparable supplement, of course!). As healthy as my own diet is, I never go a day without taking a few grams of an omega-3 fish oil supplement.

Probiotics

Grok ate dirt…all day, every day. Hey, when you never wash your hands, your food, or anything else, for that matter, you pretty much can't avoid it. But with all that soil came billions of soil-based organisms (mostly bacteria and yeast) that entered his mouth daily and populated his gut. Most were "friendly" bacteria that actually helped him better digest food and ward off infections. In fact, much of Grok's (and our) immune system evolved to depend on these healthy "flora" living in us symbiotically. Grok also ate the occasional "unfriendly" organisms that had the potential to cause illness, but as long as the healthy flora significantly outnumbered the bad guys, all was well. Several trillion bacteria live in the human digestive tract—some good and some bad. Much of your health depends on which of the two is winning the flora war.

The problem today is that not only do we avoid dirt, but we pursue sterility to the extent that we eliminate a significant amount of healthy bacteria from our diet. Of course, given the germs that prevail in the civilized world, it's probably best that we do thoroughly wash or cook everything we eat. In most healthy people, exposure to routine germs doesn't usually present a problem. As long as there are some healthy gut bacteria present (healthy, natural foods contain these probiotics inherently—even if we wash them); as long as we don't get too stressed out (stress hormones can kill off healthy flora) or too sick (diarrhea and vomiting are ways the body purges bad bacteria—but it purges good bacteria along with them), eat too much processed food (sugar, trans and partially hydrogenated fats, and chemical additives support the growth of unhealthy bacteria and yeast, while choking out healthy flora), or take antibiotics (antibiotics tend to kill most bacteria, good and bad—that's their job); and as long as we are eating well, those healthy bacteria can flourish and keep us healthy.

Of course, the healthy bacteria balance in our intestinal tract gets compromised regularly in all the ways

> *The problem today is that we pursue sterility to the extent that we eliminate a significant amount of healthy bacteria from our diet.*

mentioned (even with generally healthy people), again creating an opportunity to benefit from supplementation. You don't necessarily need to take probiotics every day, because once these "seeds" have been planted in a healthy gut, they tend to multiply and flourish easily on their own. I'd certainly take extra probiotics under times of great stress, when you have been sick or are taking (or have just taken) a course of antibiotics, when you are traveling (particularly to foreign countries, where unfamiliar bacteria—even good stuff from good foods—can overwhelm your digestive system), or when you detect any sign of compromised immune function (the digestive system is critical to immune function). The reversal of fortune from a few days of taking probiotics can be dramatic. "Better than eating dirt," I always say.

Protein Powder

Restricting your intake of processed carbs often means being at a loss for quick, convenient snacks or small meals. We are so conditioned to reach for a bagel, an energy bar, chips, crackers, and other grain-based products or sweets for snacks, we often run short of convenient, transportable, nonperishable options for an afternoon pickup snack or mini meal. While not exactly Primal, protein powders do combine the best of 21st-century technology with a true Primal intent: get me a fast, good-tasting source of protein without too many carbs or unhealthy fats. I prefer micro-filtered whey protein to obtain an impressive profile of all essential and nonessential amino acids, and I require that the product taste great when mixed only with water (so I don't have to add sugary juices or milk just to choke it down). That way I can always throw in a piece of fruit if I like for added calories or flavor. If I am in a hurry and want a quick, high-protein start to my day, my morning protein shake takes less than a minute to make and addresses by broad nutritional needs (adding some omega-3 oil covers two more critical Primal areas). Micro-filtered whey, while derived from dairy, has insignificant amounts of lactose, so it's fine for all but the most severely lactose-intolerant folks.

This list contains what I believe to be the most useful product categories to consider for supplementation, though it is by no means exhaustive. There are numerous other excellent product categories and individual supplements that address more specialized needs, such as phosphatidylserine (PS) for memory loss and moderating cortisol damage; glucosamine, chondroitin, MSM, and enzyme cofactors to support connective tissue and alleviate pain; or others that might be recommended by a knowledgeable health care practitioner. Please visit MarksDailyApple.com or PrimalNutrition.com for more discussion on supplements.

Supplement Quality

Regardless of what brand of products you choose, you should be extremely vigilant in an industry that is minimally regulated by the FDA. Good manufacturers have a tightly controlled production environment where every single raw material that goes into the finished product is easily sourced and certified by the supplier. At Primal Nutrition, we purchase our raw materials from trusted suppliers who supply a Certificate of Assay attesting to the potency and purity of each ingredient. Upon receipt, we test everything again ourselves to confirm the purity. The product is then quarantined until it is manufactured in a pharmaceutical-grade environment and sealed for distribution direct to the consumer.

Call the manufacturer of supplements you use or consider and inquire about their product-quality standards. You'll quickly discern which outfits are able to provide a satisfactory answer. Ask whether the product is made under the GMP (Good Manufacturing Practices) standards overseen by the FDA. Examine labels and choose supplements that are free of common fillers and additives, such as colorings, waxes, preservatives, and other chemicals, listed under "inactive" or "other" ingredients. You'll be surprised to discover just how prevalent these agents are in many of the leading vitamin brands and discount products available through big-box retailers and in supermarkets and drugstores. Understand that premium-quality supplements are typically far more expensive than the giant bottle of multivitamins found on the shelves of warehouse stores. The latter offer minimal potency and bioavailability and bring literal accuracy to the expression "pissing away your money."

> *Understand that premium-quality supplements are typically far more expensive than the giant bottle of multivitamins found on the shelves of warehouse stores. The latter offer minimal potency and bioavailability and bring literal accuracy to the expression "pissing away your money."*

Chapter Summary

1. Plant Foods: Plant foods should constitute the bulk of your food intake in terms of meal emphasis and nutritional benefits. Brightly colored foods have high levels of antioxidants, phenols, fiber, vitamins, minerals, and other micronutrients. Consuming fruits and vegetables helps naturally promote alkalinity in your body, boosting immune function and reducing disease risk. Dark leafy greens are an excellent choice to consume regularly as a base for any main course. Berries offer excellent antioxidant and nutrient levels. Eating fruits and vegetables liberally will still result in a satisfactory average total carbohydrate intake of 150 grams or less per day.

It's essential to select organic, locally grown plant foods for maximum nutritional value and health safety. Be strict about going organic with fruits and vegetables that have a large surface area (leafy greens) or a soft open skin (bell peppers, carrots, winter squash, berries, peaches). You can be less strict with plants that have a tough, inedible skin (bananas, avocados, melons, oranges). Certain fruits with relatively high glycemic, low antioxidant values might be consumed in moderation by devoted Primal enthusiasts (an ode to how different today's cultivated fruits are from Grok's more fibrous, less sugary wild fruits).

2. Animal Foods: Animal foods are healthy and nutritious and will help you reduce excess body fat and build lean muscle. Be sure that you choose certified organic animal products (or, failing that, certified humanely treated or 100% grass-fed/finished animal products) to avoid today's poor quality conventional animals fattened up with grains and laden with hormones, pesticides, and antibiotics. Choose only wild fish caught in remote, pollution-free waters, which offer the extremely beneficial omega-3 fatty acids. Eggs are a healthy, nutritious food that should not be avoided based on the flawed assumption that their high-cholesterol content is a heart disease risk factor. The potential budget increase for buying organic products pales in comparison to the importance of leading a healthy life and avoiding disease risk factors.

3. Nuts and Seeds and Their Derivative Butters: These concentrated energy foods offer high levels of beneficial monounsaturated and omega-3 fats, phytonutrients, fiber, antioxidants, and numerous vitamins and minerals. They are deeply satisfying—an excellent snack choice for appetite control—and have been found to minimize disease risk.

4. Herbs and Spices: Herbs and spices offer tremendous micronutrient value, especially as they pertain to antioxidants. Herbs and spices can enhance your enjoyment of meals and offer potential benefits for certain health conditions.

5. Moderation Foods: Some foods that weren't around in Grok's day are acceptable today, provided they are not overemphasized. These include certain fruits with high glycemic and low antioxidant values, coffee, dairy products (with a preference for raw, fermented, high-fat dairy products), fats and oils (choose animal fats over polyunsaturated oils or processed fats), starchy tuber vegetables, and wild rice.

6. Sensible Indulgences: Enjoy your carefully chosen indulgences with full attention and awareness, and never feel guilty. Alcoholic beverages (sensibly, of course), dark chocolate, and high-fat desserts can be enjoyed as a superior alternative to the culturally prevalent high-carbohydrate treats that have moderate to severe negative health consequences. Consume water according to your thirst instead of following Conventional Wisdom's "eight glasses per day" mantra.

7. Supplements: Supplements can play a critical role in a healthy modern diet, as we adapt our Primal recommendations to the realities of modern life. Supplements offer a convenient source of concentrated nutrition that helps account for nutrient deficiencies (e.g., depleted soil or objectionable conventional growing and production methods) in today's food supply. Choosing an extremely high-quality multivitamin, mineral, or antioxidant; omega-3 fish oil; probiotic formula; and whey protein powder will give you comprehensive protection and added support for even the healthiest of diets.

CHAPTER 5

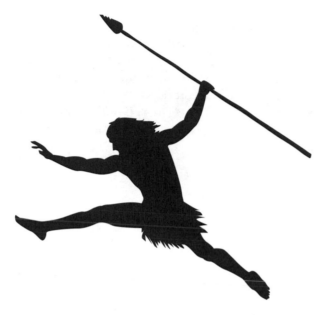

Law #2:
Avoid Poisonous Things

*"Drop Your Fork and Step Away
from the Plate!"*

In This Chapter

I detail the health risks of eating "poisonous things." In Grok's day, poisonous plants could drop him on the spot. Today we encounter factory-produced items in bright packages that kill more insidiously over decades. We explore the cultural factors that create tremendous momentum toward unhealthy choices and how to take a stand against these manipulative influences.

I pay particular attention to dispelling the Conventional Wisdom tenet that grain products (wheat, rice, bread, pasta, cereal, corn, etc.) are healthy, countering common assumptions with extensive details indicating the problems grains cause with their relatively recent (in the timeline of human evolution) introduction into the human diet. Grain consumption offers minimal nutritional value and generates a high insulin response. The phytates in grains inhibit the absorption of minerals. Glutens disturb healthy immune function and promote inflammation. Lectins inhibit healthy gastrointestinal function. Whole grains are no healthier than refined grains and have a worse impact on health in many cases due to the greater prevalence of the aforementioned agents in whole grains than in refined products

Trans and partially hydrogenated fats wreak havoc at the cellular level, promoting inflammation, aging, and cancer. Other foods to avoid include legumes, processed foods, and sugars.

When you see the golden arches, you are probably on your way to the pearly gates.
—**William Castelli, M.D.**
Director of the Framingham
Heart Study

Grok had no labels whatsoever and did a better job avoiding poisonous things than we do today, even with the trusty "Nutrition Facts" emblazoned on virtually everything with a wrapper or container. While I am admittedly sheltered from mainstream eating customs and have made fitness and health my life's work, I'd like us all to reflect for a moment on our priorities and our vision of a long, happy, healthy, fit life. When the topic of food comes up in conversation with family, friends or casual acquaintances, it's fascinating to hear the litany of rationalizations, knee-jerk defense mechanisms, self-limiting belief statements and general confusion or ignorance from otherwise intelligent folks when it comes to eating healthfully. But then again, Conventional Wisdom has often led even the best and brightest minds in nutritional science astray.

It's truly remarkable how successful Madison Avenue has been at indoctrinating eating habits that produce huge profits for giant multinational corporations—and devastating health consequences for consumers—into generations of society. The marketing message is so pervasive in modern culture that it's difficult, even stressful, to take control of your health and swim upstream against such cultural norms as fast food, the all-American high-carbohydrate breakfast, post-meal desserts, and the massive overconsumption of soft drinks. Even noble attempts to do the right thing miss the mark: mass-market "health foods" like frozen yogurt, bran muffins, poor-quality meal replacements, energy bars, and other heavily processed "fuel" marketed to athletes or purification/detox diets with clever ideas, such as eating nothing but brown rice for a week (talk about a long, hot insulin bath!). Finally, many of our eating habits are driven by social, emotional, or stress-related triggers other than hunger.

While savoring the occasional moderate serving of a rich treat is part of enjoying life, it's an entirely different story to ingest junk food habitually and mindlessly just because it's part of Americana ("baseball, hot dogs, apple pie, and Chevrolet"). If you notice yourself treading in these waters (or worse, repurposing the classic quote from Mt. Everest legend Sir Edmund Hillary—"Because it's there"—into an excuse), please give this topic some sincere reflection and take decisive action. Remember, your ancestors worked unimaginably hard to survive, thrive, and create the amazing opportunities we have today for a healthy, happy, active, and long life. As I say here often, your genes want you to be healthy and you deserve nothing less than the very best your genes have to offer.

> *Everything in moderation" is sage advice indeed, but Mark Twain best put this proverb in perspective when he said, "Everything in moderation, **including moderation.**"*

The most common retort I hear on this thread is, "Hey, everything in moderation." Sage advice indeed, but Mark Twain best put this proverb in perspective when he said, "Everything in moderation, *including moderation.*" As the Korgs prove dramatically, we live in a world where extreme measures are necessary just to avoid serious disease (remember, some three-quarters of today's American population will eventually die of heart disease or cancer), let alone enjoy optimum health, fitness, energy levels, and body composition. I strongly advocate enjoying the occasional indulgence, but why not make it from the list of approved foods of the absolute highest quality? Compare a label of a Milky Way or Snickers Bar with a high-antioxidant, organic dark chocolate bar with no additives, toxic chemicals, trans fats, or fillers. The latter, a sensible and deeply satisfying indulgence, can hardly be described as a sacrifice!

Going Against the Grain

Perhaps the most harmful element of dietary Conventional Wisdom is that grains are healthy—the "staff of life"—as we've been led to believe our entire lives. While grains enjoy massive global popularity today, they are simply not very healthy for human consumption. From two million years ago, when the first *Homo erectus* arose and began the steady evolution to the appearance of the first modern *Homo sapiens* between 200,000 and 100,000 years ago, and continuing until about 10,000 years ago, humans existed entirely as hunter-gatherers. Depending on where they roamed, early *Homo sapiens* derived their nutrition from as many as 200 different wild food sources, including animal meats, fruits, vegetables, and nuts and seeds, but grains were notably absent.

Starting about 10,000 years ago, forces conspired to create a dramatic shift in the human diet. The widespread extinction of large mammals on major continents coupled with increases in population forced humans to become more resourceful in obtaining food. Those living by water utilized rafts, canoes, nets, and better fishing tools to enjoy more bounty. On land, humans refined their toolmaking and hunting strategies to include more birds and small mammals in the food supply. Escalating competition for animal-sourced food eventually led to agricultural innovations sprouting up independently in the most advanced societies around the world (Egyptians, Mayans, etc.). As wild grains (which were a very small part of some diets but difficult to harvest for any significant yield) became domesticated, humans derived more and more calories from these readily available high-calorie sources, a trend that has continued to the present day—with dire consequences.

Loren Cordain, Ph.D., author of the 2002 best-seller *The Paleo Diet*, explains:

Cereal grains [meaning cultivated grains in general, not breakfast cereals] have fundamentally altered the foods to which our species had been originally adapted over eons of evolutionary experience. For better or for worse, we are no longer hunter-gatherers. However, our genetic makeup is still that of a paleolithic hunter-gatherer, a species whose nutritional requirements are optimally adapted to wild meats, fruits and vegetables, not to cereal grains. There is a significant body of evidence which suggests that cereal grains are less than optimal foods for humans and that the human genetic makeup and physiology may not be fully adapted to high levels of cereal grain consumption. We have wandered down a path toward absolute dependence upon cereal grains, a path for which there is no return.

Culturally, the cultivation of grains is the key variable that allowed modern civilization to develop and thrive. Families could successfully feed and raise more children. Large populations could now live permanently in proximity, and labor could specialize, leading to continued exponential advancements in knowledge and modernization. However, as Cordain elaborates, "[Grains] have allowed man's culture to grow and evolve so that man has become earth's dominant animal species, but this preeminence has not occurred without cost.... Agriculture is generally agreed to be responsible for many of humanity's societal ills, including whole-scale warfare, starvation, tyranny, epidemic diseases, and class divisions." Dr. Jared Diamond, evolutionary biologist, physiologist, and Pulitzer Prize–winning professor of geography at UCLA, and author of *Guns, Germs and Steel,* goes so far as to say that agriculture was "the worst mistake in the history of the human race" and that "we're still struggling with the mess into which agriculture has tumbled us, and it's unclear whether we can solve it."

Grain's singular benefit of plentiful calories was often more than offset by harmful aspects, including "antinutrients" (compounds that interfere with the absorption of beneficial nutrients), the high carb content, and grain proteins that were foreign to the human digestive process. Populations may have expanded, but health costs to the individual were significant. The flourishing of agriculture paralleled a reduction in average human life span as well as body and brain size, increases in infant mortality and infectious diseases, and the occurrence of previously unknown conditions such as osteoporosis, bone mineral disorders, and malnutrition. Ironically, as medical advancements have eliminated

> *The wise man sees in the misfortune of others what he should avoid.*
> —**Marcus Aurelius**
> *Roman Emporer*
> *(121-180)*

most of the rudimentary health risks faced by early humans (infant mortality, infections, etc.), we can now live long enough to develop, suffer, and die from diet-related diseases, including atherosclerosis, hypertension, and type 2 diabetes (it used to be called adult-onset diabetes until millions of kids started developing it in recent years!).

The Base of the Disease Pyramid

Grains offer the great majority of their calories in the form of carbohydrate, so they cause blood sugar levels to elevate quickly (foods that easily and rapidly elevate blood sugar are known as high glycemic foods). Because high glycemic foods, such as sugar and grains, have been recently and suddenly introduced to the human food supply (that's right, even 10,000 years ago is "recent and sudden" in evolutionary terms) and yet are consumed in massive quantities, they shock our delicate hormonal systems, which are better suited to ingesting the low-glycemic foods our ancestors ate, such as meat, vegetables, nuts, and most fruits.

A grain-heavy diet stresses the all-important insulin regulation mechanism in the body. After consuming that bagel, scone, muffin, French toast, or bowl of cereal (all derived from grains) and a glass of juice for breakfast, your pancreas releases insulin into the bloodstream to help regulate blood sugar levels. Even after the routine meal just described, many Americans technically become temporarily diabetic, with blood sugar levels soaring to clinically dangerous levels. You know the drill by now. After your meal, insulin is released into the bloodstream and stores glucose as muscle glycogen or directs its conversion to fat. Experience this often enough and it's very likely you'll gain weight and develop insulin resistance and Metabolic Syndrome.

If, instead, you were to have a *Primal Blueprint* breakfast consisting of a delicious cheese-and-vegetable omelet with some fresh berries, you would enjoy a moderated insulin response, leading to balanced energy levels for the hours after your meal instead of a sugar high and insulin crash. Furthermore, with blood sugar levels balanced, you would be able to access and burn stored body fat for energy until your next insulin-balanced meal.

Phytates We Hate

There is sufficient evidence that this overreliance on grains—as well as on simple carb and sugar products in general—leads to numerous vitamin, mineral, and nutritional deficiencies. Most grains contain substances called phytates that easily bind to important minerals like calcium, magnesium, and zinc in the digestive tract, making them more difficult to absorb. Ironically, the unprocessed—and, therefore, supposedly healthier—"whole" grains are typically the highest in phytates. Mineral deficiencies are common in underdeveloped nations that depend almost entirely on grain for their sustenance (bread accounts for 50 percent of the total calories consumed in at least half the countries in the world; some populations derive up to 80 percent of total calories from grain products).

Grains also play a role in interference with vitamin D metabolism and in related deficiencies of vitamins A, C, and B12. These nutrients are not present in grains (again, ironically, unless they have been processed and then "fortified" by adding back the missing vitamins—albeit at a much reduced bioavailability). Deficiencies of these basic vitamins are prevalent mainly in third-world countries (see the recurring theme?). However, even Western eaters with more balanced diets, but who still rely too heavily on grains, miss out on eating more nutritious foods, such as meats, fruits, and vegetables. In the United States, 45 percent of citizens get zero daily servings of fruit or juice and 22 percent get no daily vegetables.

Gluten, Lectin—Immune Affectin'

Certain grain (and also some dairy) proteins mimic those found in viruses and bacteria, triggering an immune response when ingested. Gluten—the large, water-soluble protein that creates the elasticity in dough (it's also the primary glue in wallpaper paste)—is found in most common grains, such as wheat, rye, and barley. Researchers now believe that as many as a third of us are probably gluten-intolerant or gluten-sensitive. That third of us (and I would suspect many more on a subclinical level) "react" to gluten with a perceptible inflammatory response. Over time, those who are known to be gluten-intolerant can develop a dismal array of medical conditions: dermatitis, joint pain, reproductive problems, acid reflux and other digestive conditions, autoimmune disorders, and celiac disease. And that still doesn't mean that the rest of us aren't experiencing some milder negative effect that simply doesn't manifest itself so obviously.

Grains also contain high levels of mild, natural plant toxins known as lectins. Researchers have found that lectins can inhibit healthy gastrointestinal function by damaging delicate brush borders that allow appropriate forms of nutrients (glucose, amino acids, fats, vitamins, and minerals) to travel from the digestive tract into the bloodstream. Lectin damage allows larger, undigested protein molecules to infiltrate the bloodstream. The ever-vigilant immune system sees these unfamiliar protein molecules (not necessarily lectins, but *anything* you ingest that was supposed to be fully processed in the digestive tract before entering the bloodstream) and sets up a typical immune response to deal with them. Unfortunately, these undigested protein molecules can resemble molecules that reside on the outside of healthy cells, leaving your immune system confused as to who the real enemy is. When your healthy cells come under attack by a confused immune system, you experience what is known as an autoimmune response, something experts believe is the root cause of many diseases.

The Holes in the Whole Grain Story

Many health-conscious eaters are well aware of the drawbacks of eating refined wheat flour, white rice, pasta, and other grains that have been stripped of their natural fiber and other nutrients during the manufacturing process. While a refined grain product will (in most cases) produce a higher glycemic response than a whole grain food (because fiber delays the absorption process and mutes the blood sugar effect), a whole grain might well be considered less healthy than its stripped-down cousin for many other reasons.

By definition, whole grains are those that have all three edible components intact: the endosperm (starchy), the bran (fibrous), and the germ (oily). As we learned earlier in this chapter, many whole grains contain harmful phytates, glutens, and lectins that promote inflammation and offend your immune and digestive systems. While you also get that highly touted dose of fiber from your whole grains, this, too, can be seen as a negative. Contrary to Conventional Wisdom, excessive fiber intake (practically automatic when you emphasize whole grains) can increase appetite and interfere with healthy digestion, mineral absorption, and elimination. (I detail the drawbacks of consuming too much fiber in the *Primal Blueprint* Q&A at MarksDailyApple.com.) You can obtain optimal amounts of fiber (and eliminate the risk of overdoing it) from emphasizing vegetables and fruits à la the *Primal Blueprint*.

When you ingest a refined product, such as Wonder bread, soda, or candy, you get empty calories and a big insulin hit—but that's all you get. Furthermore, the total glycemic load is the same for a slice of white bread as it is a slice of whole wheat bread. True, the wheat bread might burn a little slower, but you eventually produce the same amount of insulin to deal with the glucose load. The only thing in whole grain's favor is a very minimal amount of protein and a few micronutrients. However, the nutritional advantages of eating whole grains are simply insignificant—especially in comparison to any vegetable, fruit, nut, seed, or organic animal food with far more nutritional value calorie for calorie (and, unlike whole grains, they also taste good!)—and free of objectionable agents.

For purposes of weight control and preventing disease, a gram of carb from a whole grain is no better than a gram from a refined grain. I'm not suggesting that you choose refined grains over whole grains; I'm suggesting you ditch *all* grains in favor of *Primal Blueprint* foods. That said, the next time you are faced with the option to eat grains, and you rationalize that whole grains are a step up from Wonder bread and soda, be sure you understand the "whole" story.

Say Good-Bye to Fatigue, Illness, and Suffering

Understanding that the long-term effects of chronic hyperinsulinemia (high insulin levels in the bloodstream) are such conditions as general systemic inflammation, obesity, diabetes, heart disease, and cancer should be enough to convince you that it is critical to pursue a more natural way of eating. Eating low-carbohydrate, grain-free meals will not only result in immediate gratification in the form of regulated energy levels, but it can help you succeed with long-term weight management and quite possibly save your life.

As a reminder, insulin is a "master hormone" that regulates the metabolism of fat and carbohydrate in your body. The single most important requirement to improve your fat metabolism and succeed with long-term weight management is to normalize and balance the general amount of insulin you produce. High insulin levels promote fat storage and disease. Moderated insulin levels (typical with *Primal Blueprint* eating) stimulate fat burning and good health. It's that simple.

> *High insulin levels promote fat storage and disease. Moderated insulin levels (typical with Primal Blueprint eating) stimulate fat burning and good health. It's that simple.*

At the risk of sounding overly dramatic or redundant on this position, we must understand that the reasonable, "evolutionary" voice challenging Conventional Wisdom about grains is being battled by billions of dollars in corporate and government propaganda pushing us to conform to dietary habits that we are not suited for, that do not nourish us, and that are downright destructive to human health. As Professor Diamond reminds us, humanity is very far down a disastrous road, and righting course is incredibly problematic.

If you are one of the fortunate folks who are less sensitive to glutens, lectins, and phytates than most, you might take exception to my wholesale damning of foods that are a dietary centerpiece across the globe. Absent acute symptoms, I'll still argue that we are all genetically "allergic" in some way to foods that are not aligned with the *Primal Blueprint*. Perhaps you can try eliminating grains for 30 or 60 days, taking note of any general improvements in your condition. I'll bet your energy will be more regulated after meals, your digestion and elimination will improve, and the frequency of minor illnesses or inflammation conditions will subside, and you will be more successful controlling your weight. There simply are no good reasons to base your diet on grains—and a lot of reasons never to eat much grains for the rest of your life.

Trans and Partially Hydrogenated Fats

> *More die in the United States of too much food than of too little.*
> —*John Kenneth Galbraith*
> *Canadian-American economist*

Perhaps the most offensive and dangerous element of the modern diet is the widespread consumption of toxic processed fats: partially hydrogenated, hydrogenated, and trans fats. *Note*: the three are not quite the same but are very similar—and all evil. Throughout the book, we use the term *partially hydrogenated*, because it is more widely used in food manufacturing and a more familiar term on food labels than plain *hydrogenated*. What's more, partially hydrogenated fats are actually more objectionable than fully hydrogenated fats.

These fats are found in almost every processed food product in the supermarket, including frozen dinners, breakfast foods, sweets, and desserts; packaged snacks (e.g., crackers, chips, and cookies); deep-fried foods; pastries and baked goods (e.g., donuts, croissants, and cupcakes); and, peanut butter, soups, and even grain products (e.g., bread, cereal, pasta, and rice mixes). A commonly cited estimate is that 40 percent of all products in a typical supermarket contain partially hydrogenated oils.

As mentioned in Chapter 3, processed fat damage cell membranes and body tissue and hamper immune function. Pr fats are not recognized as foreign by the body, so they are incorporated into cell membranes and asked to function as natural fats. Of course, they don't function normally; they just take up space usually reserved for healthy fats and wreak havoc on homeostasis.

Many scientists consider the cell membrane to be the brain of the cell (as opposed to the more common assumption that the nucleus runs the show), because the membrane receives feedback from the outside environment (e.g., ingested nutrients like glucose entering the bloodstream, the presence of a virus attacking healthy cells, or increased blood flow due to exercise stimulus) and takes consequent action (e.g., triggers the expression of certain genes or the release of certain hormones).

When you have cell membranes comprising natural molecules and you replace them with synthetic dysfunctional molecules, (trans or partially hydrogenated fats), the intricate signaling system is compromised. Plain and simple, the routine and prolonged ingestion of these toxic agents is a major contributor to the alarming increase in not only diet-related cancers but many other diseases and adverse health conditions. For example, many experts believe there is a direct connection between consuming processed fats and obesity (beyond their contribution to caloric excess), theorizing that insulin resistance could be exacerbated by dysfunctional fat molecules accumulating in cell membranes.

Research suggests that consumption of trans and partially hydrogenated fats promotes inflammation, aging, and cancer. The *New England Journal of Medicine* reviewed numerous studies and reported a strong link between processed fat consumption and heart disease (including the strong tendency for processed fats to significantly raise LDL cholesterol levels and lower HDL levels). Harvard Medical School estimates that processed fats may be responsible for as many as 100,000 premature deaths each year in the United States. The United States Academy of Sciences says that there is "no safe level" of processed fat in the American diet. The good news is that when you change your diet to eliminate these toxic agents, over time your cells will repair or replace these dysfunctional molecules with healthy ones.

Other Foods to Avoid

Grains...Oh, Did I Already Mention Them?

Wheat, corn, rice, oats, breakfast cereals, pastas, breads, pancakes, rolls, crackers, and even "natural" grains like barley, millet, rye and the like. Buoyed by Conventional Wisdom, I consumed grains with reckless abandon as a major percentage of my dietary calories for some forty years. It wasn't until I completely eliminated grains from my diet that some epiphanies occurred. Those occasional stomach cramps that I always attributed to stress? They were more likely due to wheat allergies (their severity triggered by stress, of course). That sluggish feeling I had after pasta dinners that I attributed to fatigue from a hard day training or working? It was actually my brain experiencing glucose depletion from the postmeal insulin flash flood in my bloodstream. The bloating that caused me to loosen my belt buckle after big meals that I attributed to eating too much? This may have represented a mild allergic reaction to gluten. The mild arthritis in my fingers that I first began to notice on the golf course in my forties and chalked up to the aging process? Likely due to the pro-inflammatory nature of the lingering amounts of grains still remaining in my diet. These routine tribulations that I had long considered a regrettable but inevitable part of life completely disappeared once my transition to a completely Primal diet took hold.

I've met very few people who eat a lot of grains yet who also claim to enjoy ideal weight, experience perfectly satisfactory and steady energy levels, and never feel digestive distress. At the very least, it's worth conducting a 30-day test to determine your sensitivity—and get a glimpse of your potential upside—from eliminating grains from your diet. Chances are, even if you are at a decent launching point now, you will experience a noticeable stabilization of daily energy levels, improved immune function, and a reduction in minor digestive distress from reducing or eliminating grains.

Legumes

Alfalfa, beans, peanuts, peas, lentils, and soybeans. These foods, often incorrectly classified by many consumers as vegetables, are heavily domesticated and were "recently" introduced into the human food supply, much the same as grains. While legumes offer a good source of protein, fiber, potassium, and antioxidants, they also provide significant levels of carbohydrate and increase the overall insulin load of your diet. Furthermore, legumes contain those pesky antinutrients lectins. As *Paleo Diet* author Dr. Loren Cordain explains, "Most legumes in their mature state are non-digestible and/or toxic to most mammals, when eaten in even moderate quantities."

The fact that legumes need to be altered for human consumption through cooking, soaking, or fermenting should be our best clue to avoid or strictly minimize their consumption (all truly safe fruits and vegetables can be eaten either raw or cooked). To tiptoe into a sensitive subject, the beans that are consumed liberally by many world cultures (kidney, pinto, black beans, lentils) come with the annoying by-product of flatulence, caused by the fermentation of indigestible carbohydrates.

While soy has achieved great popularity as a "healthy" alternative to meat, unfermented soy products contain compounds that may interfere with thyroid hormone production and have demonstrated an estrogenic (feminizing) effect in certain tissue. That said, soy products do have decent nutritional value and certain fermented products may be less objectionable (tempeh, natto, etc.).

I understand that many people have a strong affinity for legumes and that legumes enjoy a reputation as a healthful food category, particularly among vegetarians, who otherwise have limited protein options. It will not be a disaster if you occasionally dip your vegetables in hummus at a dinner party, fry some tempeh with vegetables for a main course, or enjoy side dishes of peas, lentils or steamed beans. However, emphasizing legumes in your diet is an inferior strategy to having vegetables, fruits, nuts and seeds, and animal foods as your primary meal and snack choices.

Processed Foods

Anything with chemical additives or that's been heavily altered from its natural state requires little discussion. Realize that you have been pummeled with marketing messages your entire life to consume branded, boxed stuff that has contributed directly and tragically to the obesity, illness, and death of those in your community. As important as knowing what our ancestors ate is knowing what they *didn't* eat: Grok never touched refined sugar, trans or partially hydrogenated fats, grains, desserts, processed foods, or anything with pesticides, herbicides, fungicides, preservatives, or other chemicals.

Sugar

I recognize how addictive sweets are. After all, our genes were programmed to appreciate those rare sweet natural sugars our ancestors discovered on occasion. Unfortunately, today we are bombarded by sugar everywhere. Sugar products greatly stress your insulin sensitivity and reinforce an addiction to both sugar and all simple carbs.

No discussion of sugar would be complete without mention of HFCS (high fructose corn syrup). Fructose has long been considered a superior sweetener to table sugar (sucrose), since it is the primary sugar in fruit and generates a lower insulin response (fructose must be converted into glucose in the liver before it can be utilized in the bloodstream, thus muting both the glucose and insulin spikes). Unfortunately, the fructose that sweetens most processed foods and beverages today – HFCS - is derived from corn, not fruit. This inexpensive and extremely sweet chemically processed agent is found in the vast majority of sodas, energy drinks, teas, juices, baked goods, desserts, and snack foods in your grocery store.

It has been well-established that HFCS is even more lipogenic (fat-promoting) than glucose, since it is readily converted into either glucose or triglycerides in the liver. Diets high in HFCS have been shown to substantially increase triglyceride levels, increase risk of obesity (particularly in kids, since their soda consumption is so excessive in relation to their body weight), and contribute to the development of serious health problems like type 2 diabetes, Metabolic Syndrome and non-alcoholic fatty liver disease (NAFLD).

Many health-conscious consumers believe that honey or agave nectar are superior alternatives. Unfortunately, honey has a similar effect on blood sugar levels as table sugar, while agave has a higher fructose concentration than even HFCS (and thus prompts undesirable triglyceride production). There's no free ride here!

Artificial sweeteners are to be strictly avoided also, not only due to the health risks of ingesting chemically processed agents, but because they trick the brain into thinking you have just consumed a very sweet food or drink. As a result, your confused hormone response system stimulates an inappropriate insulin release, and the "high-low, high-low" cycle begins. Some research suggests that your brain will seek even more "replacement" calories in reaction to being tricked with a sweet food that provides no energy. Supporting this theory are the ever-increasing obesity rates despite widespread use of non-caloric artificial sweeteners in beverages and other foods (which, absent any other variables, should predict a collective decrease in caloric intake and obesity).

All forms of natural and processed sugars and sweeteners have a deleterious effect on your insulin system and general health. The less you eat sweeteners of any kind (yes, even the supposedly healthy Stevia) the less you will crave them. Try cutting way back on sweets and sodas for even a couple of days and notice how your life improves immensely. If you can do away with them, you'll be well on your way to eliminating the addiction.

Chapter Summary

1. Avoid Poisonous Things: Make a sincere effort to reject the powerful manipulative influence of corporate advertising pushing you in the direction of poor food choices and cultural traditions favoring unhealthy meal habits. Processed carbohydrates, including sugars and products derived from grains (wheat, rice, bread, pasta, cereal, corn, etc.), should be eliminated or strictly moderated due to their effect on insulin levels and immune function and their inferior nutritional value to plants and animals.

2. Grains: While grains (and legumes) have been presented as healthy staple foods for thousands of years of civilization, our genes are maladapted to ingesting them because they elicit an high insulin response compared to the foods that have sustained human life for two million years: vegetables, fruits, nuts, seeds, and animal products. The regular pattern of stimulating high blood insulin levels from a diet of excessive grain and sugar products leads to difficulty burning stored body fat (hence, lifelong weight gain) and serious long-term health problems, including heart disease and diet-related cancers.

Grains offer minimal nutritional value in comparison to Primal foods, ironically making grains a leading cause of nutritional deficiencies across the globe. Objectionable agents in grains compromise health mildly to severely, depending on your sensitivity. The phytates in grains can inhibit the absorption of minerals. Glutens can disturb healthy immune function and promote inflammation. Lectins can inhibit healthy gastrointestinal function. Whole grains can have a worse impact on health than refined grains in many cases due to higher levels of the aforementioned agents.

3. Trans and Partially Hydrogenated Fats: These chemically altered molecules found in heavily processed foods are highly toxic to the body and are a major contributor to inflammation, accelerated aging, and many cancers. Trans and partially hydrogenated fats promote rampant oxidation and free radical damage in the body and disturb the healthy composition and function of cell membranes.

4. Other Foods: Legumes are often incorrectly considered vegetables. While offering decent nutrient value, they can stimulate a high insulin response, may also contain lectins, and are best replaced with Primal foods. Processed foods and sugar are devoid of nutrition, stimulate excessive insulin, and are the leading factor in the modern decline of human health.

CHAPTER 6

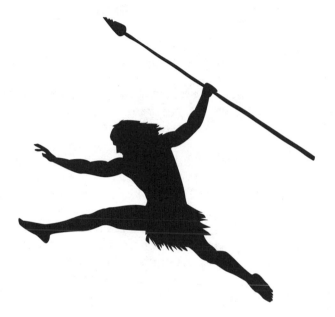

The Primal Blueprint Exercise Laws

Here's a Hint: Walk, Lift, and Sprint!

In This Chapter

I detail the rationale and benefits of the three *Primal Blueprint* exercise laws: Law #3, Move Frequently at a Slow Pace; Law #4, Lift Heavy Things; and Law #5, Sprint Once in a While. Following these laws will enable you to approximate the active lifestyle of Grok and develop what I call *Primal Fitness*. Primal Fitness represents a versatile and diverse set of abilities that allow you to tackle varied active lifestyle or athletic challenges safely and competently. In contrast, many pursue narrow, specialized forms of fitness that are minimally functional and often compromise general health (endurance athletes and bodybuilders fall in this category). Following the *Primal Blueprint* exercise laws will also help delay the aging process by preserving lean muscle mass, which correlates with enhanced organ function, a concept known as organ reserve.

I contrast the benefits of *Primal Blueprint* exercise with the many drawbacks and health risks associated with Conventional Wisdom's fitness recommendations. Moving frequently at a slow pace is superior to an exhausting routine of Chronic Cardio. These workouts often lead to sugar cravings that compromise weight-loss efforts as well as hamper immune system and endocrine function. Lifting heavy things involves brief, intense sessions (lasting 7 to 60 minutes) that promote optimal hormone secretion and prevent the catabolic effects of prolonged sessions where you leave the gym exhausted and depleted.

Few things are more Primal than running for your life once in a while! Short, intense sprints (or other maximum efforts on cardio machines, on a bicycle, or with plyometric drills) trigger optimal hormone balance, lean muscle development, accelerated fat metabolism, and incredible fitness breakthroughs. I discuss the best strategic approach for conducting workouts for each of the three *Primal Blueprint* laws, including form pointers for running and cycling and the benefits of going barefoot. Specific workout suggestions for strength training and sprinting are provided online at MarksDailyApple.com.

Those who think they have not time for bodily exercise will sooner or later have to find time for illness.

—Lord Edward Stanley
Three-time United Kingdom
Prime Minister (1799-1869)

The movements that dictated how our genes evolved were simple: squat, crawl, walk, run, jump, climb, hang, carry, throw, push, pull, and more stuff we probably don't even have names for! This primal "training program" helped Grok survive the rigors of a hostile environment, explore new territories, track and exploit new types of food, build shelters, and basically become ripped. If we simply emulated these movements with lots of low-level work and intermittent bouts of higher-intensity efforts, we'd get most, if not all, the results we seek. We would have little need for the incredible complexity of today's fitness scene—the outrageous gym equipment, obsessively detailed and regimented training programs, and fancy contraptions, such as cyclometers and GPS units. This stuff, while possessing a high "cool" factor, can also lead us astray from the benefits of having a simple, varied, and intuitive approach to exercise. By the way, most young kids will employ many of Grok's movements (squat, crawl, walk, etc.) when left outside to play in a suitable environment. If your fitness regimen consisted of simply playing with school kids at recess, you'd be in super shape!

Unfortunately, commuting, work, digital entertainment, urban living, and a to-do list a mile long hinder our opportunities to enjoy spontaneous play and get fit naturally. Furthermore, Conventional Wisdom has brainwashed us to believe that a lean, fit body comes from either lucky genes or following a regimented, physically stressful exercise routine. Accumulate endless hours and miles of vigorous aerobic exercise, hit the strength-training machines religiously for several hours a week—oh, and count every calorie that enters your mouth—and you, too, can look like a magazine cover model! It's no wonder that many well-meaning enthusiasts have become either exhausted or totally turned off to getting fit. Millions more endure with flawed approaches that leave them disappointed and discouraged when they fall far short of their ultimate peak performance potential and ideal body composition.

A healthy, fun, successful exercise program is as simple as moving around frequently at a slow pace, lifting heavy things regularly, and sprinting once in a while. At the bare minimum, you can get healthy and fit on two hours a week of walking around, one mini-strength workout a week lasting less than 10 minutes, one complete strength workout a week lasting less than 30 minutes, and a sprint session every 7 to 10 days with perhaps 10 minutes of hard work (bookended by sufficient warmup and cooldown).

Primal Fitness Pyramid

for functional, diverse athletic ability, and a lean, proportioned physique

Sprint
"All out" efforts
< 10 minutes total duration
Once every 7-10 days

Lift Heavy Things
Brief, intense sessions of
full-body functional movements.
1-3x per week for 7-60 minutes

Move Frequently at a Slow Pace
Walking, hiking, cycling, easy cardio
at 55-75% of maximum heart rate for 2-5 hours per week

Exercising according to the three *Primal Blueprint* laws will optimize gene expression and promote Primal Fitness.

- **Law #3: Move Frequently at a Slow Pace** strengthens the cardiovascular and immune systems, promotes efficient fat metabolism and gives you a strong base to handle more intense workouts.
- **Law: #4: Lift Heavy Things** stimulates lean muscle development, improves organ reserve, accelerates fat loss, and increases energy.
- **Law #5: Sprint Once in a While** stimulates the production of HGH and testosterone, which help improve overall fitness and delay the aging process - without the burnout risk of excessive prolonged workouts.

The Conventional Wisdom approach to fitness is clearly not working! Stress is excessive, weight loss goals are compromised, and many are misguided to pursue narrow fitness goals that are unhealthy.

- **Avoid Chronic Cardio** (frequent medium-to-high intensity sustained workouts)
- **Avoid Chronic Strength Training** (frequent and/or prolonged sub-maximal lifting sessions ending in exhaustion)
- **Avoid Regimented Schedules** (instead, allow for spontaneous, intuitive variation in type, difficulty and frequency of workouts)

That's less than three hours out of the 168 at our disposal each week. You don't need to invest in a gym membership or fancy equipment. You don't have to thrust yourself into uncomfortable situations, like an ear-splitting aerobics class with a bunch of hard bodies. You don't have to devote huge chunks of time to drive to the proper venue at the appointed time, change into the appropriate gear, learn complex techniques, and endure the fatigue and exhaustion that so many have suffered when following Conventional Wisdom's recommendation to adopt a consistent and unnecessarily complex exercise program. You don't even have to be consistent; in fact it's better if you are *inconsistent* with your workout routine. Heck, the old saying "All you need is a pair of shoes" doesn't even apply—you don't even need shoes! (See my sidebar "Happy Feet" later in the chapter.)

It's clear that there are many folks on the sidelines intimidated by the daunting "all or nothing" mentality of Conventional Wisdom's fitness movement. I'll assert that a 10-minute workout is not only worthwhile but can be a centerpiece of your weight-loss and peak performance efforts. Furthermore, slowing down the pace of your cardio will get your fitter, faster, and healthier, and I'll explain why in great detail in this chapter.

Pursue challenges that turn you on instead of worrying about what the magazines say is the "best" workout or the marketing hype that glorifies extreme events.

I'll also assert that you can take the *Primal Blueprint* exercise laws all the way to the top. If you are a devoted gym rat looking to get ripped, if you dream of auditioning for a swimsuit ad, or if you are competing at the elite level in team or individual sports (yep, including endurance sports), a comparatively minimal time commitment of the *Primal Blueprint* approach can produce vastly superior results (and decreased risk of injuries and burnout) to a traditional approach of frequent, prolonged strenuous workouts.

For example, an optimal exercise week for a very devoted exerciser could include a two-hour hike, another easy cardio session of one hour, two full-body strength-training sessions lasting between 30 and 60 minutes each, another lasting just ten minutes, a sprint session with about 10 total minutes of maximum effort, and a hard "play" day (e.g., a pickup soccer, basketball, or Ultimate game). This still only totals about seven hours of exercise. If you are currently racking up a dozen or more hours of Chronic Cardio each week, or hitting the gym most every day for prolonged strength-training sessions isolating specific muscle groups, I encourage you to reframe your perspective from "more is better" to "intense is better." If you find yourself bouncing off the walls with extra energy because your new Primal schedule is "too easy," make your hard workouts *even harder*…not longer or more frequent. Remember, the goal is to trigger optimal gene expression, not fill in all the blanks of your log book.

For those interested in the effects of Primal exercise on weight loss, we must start with the critical assumption that you are eating Primally (as we've discussed at length, any potential weight-management benefits of working out are significantly compromised with a high-carb, high-insulin diet). Also understand that low level cardio sessions alone do not raise your metabolic rate significantly enough to stimulate significant fat reduction. However, low level cardio workouts greatly enhance your ability to metabolize fat—both during exercise and at rest. Meanwhile, brief, intense strength and sprint sessions elevate body temperature and stimulate an increase in your metabolic rate, not only during the workout but for many hours afterward.

Put everything together and you have a formula for successful long-term weight management: eating Primally and moving frequently at a slow pace (optimizing your fat-burning system) and lifting heavy things and running really fast occasionally (stimulating lean muscle development and increasing metabolic rate). This "round-the-clock" concept of reprogramming genes (through Primal diet and exercise habits) for optimal expression is the true secret to natural, effortless, long-term weight loss and/or weight management. The story stands in sharp contrast to Conventional Wisdom's "calories in, calories out" model where you hope the 500 calories burned during your 50-minute step aerobics class will somehow lead to weight loss. (Recall that a depleted Kelly Korg inhaled double that on her quick visit to Jamba Juice!)

Primal Fitness

With a balanced regimen patterned after Grok and designed to promote optimal gene expression, you will develop what I call *Primal Fitness*. This means you have a broad range of skills and attributes (strength, power, speed, endurance) that allow you to do pretty much whatever you want (or, in Grok's case, survive the various challenges of primal life) with a substantial degree of competence and minimal risk of injury.

If the urge struck, you could complete a half-marathon or triathlon successfully on very little added specific training. On your summer vacation at the lake, you could grab a water ski rope and enjoy a few exhilarating pulls—and still be able to get dressed the next morning. During the holidays, you could hold your own with the younger generation at a family basketball, soccer, or Ultimate game. If a sudden snowstorm hit, you could fervently shovel a path through two feet of white stuff with a smile on your face—instead of a stabbing pain in your back.

Primal Fitness means you possess the unmistakable physique of an athlete, but it's hard to tell which sport! Contrast this with the Michelin Man–armed, Gumby-legged bodybuilders, the emaciated endurance athletes, or, worse yet, the droves of exercisers with flawed regimens—combined with flawed diets—who faithfully put in the hours but nevertheless fail to pare down excess body fat. While the Primal Fitness descriptions of having broad athletic ability and an impressive physique sound reasonable, they are effectively out of reach for many devoted exercisers because of poor dietary habits that hamper fat reduction efforts, poor workout choices that lead to lingering fatigue and glaring muscle imbalances, or extreme performance goals that produce one-dimensional fitness.

Speaking of one-dimensional, during my days as a marathoner, I would occasionally shock myself at how grossly unfit I was for anything besides running. I wouldn't even play ball sports or side-to-side sports, for fear of injury. If I did so much as hoist a dozen sandbags into place to prevent flooding in my driveway, I'd get a backache that would compromise my training the next day. MarksDailyApple.com has extensive commentary about how pursuing specialized athletic goals is inherently destructive to your health. We are focusing on something entirely different here with Primal Fitness. Perhaps of most interest is the improvement in body composition you can enjoy with the combination of *Primal Blueprint* eating and exercise. By breaking free from the cycle of carbs fueling stressful, carb-burning Chronic Cardio workouts, you can easily get into the ideal body fat percentage range of 8 to 15 percent for men and 12 to 20 percent for women. This is true no matter who you are or how plump your family tree is.

For women, a Primal Fitness program will tone your entire body—not just lower body fat levels but also give you some Linda Hamilton-in-*Terminator 2*-style definition in your arms, legs, and core. While many female exercisers are concerned exclusively with weight management and not inclined toward competitive athletic endeavors, you may surprise yourself—and gain some street cred with the neighborhood kids—when you display your aptitude on the soccer field or in a footrace. When you expand your horizons beyond "jogging at a strenuous pace for five songs on my iPod," your body will begin to show the effects all over, most notably by correcting the common trouble spots of excess butt, hip, thigh, and abdominal fat.

For the competitor, you can expect to branch out beyond your bread-and-butter skills to become a more complete athlete. Those who rely on bulk to hoist mucho plates or post up under the basket will become leaner and improve their power-to-weight ratio (how strong you are in relation to your body weight). This translates into more pull-ups, a higher vertical leap, and more quickness on your first step. Those who tend to be slight of frame and lacking in power will add a bit more muscle and improve pure strength and explosiveness, expanding their repertoire not only to outlast the competition but to out-power them.

Power-to-weight ratio is a critical Primal Fitness benchmark because it has a strong functional component. Bruce Lee, a skinny dude, was by reasonable definition more powerful than Hulk Hogan because of having a superior power-to-weight ratio. Bruce possessed incredible strength, power, and movement mastery, as well as the endurance to apply that strength and power to execute his martial arts moves long enough to exhaust his opponent. By contrast, a bodybuilder can flex for 30 seconds onstage and then has to recover from dehydration for a week (just kidding...sort of). An endurance runner can bust out a 20-miler and be home in time for brunch, but might walk stiff for a week after a pickup basketball game.

American Brian Clay, 2008 Olympic decathlon gold medalist, is the quintessential Primal athlete. At five feet eleven inches and 180 pounds, Clay is smaller than many of his competitors but is capable of a stunning versatility of athletic performances. While his physique is certainly impressive and looks great on the beach, it is not overly bulky nor overly defined like the vein-popping magazine cover dudes. However, Clay can sprint, run hurdles, long and high jump, pole vault, and throw such implements as shot, discus, and javelin at very respectable levels when each is considered individually. Decathletes complete five events on day one and five more on day two, a schedule requiring tremendous endurance on top of the strength, power, and speed demanded for the various events. In the SPARQ (speed, power, agility, reaction, and quickness) test commonly used to evaluate NFL prospects, Clay achieved a phenomenal score of 130. In comparison, Reggie Bush, a remarkable physical specimen who won the Heisman Trophy for USC and became a running back for the New Orleans Saints, scored a 93.

Others point to the diverse athletic demands of boxing as fodder for the greatest all-around athlete distinction. Basketball stars, such as Kobe Bryant and LeBron James, blend an incredible array of skills—speed and endurance, strength and quickness—to perform seemingly superhuman feats. (Ever try a 360-degree slam dunk—even on a low basket? It ain't easy!) CrossFit.com, a popular exercise Web site, idealizes the ultimate athlete as a combination gymnast, power lifter, and sprinter. For the last word, I'll echo the *Primal Blueprint* philosophy about dietary habits. The ideal body that you build comes down to personal preference within the broad guidelines of the *Primal Blueprint*. Do the exercises that turn you on the most—in your mind, your heart, and your genes!

Regarding the specific workout plan to reach your Primal Fitness goals, your exercise program should be like your eating style: intuitive and free of excessive struggle or regimentation. There, I have just saved you hundreds of dollars in personal training fees, magazine subscriptions, and book purchases that add unnecessary layers of complexity and confusion to your quest for fitness. Instead of following a strict schedule, you should make sure your workout decisions align with your energy and motivation levels. Sprint once in a while when you are super motivated and energized. Take a walk around the block or hike up to the radio tower on Sunday morning if you feel the urge, or stay home and read the newspaper in bed if you are dragging and just don't feel like working out.

An intuitive approach might feel uncomfortable if you are under the influence of flawed Conventional Wisdom that values consistency, gadgetry, and judging your fitness progress by the obsessive tracking of quantifiable data such as miles covered, calories burned, reps completed, time in target heart rate zone, or placing in the race. Grok knew nothing of this superficial silliness. His motivation to exercise was completely pure: to acquire his basic needs of food and shelter or to satisfy the innate human desire for adventure, competition, and play and for exploring the boundaries of the human spirit, regardless of what measured results came of it. I urge you to determine the success of your fitness program by *how much fun you are having*! Pursue challenges that turn you on instead of worrying about what the magazines say is the best workout or about the marketing hype that glorifies extreme events, such as the marathon or ironman triathlon, as the ultimate athletic accomplishment.

> *Instead of following a strict schedule, you should make sure your workout decisions align with your energy and motivation levels. Sprint once in a while when you are super motivated and energized…or stay home and read the newspaper in bed if you are dragging and you just don't feel like working out.*

Organ Reserve: The Key to Longevity

If you fall somewhere short of fitness freak on the continuum, keep in mind that the benefits of a sensible exercise program extend far beyond competitive success and looking good. The more lean muscle you maintain throughout life, the better your organs will function (up to a point of diminishing returns; e.g., a bodybuilder has heaps of excess muscle that serve little or no functional purpose and requires a lot of caloric energy to sustain). Optimal organ function correlates with maximum longevity and excellent health. Organs, like muscles, adhere to the "use it or lose it" natural law. When you hit the deck for 50 push-ups, the conscious decision to engage these muscles in a work effort calls your heart, lungs, liver, adrenals, and other organs into action. Blood chemistry changes as you burn glycogen and fat, process oxygen, and produce metabolic by-products (e.g., lactic acid) at an accelerated rate. You are asking your organs to keep up with your active lifestyle, in the process strengthening them to better withstand the demands of daily life and the natural aging process.

In contrast, when your activity diminishes, as in the classic paradigm of aging, you send signals telling your muscles and organs to atrophy. Their function decreases because they are given no reason to remain at 100 percent efficiency. An unfit person has lower bone-density, less lung capacity (the quantity of air you can exchange on each breath) and stroke volume (the amount of blood your heart pumps with each beat) than a fit person. The aging process—at least in America—should really be called the "process of physical decline largely due to inactivity."

Because all of your organs and body systems work synergistically, you are vulnerable to the often fatal effects of your weakest link. For example, an unfit accident victim or a surgery patient who loses a lot of blood and has a heart operating at only 45 percent of potential capacity will often fare differently than a fit person with superior heart function suffering the same trauma. Bones break more easily among the unfit. Pneumonia is a common cause of death among the elderly often due to the inability of their weakened lungs to help clear the germ-laden mucus effectively through coughing.

Primal Blueprint Law #3: Move Frequently at a Slow Pace

> The aging process should really be called the "process of physical decline largely due to inactivity."

While you can benefit from low-intensity aerobic exercise almost indefinitely (e.g., hiking the Pacific Crest Trail or Appalachian Trail all summer is pretty darn good for your overall health), you can obtain outstanding health and fitness benefits by engaging in a moderate amount of low-intensity aerobic movement (hike, walk briskly, cycle gently—or jog if you are really fit). Everyone should shoot for a bare minimum of two hours of low-intensity aerobic movement per week. Obviously, Grok did much more than this and ideally we would, too. I'd consider three to five hours per week an optimal range for most people with busy lives. If you can manage a single long hike on the weekend and a few short walks or cardio machine sessions during the week, you will dramatically reduce your risk of heart disease (in comparison to being sedentary), support optimal metabolism, better control your weight, and, in conjunction with the other two types of workouts, achieve Primal Fitness.

Remember that these recommendations are averages. I will occasionally go for extended periods of time (for instance, when I travel for business or pleasure) doing much less exercise than normal. I suffer no ill effects, experience no change in body composition, and invariably pick up right where I left off when I resume normal training. At other times, when the stars align and I have the free time, I'll benefit greatly from doing vastly more than the recommended average (e.g., when going on a backpacking trip or another active vacation).

My definition of *low intensity* is working at 55 to 75 percent of maximum heart rate (I will discuss in detail just what this means shortly). With this casual aerobic exercise, your heart and other energy systems work a little harder to handle the extra fuel and oxygen delivery demands, but not so much that you are overstressed. The specific biochemical signals created by this low-level aerobic activity produce numerous health and fitness benefits:

Improved Fat Metabolism: Low-level aerobic exercise trains your body to efficiently utilize free fatty acids for fuel, a benefit that is realized 24 hours a day, with a higher metabolic rate and a preference for fat over glucose (provided you follow the *Primal Blueprint* low insulin–producing diet). Low-level aerobic exercise has also been shown to help balance blood sugar levels and regulate appetite.

Improved Cardiovascular Function: Aerobic exercise increases your capillary network (blood vessels that supply the muscle cells with fuel and oxygen), muscle mitochondria, and stroke volume of your heart (more blood pumped with each beat) and also improves oxygen delivery by your lungs.

Improved Musculoskeletal System: Aerobic exercise strengthens your bones, joints, and connective tissue so you can absorb increasing stress loads without breaking down. This is critical to your ability to perform and recover from the occasional intense workouts that are a key component of the *Primal Blueprint* program.

Stronger Immune System: Aerobic exercise enhances immune function by stimulating beneficial hormone flow and building a more efficient circulatory system.

Increased Energy: Low-level aerobic exercise leaves you energized and refreshed, rather than slightly fatigued and depleted from more intense workouts.

Zoning: "In" and "Out"

My discussion about Law #3 repeatedly references the optimal low-level exercise zone of 55 to 75 percent of maximum heart rate. Fifty-five percent of maximum reflects the bare minimum exertion level to legitimately consider your effort "exercise." An unfit person can reach this walking to the mailbox. If you aren't familiar with heart rate training, you may be surprised to discover just how easy even the upper limit of 75 percent of maximum heart rate is. At this pace, you break a light to moderate sweat, can easily converse without getting short of breath, and finish feeling refreshed and energized instead of slightly fatigued and hungry, as you might after more strenuous workouts.

> *Walking is the best possible exercise. Habituate yourself to walk very far.*
> —**Thomas Jefferson**

The increasingly popular (and affordable—an excellent model can now be had for about $70) wireless heart rate monitors can help you accurately determine your exercising heart rate to ensure you stay in optimal range. While I won't say monitoring your heart rate is mandatory, this is one area where technology can play a valuable role, especially to ensure the success of your low-level workouts. Even for experienced athletes, it's quite easy to exceed 75 percent (and thereby sabotage the benefits of your session) because perceived exertion at that level is so minimal.

The most accurate way to determine your maximum heart rate (and thus calculate your numeric ranges for your 55 to 75 percent exercise zone) is with a maximum heart rate test. No fancy laboratory wires needed; you simply warm up, exercise all-out for a couple of minutes and then sprint the last 15 seconds and note your heart rate (or have someone note it for you if you become cross-eyed…or horizontal!). All kidding aside, conducting a max heart rate test requires full medical clearance from your physician and is best done under supervision from a fitness professional. The next best option is to use these formulas to generate an accurate estimate for the vast majority of the population:

- **220 – age = estimated maximum heart rate for males**
- **226 – age = estimated maximum heart rate for females**

For example, Ken Korg at 40 would have an estimated max of 180 beats per minute (220-age 40). His low-level aerobic workouts should thus be conducted in a heart rate range of 99 beats per minute (180 max × 55 percent) to 135 beats per minute (180 max × 75 percent). The "Primal Fitness Heart Rate Zones" sidebar will help you understand the perceived exertion equivalents to various heart rate zones, as well as the metabolic effects of working out at these intensities. The workout descriptions in each zone based on fitness level are purposefully vague and are meant just as a rough guideline.

Heart rate training individualizes your experience to ensure you get an optimal workout, particularly when you consider the benefits of staying under 75 percent versus the drawbacks of exceeding 75 percent routinely. This critical "individual" element—one that can make or break your entire exercise program—has long been ignored by group class instructors, Team in Training coaches, and other social or competitive workout groups. Generally speaking, asking a class or group of workout partners to keep pace together is a recipe for failure, *for all but the fittest members of the group*. Sure, the camaraderie aspect is motivating and enjoyable, but those with inferior conditioning will become overstressed. There are many ways to still achieve a beneficial group workout (i.e., with each person staying in the optimal heart rate zone) with exercisers of disparate fitness levels, including something as simple as having the faster athletes loop back time and again to retrieve slower members of the group.

The Primal Fitness Heart Rate Zones

20 to 30 percent of maximum: resting heart rate for the extremely fit athlete. Athletes have a higher stroke volume (more blood pumped per beat) than an unfit person. In my marathon days, my resting heart rate was 38 beats per minute. So much for astronaut Buzz Aldrin's quote about not doing exercise because "the heart only has so many beats and I don't want to waste any!" The finite capacity of the heart is literally true, but a fit person will save about 72,000 beats a day, 26 million over a year, and a couple of billion over a lifetime.

40 to 50 percent of maximum: resting heart rate for the unfit person. The average resting heart rate for adults is 72 beats per minute. Smokers and completely sedentary folks can have resting heart rates that exceed 100 beats per minute. (Lance Armstrong can ride in the pack at 25 mph during the Tour de France at about this rate!)

55 percent of maximum: lower limit of zone for Law #3, Move Frequently at a Slow Pace. This is the minimum heart rate for an activity to be considered a workout.
Energy source: primarily fat.
Fit person: slow to medium hike, slow bike ride, very easy to easy cardio machine.
Unfit to moderately fit person: casual walk around the block.

75 percent of maximum: upper limit of zone for Law #3, Move Frequently at a Slow Pace. This is the optimum heart rate for maximum aerobic benefits to occur with minimal stress response or glucose metabolism.
Energy source: still primarily fat.
Fit person: vigorous hilly hike, moderately hilly bike ride, medium-intensity cardio machine, medium intensity group gym workout, or slow to medium jog.
Unfit to moderately fit person: slow to medium hike, minimal to moderately hilly bike ride at slow pace, easy to medium intensity cardio machine, easy to medium intensity gym workout, or very slow jog.

80 percent of maximum: upper limit of zone for Law #3, Move Frequently at a Slow Pace—*for accomplished endurance athletes.* With an excellent aerobic base present, 80% workouts will still rely primarily on fat metabolism with minimal stress response.

85 to 90 percent of maximum: Chronic Cardio "no-man's-land." These workouts stimulate anaerobic metabolism with glucose as the preferred fuel, lactate accumulation in the bloodstream (waste product from insufficient oxygen that causes the familiar "burn" and postexercise soreness), and excessive cortisol production.
Energy source: primarily glucose
Fit person: brisk pace or hilly bike ride, vigorous cardio machine or group gym workout, brisk paced run
Unfit person: vigorous hilly hike, medium speed or moderately hilly bike ride, medium to vigorous intensity cardio machine, medium to vigorous intensity group gym workout, or slow to medium jog. Intensity too high to be considered aerobic but too low (or too lengthy in duration) to be considered an effective sprint session. Occasional sustained workouts in this "race pace" zone can produce outstanding fitness benefits; damage occurs when these cardio workouts are conducted too frequently (i.e. Chronic Cardio).

continued

90 to 100 percent of maximum: high-intensity zone for Law #5, Sprint Once in a While. This is the optimal zone for occasional brief, all-out efforts. These workouts build muscle, support enhanced organ function, accelerate metabolism, and delay aging via the "use it or lose it" principle.

Energy source: glucose (for sprints over 30 seconds), lactate (8-30 seconds), or Adenosine triphosphate ("ATP"; for efforts under 8 seconds). Cortisol is released briefly in line with the genetic fight-or-flight response.

A Case Against Cardio

> *Chronic Cardio—a program I followed for nearly 20 years as a marathoner and later as an ironman triathlete—is bad for your health, period.*

In contrast to the comprehensive benefits of a frequent, comfortably paced exercise, getting more serious about working out can really mess you up if you have a flawed approach. Chronic Cardio at heart rates above 75 percent and up to 95 percent of maximum places excessive stress on your body to which you are not genetically adapted. I'd estimate that the vast majority of folks you see working out on cardio machines, jogging through the neighborhood, or keeping pace in the group class are exceeding 75 percent (often by a wide margin) for the duration of nearly every session.

While an aerobic workout at the typical intensity of 75 to 95 percent might not feel terribly difficult at the time, a sustained pattern of Chronic Cardio can lead to numerous problems with metabolism, stress management, immune function, and general health. As exercise intensity increases, your preferred fuel choice shifts from primarily fat at intensities below 75 percent (fat burns well in the presence of oxygen, and supplies are abundant—even in the skinniest marathoners!) to an ever-increasing percentage of glucose (quicker and easier to burn when oxygen is lacking due to your quickening pace).

A routine of Chronic Cardio requires large amounts of dietary carbohydrates each day to support it. While the risks of excess fat storage and hyperinsulinemia (overproduction of insulin) are moderated somewhat by a heavy exercise schedule, they are still significant because of your altered dietary habits throughout the day. When muscles are depleted of glycogen (remember, stored glycogen is converted back into glucose for exercise fuel), your brain sends a powerful signal to replenish with quick-energy carbohydrate foods. Our brains have a tendency to tell us to overcompensate by eating a little too much. This is a genetically programmed survival adaptation against starvation risk, handed down to us from Grok. If you are looking to reduce body fat primarily through vigorous cardiovascular exercise (as Conventional Wisdom promises), you are quite likely to fail unless you slow down your pace and alter your diet to limit your carb intake.

Besides the weight-loss challenges, Chronic Cardio increases the production of cortisol (in all but the most genetically gifted endurance athletes), which breaks down muscle tissue and suppresses production of key anabolic hormones, such as testosterone and human growth hormone. This hormonal imbalance caused by overexercising contributes to fatigue, burnout, immune suppression, loss of bone density, and undesirable changes in fat metabolism. Furthermore, the stress of Chronic Cardio increases systemic inflammation (a strong contributing factor to heart disease, cancer, and nearly all other health problems) and increases oxidative damage (via free radical production) by a factor of 10 to 20 times normal. This can lead to acceleration of the aging process. It's ironic that many in their 40s and 50s start engaging in marathon or triathlon training in hopes of improving health and delaying the aging process, when, quite often, it has the exact opposite effect.

Why Run When You Can Grok?

For those heavily indoctrinated into the Conventional Wisdom that Chronic Cardio is the path to health, fitness, and weight control, consider again the premise of the *Primal Blueprint*. Because Grok was a lean, strong, extremely active dude, he probably was capable of running long distances, similar to today's gung-ho endurance athletes, but he most likely very rarely decided to do so. When the concept of organized hunting came along, it appears that Grok relied more on superior tracking ability (using his highly evolved brain) and walking or slow jogging (using his superior fat-burning system), rather than literally chasing down his prey. In fact, squandering valuable energy reserves (and increasing glucose metabolism by a factor of 10) by running hard for long periods of time would have hastened his demise. Imagine Grok chasing some game animal all-out for a few hours and—oops—not succeeding in killing it. He's spent an incredible amount of energy yet now has no food to replace that energy. He has suddenly become some other animal's prey because he is physically exhausted.

A 2007 Taiwanese study published in the *British Journal of Sports Medicine* revealed that a single intense *sustained* workout (working at 85 percent of maximum effort for at least 30 minutes) disrupted immune system function, destroyed some white blood cells, and triggered whole body inflammation for up to 72 hours. In contrast, there are literally hundreds of scientific studies confirming the benefits of conducting occasional short-duration, intense workouts (such as interval workouts—spacing work efforts by a particular rest interval). Intervals and sprints quickly and time-efficiently improve key performance factors including VO2 Max (how efficiently you process oxygen during peak exercise effort), competitive performance, and body composition.

I cannot emphasize strongly enough the importance of slowing down the pace of your cardio workouts to improve your health and fitness. (Note that I'm speaking to the vast numbers of fitness enthusiasts in the gyms and on the roads who generally take their pace to "slightly uncomfortable" in the name of pursuing Conventional Wisdom's definition of "getting a workout.") If you already like to take your time and smell the flowers on your walks, hikes, and bike rides, congratulations! Just get ready to add a few sprint workouts into the mix. That's where huge benefits will accrue for little investment.

> "You have to stay in shape. My grandmother, she started walking five miles a day when she was 60. She's 97 today and we don't know where the hell she is.
> —**Ellen DeGeneres**"

As I will detail shortly, slowing down (and adding workouts from Laws #4 and #5) will not only improve health but will lead to outstanding fitness breakthroughs.

I am fully aware of the many loud and passionate voices extolling the psychological and lifestyle virtues of devoted endurance training and agree that pushing and challenging your body with inspiring competitive goals supports mental, emotional, and also physical health (albeit with the significant caveats already discussed). An exercise physiologist friend of mine countered my "case against cardio" position recently by reminding me that Hawaii Ironman finishers are vastly healthier than the average population. While true, let us not forget, in the words of Jay Leno, the "average" we are dealing with: "Today there are more overweight people in America than average-weight people. So overweight people are now average. Which means you've met your New Year's resolution."

Furthermore, I'll assert that an old has-been like myself (goals: eat Primally, with no processed carbs; visit the gym several days a week, for sessions of widely varied difficulty; and hang with teenagers for two hours of Ultimate on weekends) possesses far superior health and Primal Fitness to the lean, ripped (but often emaciated), super "fit" physical specimens that strut in their Speedos down the main drag of Kailua-Kona, Hawaii, every October during Ironman week. Yes, they can all drop me like a shot in a long-distance swim, cycling, or running race (it mighta been a different story back in the day), but their endurance superiority comes at great cost. Collectively, they tend to suffer from recurring fatigue and adrenal burnout, frequent overuse injuries, too-common minor illnesses from suppressed immune function (I get a cold maybe once every five years; a fair number of ironman triathletes probably get five every year), and, last but certainly not least, high overall life stress factor scores—something often touted as the number one heart attack risk factor.

Having spent many years immersed in the type A community of driven fitness enthusiasts and competitive endurance athletes, I am aware that many heads will nod in agreement with my message—and then turn around and plug along with their familiar exhausting training regimens. If serious endurance exercise is a centerpiece of your life, I don't wish to deprive you of your passion. That's right, go ahead and hammer that three-hour group ride or that 15-mile trail run with the big boys or big girls *once in a while*. If you follow my plan, you'll certainly be fit enough to do it occasionally. Just don't do it every weekend, or even every other weekend. Going long and hard once in a while (the specifics are quantified by your fitness level) produces far superior fitness benefits and eliminates the risk factors of repeating highly stressful workouts too frequently.

If the New York City Marathon or Hawaii Ironman is calling your name, enjoy the process as a twice-in-a-lifetime experience. That's right—the first one is to say you finished, and the second one is to improve your previous time! The droves of folks with framed race numbers commemorating a dozen consecutive finishes of their signature event have in many respects achieved their superficial prizes at the expense of their health. Doing a marathon or an ironman triathlon won't kill you, but continuing to follow a stressful, regimented training program for the six months afterward—or doing dozens of extreme events over the years—will likely create significant to extreme stress-related damage in your body. Don't be afraid to rest completely for three days after your big weekend hammer session, take an entire calendar year away from your competitive schedule, or simply step away from the cultural pressure to prove your athletic worth with measured results—in favor of more esoteric fitness goals. This is what Primal Fitness is all about.

> *If you start to feel good during a marathon, don't worry, that will pass.*
> —**Don Kardong,** *U.S. Olympic marathoner and author*

Chronic Cardio Drawbacks - Pocket Reference

A consistent schedule of frequent medium-to-high–intensity (75% of maximum or higher) sustained workouts can overstress the body and lead to these negative consequences:

Hormones: Chronic Cardio raises cortisol and lowers testosterone and growth hormone. This hormonal imbalance compromises optimal fat burning, muscle development, energy levels, and sex drive. Burnout is a common consequence of pursuing the "runner's high" too frequently.

Injuries: Recurring muscle fatigue, repetitive impact, restrictive footwear, and inflammation arise from excessive catabolic hormones released in response to Chronic Cardio. This traumatizes joints and connective tissue, increasing risk of injury.

Metabolism: Burning more sugar (at above 75 percent of maximum heart rate) drives eating more sugar drives producing more insulin drives storing more fat.

Stress: Excessive oxidation and triggering of the fight-or-flight response compromise the immune system and accelerate aging and disease risk.

Use It or Lose It: Chronic Cardio compromises development of power, speed, strength, and lean mass and leads to muscle imbalances and inflexibility. Total fitness is sacrificed in favor of narrow, minimally functional aerobic endurance.

"But This Feels Too Easy!"

Granted, those with competitive endurance goals may not be satisfied to putter along exclusively at a slow pace and think they can take down the competition with that approach. The most direct performance benefits occur from the intense workouts that approximate the challenge of your competitive goals. However, whether you are a casual fitness enthusiast or a professional athlete, you must establish a strong base of low-level aerobic conditioning before you can introduce more stressful, higher-intensity workouts. With a strong aerobic conditioning base in place, you then have the ability to absorb and benefit from the *occasional* intense workouts that lead directly to competitive success—if you've chosen such goals. The tertiary benefits of low-level work (better balance, strong postural muscles, increased mitochondria development and capillary profusion, and strengthening of bones, tendons, and ligaments to prevent injury) might not be as readily apparent as the direct competitive application of beating your personal record at a time trial, but one cannot happen without the other.

This concept of base first, then intensity has been proven successful by the training regimens of the world's greatest endurance athletes of the last 50 years, beginning with the pioneering work of New Zealand running coach Arthur Lydiard. Lydiard's prize students, including 1960 and 1964 Olympic track gold medalist Peter Snell (today one of the world's leading exercise physiologists, in Dallas, Texas), showed that long-duration, low-intensity training, coupled with intense interval training and adequate rest (rest was another far-out concept for the '60s), could lead directly to Olympic gold medals and world records at races as short as 800 meters (which lasts less than two minutes).

When I completed my career as an elite marathoner and triathlete and transitioned into a career as a personal trainer, my training regimen shifted dramatically. I was still out there moving for several hours a day, but I went from banging my brains out with super fit training partners to dawdling along with a succession of clients on my daily calendar. Unlike many of today's fitness trainers who stand there and count reps, I got outside with my unfit to moderately fit clients and did their workouts with them. Bike rides that I previously hammered at 20+ mph for hours were now conducted at 13 mph (it seemed like any slower and we'd tip over!). The long, hard trail runs of my marathon days were replaced with easy jogs where my heart rate barely exceeded 100 beats per minute (only 50 percent of my max). With a young family and a career filling my days, I rarely had time to do my own specific workouts. I made the most of these opportunities by conducting extremely intense interval sessions once or twice a week—on cardio equipment or with a few quick laps around the track. Usually these sessions lasted around 20 minutes—until my next client came strolling in!

When I jumped into the occasional long or ultra-distance endurance race, the results were shocking to me. My "by chance" regimen of very, very slow workouts coupled with occasional very short, intense workouts allowed me to place among the top competitors in the world in my age group and very close to the standards set by top professionals of that era! Indeed, the *Primal Blueprint* parameters literally took shape in my mind as I blew by my rivals (who were putting in big Chronic Cardio miles, just like I used to) at races despite what most experts and prevailing Conventional Wisdom would deem ridiculously inadequate preparation.

Mike Pigg and Mark Allen, world champion professional triathletes who dominated the sport in the late '80s and early '90s, both claimed their careers were elevated to the next level—and extended by several years—when they moderated their training pace to stay below an individually determined maximum *aerobic* heart rate with great discipline. Guided by applied kinesiologist and endurance training pioneer Dr. Phil Maffetone, they were able to improve their aerobic conditioning in each discipline (swimming, biking, and running) by training at a sensible, comfortable pace that represented about 80 percent of their maximum heart rate. (I advocate an upper limit of 75 percent for all but the most highly trained endurance athletes.)

By limiting the majority of their efforts to the aerobic zone, they could exercise for long hours without breaking down or succumbing to the fatigue that is so common among elite triathletes. At their peak, Pigg or Allen could maintain a running speed of better than six minutes per mile for a half-hour or cycle at 25 mph for hours on end with a predominantly aerobic, fat-burning metabolism. In contrast, a lesser-trained individual training side by side would quickly become depleted and exhausted due to the *relatively* intense pace of the session. When it came time to race, Pigg and Allen could dispose of the competition because their aerobic efficiency allowed them to maintain an unmatched all-out race pace. It follows that if running a six-minute mile is "easy" for a superior endurance athlete, he or she has more room to escalate pace until reaching maximum effort than an athlete who struggles at a pace of six-minutes per mile.

Primal Blueprint Law #4: Lift Heavy Things

The popular Conventional Wisdom concept of following a strength-training routine that involves repeating the same workout several days a week is flawed. Your body thrives on intuitive, spontaneous, and fluctuating workout habits—not ego-driven regimentation organized around an arbitrary time period of seven days that has no special relevance to your fitness progress. In asking, "What would Grok do?" (that is, what is best for your genes), you'll realize that intermittent workouts that continually vary in type and intensity level will bring the best results. Some researchers refer to this as shocking or surprising the muscles, so they don't get used to doing the same things over and over. Others have called it muscle confusion. Remember, it's the signals created when your muscles are challenged beyond what they are used to that prompt genes to make those muscles stronger. Get creative and integrate the "lift heavy things" law into daily life, aside from your formal sessions. For example, come fall, try raking your leaves vigorously—it's an unsurpassed shoulder, core, and abs session, and it will get your yard clean to boot!

Regarding the particulars of how to balance upper- and lower-body efforts, "push and pull" workout groupings, light weight with high reps or heavy weight with low reps: *it doesn't matter that much!* This is not rocket science. The idea is to challenge your body on a regular basis with brief, intense resistance workouts of any kind that you desire—in a fancy gym; in your garage with a few basic weights or stretch cords; using creative "Primal" implements like kettlebells, slosh tubes, and sandbags; or in a hotel room with nothing more than a chair and some floor space. (Check out MarksDailyApple.com for hundreds of interesting and challenging resistance workout ideas.)

Personally, I'm a devoted gym rat, but my faithful appearance at the local gym four or five days a week has a heavy social element. Some days I'll be in there for an hour and 15 minutes, shooting the breeze, preening, and trash-talking with my pals—interspersed with some embarrassingly low-effort exercises where I barely sweat. Other days, when I'm feeling fired up, I'll push it hard for 25 minutes of maximum effort sets with short rest. After these workouts, I have trouble slipping my sweatshirt on and sticking my key in the ignition to drive home, but I am exhilarated and recovery is quick. These hard days are few and far between, but they make a big difference. Overall, it honestly does not require that much time to maintain excellent all-around functional muscle strength and an impressive physique. It's simply a matter of establishing a reasonable baseline commitment of regular workouts, with the occasional super effort that stimulates a fitness breakthrough.

A high-intensity, short-duration workout will stimulate the release of adaptive hormones—particularly testosterone and human growth hormone—that get you lean, energetic, and youthful. Work hard and complete your session in less than an hour, even (or especially) if you are an experienced lifter. That's right—go against the Conventional Wisdom of long, drawn-out workouts of the same old sets with the same weight and repetitions. A 30 to 45-minute session is actually plenty for most people.

As you improve your fitness, keep your focus on increasing intensity (more resistance, shorter rest periods, and tougher exercises) rather than extending the duration of your workouts. Repeated workouts that extend beyond an hour (I've seen some hardcore lifters routinely go for two hours or more!), where you lift moderate weights to failure again and again, can stimulate the excessive release of destructive (also called catabolic) hormones like cortisol that lead to fatigue, breakdown, and the metabolic problems already discussed at length. Again, think about Grok: he moved some big rocks, which gave his body a shock. But when the quick job was done, he could relax and have fun, basking in the sun.

Always align the difficulty of your sessions with your energy level, and don't push yourself beyond what you are motivated and inspired to do. You will notice after your first couple of sets whether your performance is worse or better than normal. If you are feeling—and performing—significantly worse than normal, consider skipping or sharply curtailing the workout. On the other hand, if you feel energized and ready to ramp it up a notch, go for it!; push yourself beyond your typical routine to achieve a fitness breakthrough.

I should point out that if you are new to strength training, you might get too tired to actually complete even 25 minutes of high-intensity effort. Instead, you can work up to it by either compressing your workout time further or taking longer rest intervals between your hard efforts. Even a workout as short as seven minutes can produce outstanding benefits. I know of an ex-collegiate gymnast, still in competitive shape with an amazingly cut physique, who claims only to work out for seven minutes a few times a week, with no resistance equipment, in a tiny floor space in his living room.

> *Always align the difficulty of your sessions with your energy level, and don't push yourself beyond what you are motivated and inspired to do. On the other hand, if you feel energized and ready to ramp it up a notch, go for it!*

Impossible? Get a load of his routine: three sets of 10 handstand push-ups, followed by three sets of 20-clap push-ups and 20 one-armed push-ups (for each arm), transitioning immediately into 3 sets of 10 leg flairs, then five handstand push-ups, followed by….well, you get the picture! His many years of intense daily training have given him a fitness base to accomplish a phenomenal amount of work—and maintain exceptional fitness—with a minimal time commitment. Oh, and he walks a lot and eats right, too!

If you are spent after a 10-minute workout, congratulations! You've pushed yourself to the max and elicited a desirable fitness response in your body. By the way, those seemingly inconsequential hikes and walks will actually contribute substantially to your ability to hit it hard in the gym, thanks to the well-established connection between the cardiorespiratory and musculoskeletal benefits of comfortable aerobic exercise and your ability to perform at peak intensity (as illustrated with the Peter Snell example of his heavy overdistance training preparing him for intense track competitions).

I suggest you shoot for an average bare minimum of one comprehensive 25-minute session and an abbreviated seven-minute session per week. Even for devoted strength trainers, I believe an optimum schedule would be to average a couple of half-hour sessions and an abbreviated intense session of under 10 minutes per week. If you are a "more is better" gym rat, I'll argue in favor of increasing the intensity of these three sessions rather than adding additional workouts.

Feel free to experiment with the types of exercises that are most fun for you and with a routine that fits most conveniently and comfortably into your daily lifestyle. Be sure to alter your routine constantly, not only to account for your improved fitness level but to enjoy the psychological and physical benefits of evolving your fitness goals and interests. The Lift Heavy Things Workout Suggestions appendix at MarksDailyApple.com offers an ever-expanding list of workouts, featuring not only descriptions but photos and videos.

Realize that this concept of sporadic, intuitive exercise means you have permission to take—and will, in fact, greatly benefit from—vacation time. The more extreme your goals and training regimen are, the more effort required to balance your overall stress levels on both a micro (daily or weekly) and macro (annual) scale. As I discovered for myself (the hard way), trusting the body's need for balance and intermittent stress can lead to results that are superior—in weight loss or peak competitive performance—compared to the die-hard trainaholics who never miss a workout and never get sufficient rest.

> *Trusting your need for balance and intermittent stress can lead to superior results compared to the die-hard trainaholics who never miss a workout*

To make sure you are adhering to the Primal philosophy, I suggest paying close attention to your energy level and even your emotional state in the hours after a strength workout. After even my toughest sessions, I feel alert, energized, and positive—basically a natural buzz—for hours afterward. My muscles, while certainly not eager to repeat the workout in the immediate future, feel pleasantly relaxed, loose, and warm. In contrast, if your muscles feel stiff and sore after strength sessions, or you feel like taking a nap, raiding the fridge, or snapping at your loved ones, I recommend conducting fewer, shorter, more intense—more Primal—workouts. If you can only maintain high-intensity effort for seven minutes, then end your workout there and work up to more sets in the future.

In regard to body composition, remember your strength training efforts fall into the fine-tuning 20 percent category, while 80 percent of your success is determined by how you eat. This is a sobering stat if you are working hard at the gym, eating poorly, and praying for results. In this scenario, all that hard work in the gym will contribute mostly to a higher grocery bill (okay, and more fleeting pleasure from unrestricted caloric intake), but you'll be wearing the same size clothing on your trips to the market.

Strength Workout Strategy

The particulars of your strength-training routine are less important than your strategic approach (intermittent, fluctuating, intuitive, and balancing effort with energy levels). Remember that you are striving to achieve a high power-to-weight ratio and balanced, functional, total-body strength. You want to be lean, well muscled, and fit enough to perform reasonably well at any physical challenge that comes along, Consequently, your routine should be focused on exercises that engage a variety of muscles with sweeping, real-life movements (squats, pull-ups, push-ups, etc.) instead of a series of isolated body part exercises (this includes those ever-popular, narrow-range-of-motion abs machines!).

This approach is a simpler and safer alternative to popular routines designed to pack on more muscle than your body is naturally suited for or to produce disproportionate muscles ("Develop huge guns in six weeks!") in the interest of vanity over functionality. For example, to work my calf muscles in a functional manner, I like to run on an inclined treadmill for five to seven minutes in stocking feet, without letting my heels touch the ground. This offers a real-life functional test for my calves and works the small muscles, tendons, ligaments, and connective tissue in my lower extremities that are otherwise artificially protected and unchallenged when wearing high-tech running shoes. I gradually incline the treadmill to reach from two to five degrees and then steadily increase the speed. I try to make sure my heels don't bear any significant weight or provide propulsion.

Keep in mind that I just made this workout up one day, and you may or may not like it. However, I think it offers an important counter to the time spent working out and walking around in overly cushioned and arch-supported running shoes. Contrast the broad benefits of this exercise with something like donkey calf-raises. This narrow-range-of-motion exercise (sit with a weighted bar across your knees and lift your toes off the ground repeatedly) has minimal functional benefit; besides, I'll stack my calves up against any bodybuilder's!

Grok probably never warmed up for his "workouts," and I'm just not a big fan of using cardio to warm up extensively. (Sorry about that, Conventional Wisdom. I know I keep pissing you off!) That said, because you will usually be starting your workout "cold" (maybe you just left an office where you were sitting all day or you just got out of bed), it does make sense to get a little blood flowing into your muscles before hitting the intense stuff. Therefore, your strength sessions should generally start with a brief three- to five-minute warm-up using light weights or calisthenics specific to the muscle groups you'll be working that day. A few sets of easy push-ups and some jumping jacks might be sufficient.

Because Primal Fitness training is intended to recruit as many muscle fibers as possible and to build functional strength rather than sheer bulk, I wouldn't worry about following some predetermined and deliberate effort-recovery cycle. Instead, try to be slightly explosive with most of your movements. By that I mean you should apply a controlled dynamic force to each repetition such that you complete it at a speed that allows you to maintain form and a reasonable pace for the number of reps you intend to complete. Do that and, believe me, you'll slow down naturally on that final rep or two! This method will fully load the muscle and trigger the biochemical signal to grow stronger by recruiting new fibers.

While there are disparate schools of thought on the best strength-training techniques, I make this general suggestion here to align with the concept of optimal gene expression and prevention of the all-too-common "Chronic Strength Training" burnout syndrome. If you have specialized fitness goals or an expert personal trainer suggesting a different technique, I wouldn't be overly concerned. I'll default here to the big picture and assert that short, intense workouts are the key to Primal Fitness success.

Much has been written about breathing while lifting weights, some of it relevant (to protect your back from damage) and some of it conjecture. When you apply force, you should generally be either exhaling or holding your breath. This will form a sealed air space behind in the transverse abdominal muscles of your lower core that protect your lumbar spine. While some caution against holding your breath, there is no scientific support to affirm this is harmful. In fact, I find I can bang out two or three reps in a row more effectively when holding my breath and then can catch my breath during a recovery phase.

There are many excellent resources—from certified personal trainers, magazine articles, books, video Web sites like CrossFit.com, articles on MarksDailyApple.com, and even your imagination (observing certain obvious safety rules, such as spine stability)—to help you create an ideal total-body routine for your needs. The possibilities are nearly limitless if you observe the strategic rules of *Primal Blueprint*–style training. The Lift Heavy Things Workout Suggestions appendix at MarksDailyApple.com details a comprehensive session in the gym, a quick workout using only your body weight for resistance, and also a challenging "Grok" session you can do anywhere—all you need is a chair or a bench.

Stretching: If You Don't Know Squat, Try Hangin' with Grok

"What would Grok do?" It's hard to imagine Grok stretching much beyond a yawning feline-style spine elongation upon awakening, hanging lazily off a branch, or engaging in the timeless, all-purpose stretch of squatting down to the ground. Furthermore, recent research (visit the *Primal Blueprint* Resources appendix at MarksDailyApple.com to find relevant materials) seems to refute the benefits of conducting a traditional static stretching routine before exercising. It's now believed the central nervous system may be disturbed by such activity, resulting in what scientists call a neuromuscular inhibitory response. In plain-speak, your muscles might actually get weaker (by up to 30 percent) for up to 30 minutes after an inappropriate stretching session (poor technique and/or bad timing—like stretching "cold" muscles before exercise), and stretching might contribute to more injuries than it prevents.

If you follow a Chronic Cardio or Chronic Strength Training program that causes recurring muscle fatigue and tightness, you will probably feel an inclination to stretch frequently before and after workouts, even while sitting at your desk. I have a better idea: *back off!* If you are exercising according to the *Primal Blueprint*, your muscles should feel supple and strong nearly all of the time. Sure, occasionally you will place extreme challenges on your body (yep, that's a good thing) and become sore and stiff. This is nature's way of telling you you're overdoing it. By the way, the old runner's adage that stretching and light exercise the day after a race or tough workout will "flush the blood" and speed the healing of stiff, sore muscles is questionable. There is strong support for the idea that muscle tissue repair is best accomplished through inactivity, extra rest and sleep, good nutrition, and brief, repeated exposure to cold water (particularly immediately after strenuous exercise; read more details about cold water therapy in the Chapter 2 Endnotes).

As mentioned previously, the best way to prepare your body for any workout is with some brief, low-intensity exercise to help shift blood into your extremities from the organs in your working muscles. Even for something like all-out sprints, a brief low-intensity cardio warm-up of a few minutes, followed by some long, easy strides at 75 percent effort will prime you for your maximum efforts (as detailed in the Sprint Work-

continued

out Suggestions appendix at MarksDailyApple.com). It's clear that Grok didn't have time to warm up when he had to run for his life, and yet I don't think he sat out too many primal battles with muscle pulls.

On the other hand, some benefit may be obtained with a few very brief basic stretches after workouts or to otherwise help transition between active and inactive states. My two favorite stretches are (poise your notepad): the *Grok Hang* and the *Grok Squat*. The Grok Hang offers a safe, full-body stretch that leaves you feeling exhilarated every time. It's also an effective strengthening exercise—as Primal as they come. It's as simple as grabbing hold of a bar or tree branch (with overhand grip) and hanging for as long as you can support yourself.

The Grok Squat involves placing your feet approximately shoulder-width apart, bending your knees with a straight or slightly arched back and lowering your torso all the way down until your butt is nearly touching the ground. Your torso is between your knees, and arms are extended in front of you. This natural movement provides a safe, gentle, efficient stretch for your feet, calves, Achilles, hamstrings, quadriceps, buttocks, lower and upper back, and shoulders. For thousands of years people have squatted as a natural "sitting" position in the absence of chairs (to say nothing of Barcaloungers!). For Grok—and millions of people today in the undeveloped world—squatting is the default position for resting, socializing, eating meals, and even eliminating.

Try a Grok Squat for 20 seconds and notice what a comprehensive effect you get from such a basic movement. If it's first thing in the morning or when you're a little stiff from some intense activity or other stressor (e.g., jet or car travel), simply lowering into the position provides a good stretch. When I'm feeling warm and loose, I'll gently rock back and forth and/or extend my arms out farther to obtain a deeper stretch. One caution: if you haven't done this for a while, are overweight, or have joint issues, you can begin to ease into this stretch (and keep yourself from going too low or falling over) by holding on to a post or another stationary object.

Note: I know there are many passionate enthusiasts of yoga, Pilates, and other well-designed workouts that emphasize a balance of strengthening and stretching, and I don't wish to critique these here. I'm simply saying that extensive stretching before—or even after—workouts may not provide much benefit and could even be counterproductive. If you have injuries, joint issues, or a rehab protocol designed by a medical professional, you will certainly want to override these general suggestions to address your particular needs in conjunction with your workouts. Even with stretches as simple as Grok's, be wary of any discomfort, skip or adapt the movements accordingly, and ease into and out of stretching positions.

> *My own prescription for health is less paperwork and more running barefoot through the grass.*
> —**Leslie Grimutter**

Primal Blueprint Law #5: Sprint Once in a While

Obviously, Grok's life featured the occasional brief all-out sprint, not for sport but rather to kill or avoid being killed. These bursts of speed were enhanced by the immediate flooding of the bloodstream with fight-or-flight adrenaline-like chemicals. When Grok survived a run to safety from a charging bear unhurt, the resulting biochemical signals prompted a cascade of positive neuroendocrine, hormonal, and gene expression events, the net effect of which was to build stronger, more powerful muscles and an ability to go a little faster the next time.

Modern research confirms the *Primal Blueprint* premise: the occasional series of short, intense bursts can have a more profound impact on overall fitness—and especially weight loss—than a medium-paced jog lasting several times as long. This is because of increases in metabolic rate and appetite suppression (both due to elevated body temperature in the hours after workouts), development of more calorie-burning lean muscle tissue, and improved insulin sensitivity (working muscles learn not only to burn glucose efficiently but also to absorb glucose—transported by insulin—after workouts).

The profound benefits of sprint workouts really hit home for me back in the early 1990s, when my personal training clients and I would share the Santa Monica College running track with some of the world's greatest Olympic sprinters. These physical specimens were a sight to behold. Obviously, they were blessed with remarkable genetic gifts, but it was also clear they were training and living in a manner that brought out the best of their genetic potential. In getting to know some of these athletes and their coaches, it became apparent how remarkably different their training methods were to the prevailing templates of the fitness and nutrition industry.

These Olympians were not out there all day circling the track to exhaustion: their workouts consisted of minimal amounts of very slow jogging, casual stretching (between competition-specific drills), unhurried efforts to fuss with their equipment (e.g., starting blocks or resistance tools), and, finally, a brief series of explosive efforts—lasting seconds, not hours. Their banter during these sessions was light; they were always smiling, laughing, joking, and clowning around in between the intense focus of their main sprint sets. They also spent some serious time in the gym working very hard with the weights, but these track and gym sessions were interspersed with frequent easy or rest days, including occasionally sleeping in until double figures and taking daily naps. Their training diets were not laden with tofu, frozen yogurt, and power bars; they were more likely to feast on chicken and ribs after a workout. Carl Lewis, considered by many to be the greatest Olympic athlete of all time, with nine sprint and long jump gold medals to his credit, reportedly trained only an hour per day at his peak. And yet sprinters are among the leanest, most well-muscled people on the planet.

Introducing sprinting into your exercise routine is not as easy as lacing up a pair of shoes and heading out the door to go jogging. Sprinting is a physically stressful activity that requires a significant fitness base, muscle strength, and flexibility. You'll want to start the first few sessions gently, gradually increasing the speed and intensity of your sprints over time. You also need significant recovery time after sprint workouts. I recommend conducting a sprint workout approximately once every seven to ten days, and only when you have high energy and motivation levels. That's right, even as little as two to three sprint sessions *per month* can produce outstanding fitness benefits and break you out of Chronic Cardio ruts that may have lasted years. You can choose running, cycling, or any other exercise where you are comfortable producing a series of brief, all-out efforts. Running is the best but comes with a higher risk of injury if you are out of practice (i.e., you haven't chased down any animals or scored any touchdowns in the last few decades).

To reduce injury risk, beginners are advised to choose exercises that are low or no impact. Sprinting up a steep hill (and walking down to commence repeat efforts) offers a lower-impact option than flat running, while stationary cycling presents a no-impact option. I don't recommend outdoor cycle sprints (except for expert riders) due to the danger factor. You can also choose cardio machines (VersaClimber, elliptical, StairMaster, etc.), but I prefer running because the weight-bearing nature (and thus the increased degree of difficulty) of the activity offers maximum benefits, such as improved bone density and greater stimulation for muscle gain (or toning for females) and fat loss. If you are significantly overweight as you start this program and/or your knees aren't strong enough, cycling or using an elliptical machine might be the best way to start.

Novices can start with three to four sprints, short of full speed, with long rest periods in between efforts. You will likely experience some muscle soreness in the days after these efforts, but your body will quickly adapt to your new workout routine. You can then build up to a workout that includes six to eight all-out sprints—or even a few more as you become stronger. You should never push your body through an intense workout if you have any symptoms of fatigue, soreness, compromised immune system, or another malaise. As discussed with strength training, your sprint sessions should be intuitive, intermittent, and spontaneous—just as they were in primal life for Grok. The *occasional* sprint workout will elicit the more desirable gene expression effects than performing these workouts come heck or high water just because it's Tuesday.

One final note: this isn't about speed—it's about effort. It doesn't matter if you aren't covering ground quickly, as long as you exert yourself to the point of going all-out for that brief interval. Age is not an issue here. Whether you are 20 or 75, you can find a form of sprint workout that fits your style. For some people, it's simply walking fast up a steeply inclined treadmill for 30 seconds.

Clouseau-Robics and Doberman Intervals

While I've discussed the fight-or-flight response in the negative context of excessive aerobic exercise or hectic modern life, you should realize that eliciting a stress response is desirable with your sprint workouts. The difference here is that the brief, intense stress is exactly what your genes crave to build fitness and strength and to optimize metabolic function.

Imagine if every so often someone rudely interrupted your jog around the track by turning a vicious Doberman loose! I guess now you'd run as fast as possible, right? Or, like Inspector Clouseau, say you hired a martial arts master as a personal assistant to launch surprise attacks when you least expect it. Preposterous as it sounds, this type of sporadic intense "life-or-death" stimulation just might produce far superior fitness benefits than filling in all the blanks in your training log.

Sprint Workout Strategy

Your sprints should last between eight and 60 seconds, with duration, recovery, and number of repetitions determined by your ability level. While the scientific particulars of your workout choices may only be relevant to athletes trying to hone sport-specific skills and mimic competitive circumstances (track-and-field events of varied distance, football, soccer, etc.), you should vary your routine over time to include short, medium, and longer sprints.

You can also vary rest periods and number of reps to account for your fitness level and stimulate different fitness adaptations and energy production systems. Longer sprints with short rest develop your anaerobic lactic acid buffering system (a desirable ability for a half-mile or mile race), while the shorter sprints with long rest periods develop your pure speed and explosiveness (such as for a 100-meter race). All types of sprint training will stimulate your fat-burning system, lean muscle development, and beneficial hormone flow, particularly the release of testosterone and human growth hormone (HGH).

Running sprints should be shorter than cycling sprints because the weight bearing aspect makes them more difficult. I prefer going all-out for about 15 seconds (after gradually ramping up my speed) and then taking a full rest period of one minute between efforts. I'll complete six to eight reps, typically on grass or on soft or hard sand at the beach. Using different surfaces helps me enjoy a cross-training effect (e.g., I have to lift my knees higher in soft sand to generate maximum turnover). My cycling sprints might consist of six to eight times of one-minute all-out with a two-minute recovery. Your entire sprint sessions—including brief warm-up and cool-down periods—will require less than 20 minutes. The Sprint Workout Suggestions appendix at MarksDailyApple.com offer an ever-expanding list of novice, intermediate, and advanced workouts, including an exciting plyometric workout, a stadium steps workout, and a couple of low- or no-impact sprint options, such as sprinting up steep hills or on a stationary bike.

Ideally, you should sprint on a natural surface with excellent footing, such as a grass athletic field or the beach; use a running track or cement road if you can't find a suitable natural surface. I strongly recommend making an effort to minimize your dependency on bulky running shoes and strengthening your feet by going barefoot, if possible, or using specially designed shoes that encourage a fuller range of motion (see the forthcoming "Happy Feet" sidebar).

Proper Running and Cycling Form

While form concerns are relatively minimal in running and cycling compared to other sports, you must respect these important basics:

Running: Torso faces forward at all times, shoulders and pelvis square to your forward direction. Refrain from side-to-side swiveling of the hips or the shoulder girdle. Arms and hands are relaxed and pumping forward, with elbows bent at 90-degree angles. Don't let arms or hands cross the center line of your body. Drive knees high while keeping the pelvis facing forward. While sprinting, maximum force and drive are generated from the front part of the foot, with the heel rarely touching the ground, if at all. When you experience the inevitable tightening up midway through your sprint, focus on keeping your face, arms, and hands loose and relaxed. Notice in videos or photographs of Olympic sprinters how their jaws are slack and their hands are soft and open. Be aware of your breathing rhythm and resist the temptation to hold your breath or pant shallowly. Take deep, powerful breaths by focusing on a forceful exhale.

Cycling: Strive for a rhythmic cadence in a range of 80 to 100 revolutions per minute. Most recreational cyclists pedal at far too low a cadence, putting excessive strain on the muscles instead of balancing the cardiovascular and muscular load. Apply circular force to the pedals rather than stomping down. I highly recommend a clip-in pedaling system to achieve a proper circular stroke. Maintain a level pelvis at all times. Do not rock your pelvis from side to side in an effort to impart more force. Keep your upper body virtually still, with arms, chest, neck, and head relaxed and supple especially when the effort becomes difficult.

Ensure that your seat height is appropriate by placing your heel (unclip it from the pedal) on the pedal axle when it's at the very bottom of the pedal stroke. You should be able to extend your leg fully (with pelvis level) and barely touch (or barely miss) the pedal axle. A seat that is too high or too low will stress the knees and also lead to rocking. Breathe deeply by inflating your diaphragm fully on inhale. Because you are bent over, you should feel your diaphragm pressing against your rib cage when you inhale; then relax and allow a natural exhale.

Happy Feet

One of the most annoying non-Primal elements of today's fitness movement is shoes. You heard me, shoes are lame. Sure, typical athletic shoes provide substantial support, cushioning, and general protection, and are essential for many sports, but they also immobilize your feet—much like being in a cast. Hence, the complex network of 52 bones (a quarter of the total in your entire body) and dozens of tendons, ligaments, and small muscles cannot work their magic to provide balance, stability, impact absorption, weight transfer, and propulsion. Constantly wearing shoes during exercise and daily life leads to weakened feet, fallen arches, shortened Achilles tendons and calf muscles, imbalances between the hamstrings and quadriceps, an inefficient gait, and, of course, recurring pain and injury (like the old song goes, "The ankle bone's connected to the knee bone; the knee bone's connected to the hip bone"). The 43 million Americans who experience foot problems daily (we will spend an estimated $900 million annually on foot-care products by 2011) offer another disturbing example of living in conflict with the *Primal Blueprint*.

Going shoeless on occasion (and gradually increasing frequency over time) for your Primal Fitness activities can strengthen feet, improve balance and reduce injury risk. Keep in mind that a lifetime spent in "casts"—desensitizing and weakening your feet for their primary functional purpose—will require that you proceed with extreme caution with your barefoot endeavors.

Here again I'll make a concession for modern life (I don't think Grok had any broken glass to worry about on *his* hikes) by recommending the use of a unique and excellent product called the Vibram FiveFingers shoe. The Vibram "shoe" consists of a lightweight, form-fitting rubber sole sewn to a nylonlike sock with a hook-and-loop closure system. Vibrams slip onto your bare feet like fingers into a glove (with a hole for each toe) and offer excellent grip as well as protection from sharp objects and debris. Duly protected, you can simulate a barefoot experience by giving your feet a complete range of motion during activity. Search MarksDailyApple.com or VibramFiveFingers.com for details. Another option is the Nike Free product line. These are actual shoes, but designed to offer minimal support and maximum flexibility—basically the opposite of what Conventional Wisdom has advocated for runners since the running boom started in the late 1970s.

Make an effort to gradually introduce barefoot time into your workouts and everyday life, providing ample time for your feet to adjust and get stronger without undue shock. Some mild next-day soreness in your arches is to be expected after your initial barefoot endeavors and is a natural part of the strengthening process (just as with muscle work). However, make sure you don't experience any pain during your efforts to get your feet more Primal. Be particularly careful if you are minimally active or overweight or if you have a history of foot problems or other medical issues. Hopefully, one day you'll work up to running some sprints barefoot—it doesn't get any more Primal than that!

> *Going shoeless on occasion can strengthen feet, improve balance and reduce injury risk.*

Chapter Summary

1. Primal Blueprint Exercise Laws: Mirroring the active lifestyle of Grok is not a complex endeavor requiring the extensive time, money, or specific equipment that Conventional Wisdom suggests. In particular, you can get extremely fit in as little as a few hours a week, provided you exercise strategically with a balance of extensive low-intensity movement, periodic high-intensity, short-duration strength-training sessions, and occasional all-out sprints.

Best results will come when your exercise routine is unstructured and intuitive, and workout choices are aligned with your energy and motivation levels. Always allow for sufficient recovery and pursue goals that are fun and inspiring. Weight-loss goals can succeed by combining Primal eating and frequent low-level exercise (fine-tuning your fat-burning system), with occasional brief, intense strength and sprint sessions (to stimulate an increase in lean muscle and metabolic rate). Novices and elite competitors alike can succeed with the *Primal Blueprint* exercise laws, by focusing on intermittent efforts instead of consistency and blending low-level work with brief, high-intensity efforts in between.

2. Primal Fitness: Primal Fitness means you have a broad range of skills and attributes (strength, power, speed, endurance—with power-to-weight ratio as a critical benchmark) that allow you to do pretty much whatever you want with a substantial degree of competence and minimal risk of injury. In contrast, narrow, specialized fitness goals are popular today (e.g., for endurance athletes and bodybuilders). These goals often compromise functional fitness and general health. By exercising—and eating—*Primal Blueprint* style, you will develop the unmistakable physique of a well-balanced athlete and eliminate the drawbacks of narrowly focused, overly stressful exercise programs.

3. Organ Reserve: Leading an active lifestyle and maintaining ample lean muscle mass correlates with optimal organ function and longevity, because your organs must keep up with the physical demands you place upon your body. In contrast, inactivity will accelerate the aging process to the extent that it becomes a greater risk factor than simply getting older.

4. Move Frequently at a Slow Pace: Two to five hours per week of low-intensity aerobic exercise (heart rate zone of 55 to 75 percent of max heart rate), such as walking, hiking, easy cycling, cardio machines or (if you are fit) jogging offer excellent health benefits, including improved cardiovascular, musculoskeletal, and immune function and fat metabolism. In contrast, Chronic Cardio workouts (75 percent of max heart rate and up) can place excessive stress on your system, deplete the body of energy (leading to increased appetite for quick-energy carbohydrates), inhibit fat metabolism, promote overuse injuries, and generally result in a burnout condition. Slowing down workout pace and moving around more in daily life will lead to improved fitness and health.

5. Lift Heavy Things: Best results in strength training come from a sporadic routine of varied workouts that are brief and intense. These workouts will stimulate the release of adaptive hormones, such as testosterone and human growth hormone, helping improve body composition and delaying the aging process. Exercises should focus on real human movements (lunges, squats, plyometrics, push-ups, pull-ups, and other body weight resistance exercises) instead of isolations on narrow-range-of-motion gym machines. Session difficulty should be aligned with energy and motivation levels: push hard when you feel like it and take it easy or skip workouts when you are tired. With this approach, you will avoid the risk of injury, exhaustion, and burnout that comes from trying to follow a consistent schedule of long-duration workouts several times a week. Complete sessions should last under an hour, with 30 minutes sufficient for most. A mini-session of as little as seven minutes can be extremely beneficial.

6. Sprint Once in a While: No workout is more Primal than an all-out sprint. Efforts like these fueled human evolution directly in the survival-of-the-fittest paradigm. Today we can enjoy excellent fitness, body composition, and health benefits from intense sprinting, modeling the "use it or lose it" principle. Sprint sessions should be conducted sporadically when energy and motivation levels are high. Intensity is the key— efforts should last between eight and 60 seconds, with complete rest between efforts to ensure maximum performance. Novices can do low-impact options, such as uphill sprints or stationary bicycle sprints.

7. Form and Feet: Proper form in running and cycling is imperative. For running, the body should always face forward, the center of gravity should be stable, and wasted motion (i.e., side-to-side movement) should be eliminated. For cycling, ensure proper seat height and apply circular force while pedaling at a rapid, efficient cadence of 80 to 100 rpm. Make an effort to minimize bulky shoes that restrict natural foot motion and weaken stabilizing and propulsion muscles. Spend more time barefoot in daily life, and gradually integrate some "barefoot" time into your workouts. Utilize innovative footwear like Vibram FiveFingers or Nike Free to protect feet while simulating a barefoot experience.

CHAPTER 7

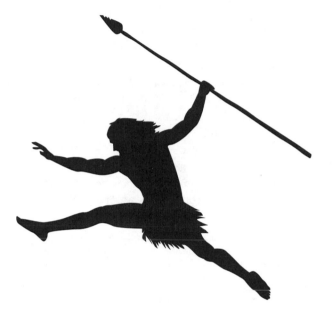

The Primal Blueprint Lifestyle Laws

"If You Don't Snooze, You Lose"

In This Chapter

I detail the five lifestyle laws of the *Primal Blueprint*: Law #6, Get Adequate Sleep; Law #7, Play; Law #8, Get Adequate Sunlight; Law #9, Avoid Stupid Mistakes; and Law #10, Use Your Brain. While Grok's diet and exercise patterns were clearly major influences in shaping how his (and our) genes evolved, there were other environmental and behavioral forces that were no less important in perfecting the DNA recipe for a healthy, vibrant human being. It would be a mistake for us to underemphasize these other lifestyle habits, because they also play a significant role in whether or not we lose fat, build muscle, and stay focused, energetic, productive, and disease-free.

Law #6, Get Adequate Sleep, delivers obvious benefits but is widely compromised today. Good sleep involves understanding the physiology of sleep cycles, establishing consistent habits, taking advantage of the profound benefits of napping (when you need one), and applying effective time-prioritization skills. Law #7, Play, requires minimal analysis or specific instruction. Again, it's an obvious but widely neglected lifestyle law that can deliver widespread benefits and make you quantifiably more productive when balanced effectively with work. Law #8, Get Adequate Sunlight, is an area where Conventional Wisdom has let us down, scaring us into avoiding the outdoors due to the misinterpreted risks of skin cancer. Obtaining optimal levels of vitamin D, synthesized from sun exposure on your skin, is critical to cellular health and cancer prevention.

Law #9, Avoid Stupid Mistakes, details how our obsessive desire to control or eliminate all sources of potential danger has made us lazy and inattentive. Cultivating the skills of hypervigilance and risk management is essential to avoid self-inflicted trauma and unnecessary suffering. Law #10, Use Your Brain, may seem counterintuitive to many of us who are hyperstimulated all day long. Actually, the unrelenting pace of modern life and intense pressure to achieve and consume strongly conflict with our genetic makeup and can lead to feelings of restlessness and discontent. Pursuing creative intellectual outlets unrelated to your core daily responsibilities and economic contribution will keep you refreshed and excited about life.

I am two with nature.

—Woody Allen

Primal Blueprint Law #6: Get Adequate Sleep

In the hierarchy of the most important ways to get Primal, sometimes sleep gets left in the dust in pursuit of more sexy and intellectually complex efforts such as tracking average daily carbohydrate gram intake or monitoring workout heart rate zones and interval sequences. Yet after all the macronutrients and workout reps are counted, virtually nothing is more critical to the success of your peak performance, weight loss, and longevity goals than getting adequate sleep. Admittedly, it's one of the most difficult *Primal Blueprint* laws to observe in modern life.

For billions of years, the evolution of nearly all life forms on earth has been driven by the consistent rising and setting of the sun. This circadian rhythm (from Latin: *circa*, meaning "around"; and *dia*, meaning "day") governs our sleeping and eating patterns as well as the precise timing of important hormone secretions, brain wave patterns, and cellular repair and regeneration based on a 24-hour cycle. When we interfere with our circadian rhythm (via excessive artificial light and digital stimulation after sunset, irregular bed and wake times, jet lag, graveyard shift work, etc.), we disrupt some of the very processes we depend upon to stay healthy, happy, productive, and focused.

Unlike Grok's dietary and exercise habits—which you can mimic well today by food shopping carefully or finding a smooth neighborhood tree branch for pull-ups—obeying your human circadian rhythm to be active when the sun is up and sleep when it's dark is a bit more of a hassle. Depending on where you live and the time of year, your efforts to follow a Primal sleep schedule could easily get pinched to the tune of two to eight hours a day. Can you say, "Ain't gonna happen anytime soon?"

This is not to say you have to turn in at sunset in order to be healthy. For one thing, modernization has substantially lowered our activity level and the overall degree of difficulty of daily life. (I know commuting is tiring, but imagine *walking* home from the office every day!) Experts' opinions vary on the amount of sleep you need, but the general consensus is that seven to eight hours per night is sufficient for most people, provided the sleep is of high quality (uninterrupted and not influenced by sleep medications, alcohol, or poor food choices) *and* that you observe a consistent pattern of bed and wake times.

During sleep, the recovery and rejuvenation of the muscles, organs, and all the systems of the body are accelerated. This is all guided by the sleep hormone melatonin, which is manufactured in the pineal gland near the center of the brain. As light diminishes, the pineal starts to convert the feel-good hormone serotonin, which has kept your mood elevated all day (and which is why so many of us take SSRIs—to avoid depleting serotonin), to increasing amounts of melatonin, so that you can get that good night's sleep. As light increases in the morning, melatonin production is then suppressed and serotonin begins to increase. You wake up happy and refreshed. It is a beautiful balance that allows you to sleep deeply yet helps improve and stabilize your mood during waking hours.

Resting the areas of the brain involved in emotional and social function helps you face the day refreshed. A study from Dr. Sophie Schwartz and colleagues presented at the 2008 Forum of European Neuroscience suggested that getting a good night's sleep can help the brain "harden up weak memories which otherwise might fade in time." Other hormones released during sleep, such as human growth hormone, help your body burn fat.

While these and many other perks of quality z-time are obvious to everyone, we are not walking our talk in modern life. A recent study cited by the Harvard School of Public Health found that an increasing percentage of Americans are seriously deficient in sleep (40 percent of Americans get less than five hours of sleep per night), and an incredible 75 percent of us suffer from some form of sleep difficulty each night. Chronic sleep deficit may lead to weight gain by affecting how your body processes and stores carbohydrates and by altering hormones that affect your appetite and metabolism. It can negatively affect your mood, concentration, and memory retention during the day, making you less productive and more irritable, impatient, and moody. Insufficient sleep can also lead to hypertension, elevated stress hormone levels, irregular heartbeat, compromised immune function, and drastically increased risk for obesity and heart disease.

Opportunity Costs—What Is Your Best Buy?

When we look at the prevalence of late-night digital entertainment, insulin-producing dietary indulgences, central nervous system stimulants, and morning alarms knocking us off our waves (be they alpha, beta, delta, or perhaps a vivid dream about paddling out on the North Shore), we must again pause and ask, "What's going on here?" I'm certainly not immune to the distractions. Even when I'm fatigued after a long week or returning from business travel, I can't wait to hang out with my wife and kids, watch a DVD, surf the Internet for interesting blog fodder, catch up on some great books stacked at my bedside, and so on. Our natural (or actually I should say, "learned") inclination to be constantly entertained is difficult to balance with our need for adequate restoration. It's not until we are truly exhausted that sleep moves up the hierarchy of wants and needs. It shouldn't have to be that way.

With a sincere dedication to health and balance, you can get away with some occasional departures from your routine with no ill effects. Just as with your dietary choices, if you can observe a consistent bedtime 80 percent of the time (there's that 80% Rule again), the 20 percent of the time where you stay up late, wake up super early, or otherwise skimp on perfect rest will probably be handled by your body more easily. On the other hand, if you have a habit of disrespecting consistent sleep time habits, you create momentum in the wrong direction and will struggle to achieve basic health and fitness goals.

Get Primal with TiVo? You Bet!

While the admonition to avoid television at night and limit television in general is likely quite familiar to you, the reality is that television is a central component of modern life. (Try 28 hours a week average American viewing time!) This is a good opportunity to put in a plug for the DVR (digital video recorder, like TiVo). When we collapse onto the couch to spend some precious time vegging out in front of the TV, we often fail to discipline ourselves to stick to quality programming and a strictly observed bedtime. We are also forced to endure commercials (accounting for 30 percent of total airtime and with often annoying, in-your-face, repetitive messages) and programming options appealing to the lowest-common-denominator. (A TV Free America study revealed that 54 percent of local news programming is devoted to crime, disaster, and war, not to mention those ridiculous fear-eliciting lead-ins: "Could toxic school playground bark be lowering test scores? Story at 11.")

The DVR empowers you with incredible freedom and control of your entertainment options, making for a far more enriching and time-efficient television experience. You can zip through commercials, store desired programming for later viewing at your leisure, and even automatically record your favorite shows around the clock. DVR service costs only about 12 extra bucks a month, and most cable and satellite operators will give you the expensive DVR machine for free on a subscription contract.

During the 2008 Beijing Olympics, the four-hour prime-time broadcasts that extended to midnight each evening led to headline stories about widespread sleep deprivation across America. For my part, I breezed through the stored broadcasts a day later (psst: the prime-time shebang was delayed half a day anyway), picking and choosing my favorite action with my four-speed fast-forward remote, in about an hour and 20 minutes. I saved loads of time...and didn't get completely sick of beach volleyball like some regular viewers!

Surf the Internet or Surf the Waves—Understanding Sleep Cycles

Sleep was long thought to be a passive state, but we now understand sleep to be a dynamic process. The brain is active during sleep (but responding to internal stimuli, not external), and it drifts in and out of various sleep stages, or cycles. Our natural sleep pattern is to progress from light sleep (rapid eye movement [REM], when you dream and can be woken easily) into escalating stages of deeper sleep cycles (non-REM sleep, when you are out like a light and experiencing maximum restorative hormone flow, balancing of brain chemicals, and cellular repair). This cycling of REM into non-REM sleep is repeated throughout the night, with each complete cycle believed to last about 90 minutes.

If you divide your night's sleep into three equal time periods, your first third is characterized by the highest percentage of non-REM sleep, while the final third of your sleep time is characterized by a lengthening of the REM cycles and a shortening of the deep sleep cycles (the middle cycle is a balance between the first and the last). Waking up naturally involves letting the cycles play out until finally, after a period of exclusive REM sleep, you wake up effortlessly. (REM sleep is characterized by increases in heart rate, respiration, and muscle and brain wave activity, making it easy to rise from this more alert state.)

Sleeping success is not as simple as merely accumulating the hours (hey, reminds me of exercise!). The Center for Applied Cognitive Studies in Charlotte, North Carolina, and many other experts report that in order for a person to feel refreshed, the number of complete sleep cycles achieved is more important than total sleep time. Achieving these ideal sleep cycles as described is a delicate process guided by hormone flows that can easily be disturbed by outside influences. Cortisol levels are sensitive to light, gradually peaking in the morning to help you summon the energy to start your day. Kelly Korg's predawn alarm arousal resulted in an unnatural, excessive, and therefore destructive spike of cortisol. I'm completely serious when I say she would absolutely be healthier and fitter by all measures (including the pinch test for body fat) if she replaced the majority of her early-morning strenuous workouts with an extra hour of sleep and a moderate 20-minute walk around the neighborhood.

Melatonin release is triggered by darkness, and levels of growth hormone and other restorative substances achieve peak levels while you are sleeping. Throwing artificial light and digital stimulation at your circadian rhythm, as seen with the late-night habits of Ken and Kenny Korg, will create hormonal stresses and imbalances that mess up metabolism, cognitive function, mood stability, and overall enjoyment of life. For example, staying up past your bedtime buoyed by artificial light and stimulation (say, a late movie or a bunch of teenagers going on a toilet paper raid) triggers a cortisol release. Remember, your genes desperately want you to achieve peak performance; melatonin flows to get you some sleep, and cortisol flows if you need to rally. The cortisol release gives you a "second wind," but it also increases your overall life stress. It doesn't matter if the stress is fun and exciting or whether it's negative and upsetting—it all goes on the opposite side of the balance scales to rest. Observing regular bed and wake times will help regulate cortisol production, something that is essential to good health.

How to Get an "A" in "Z's"

Here are some important measures you can take to get optimum amounts of high-quality sleep. Visit MarksDailyApple.com for more discussion on this topic, including some helpful tips to beat jet lag.

Create an Ideal Sleeping Environment: It's critical to make your bedroom an area of minimal stimulation and maximum relaxation. Your bedroom should be used only for sleeping (well, okay, that other stuff, too)—with absolutely no computer, television, or work desk present. You should have a clear physical and psychological separation between your bedroom and other areas of the house where you do work or enjoy entertainment. Eliminate any clutter, such as excess clothing, books, magazines, and tabletop stuff (car keys, cell phone, mail, spare change, etc.). Browse the Internet or page through design magazines to get a feeling for the beauty of contemporary minimalist bedroom styles.

In his book *The Tao of Health, Sex and Longevity*, author Daniel Reid relates an ancient Tao maxim called the Four Empties. Taoist theory says that restraint and moderation are the keys to longevity and that we should strive to avoid excess in our lives by pursuing an Empty Mind (focus on the present, meditate daily), Empty Stomach (eat when hungry and finish when satisfied, avoid overeating), Empty Kitchen (eat primarily fresh foods and minimize processed, preserved, and frozen foods), and Empty Room (avoid excessive noise, clutter, and distraction in your private sleeping quarters).

Follow Consistent Bed and Wake Times: Just like with exercise, think quality over quantity. Establish a consistent, circadian-friendly routine to optimize hormone flows and ensure you enjoy complete sleep cycles. Remember that melatonin floods your bloodstream on circadian cue triggered by darkness. More accurately, it's the time when you typically "make it dark" (e.g., when you turn out the light at your typical bedtime or when the sun sets if you're camping) and that you experience the highest percentage of deep sleep at the outset of your night. Sorry, but if you miss bedtime, sleeping in to reach your typical hourly total will not completely catch you up.

If you are a night owl, you can probably develop some level of tolerance and effectiveness for a consistent, artificial light–induced late-night bedtime and late-morning awakening. This is certainly less stressful to the body than the more common practice of fluctuating your bedtime—fighting the natural melatonin release occasionally or regularly with various artificial stimuli (TV/movie/computer, caffeine, etc.). The latter is akin to Kelly Korg's forcing her body out of bed too early and triggering a stressful cortisol release. The bottom line is that the more artificial light and stimulus you throw into your circadian equation, the farther you get from Primal, period.

Wind Down the Night and Ease into the Day: Because everything you do after sundown is technically non-Primal, it's important to wind down calmly in the hours preceding your bedtime. Minimize your central nervous system stimulation before going to bed, so you can have a smooth, relaxing transition from your busy day to downtime. Reading is a time-tested popular method to wind down, but even the subject matter should be chosen carefully. In *The 4-Hour Workweek*, author Tim Ferriss argues that we should avoid reading newspapers, something related to work, and even nonfiction, instead promoting maximum relaxation of the mind by sticking with fiction for our leisure reading.

It may also be helpful to decompress your busy brain by writing down your thoughts before bed. Take five or 10 minutes to write out everything from your day: accomplishments, to-do tasks, stresses, and worries. It's easier to arrive at solutions if you don't try consciously to force them. Get them down on paper, and then let your sleeping mind do the work for you. You'll wake up feeling clearer and more positive.

In the morning, awaken gradually and naturally coming off a complete REM-dominant sleep cycle. Staying in bed for a few minutes to read or talk ("Again, your name was…?") or starting your day with some light breathing and stretching exercises is preferable to springing up after the fourth snooze alarm and rushing into action. A brief warm shower can help stimulate your central nervous system naturally and get blood circulating—a particularly good idea if you are going to exercise soon after awakening. Hard-core Grok disciples can even try a cold-water plunge upon awakening in the summer months—beats a high-carb breakfast any day as a morning energizer.

Eat and Drink the Right Stuff: What you eat and drink before bed can have a significant impact, either positive or negative, on your ability to achieve restful sleep. In contrast to the folly of Ken Korg's ingestion of sugary foods and sleep medication, it's better to eat lightly before bed so that blood sugar fluctuations and potential digestive complications from lying down with a full stomach do not interfere with your sleep process. If you are a wine drinker, one fine glass with dinner may help you relax and unwind in the evening hours. The same goes for herbal teas. Chamomile in particular is touted for its mild sedative effect. A handful of nuts can also be helpful, thanks to their ample levels of magnesium (helps relax muscles) and L-tryptophan (promotes the production of serotonin, the potent neurotransmitter that becomes melatonin as darkness triggers sleep). Other tryptophan-rich foods that can be eaten in moderation before bed are eggs, meat, fish, and cheese.

> *No day is so bad it can't be fixed with a nap.*
> —*Carrie Snow*
> *Stand-up comedian*

Avoid the Conventional Wisdom that promotes carbohydrates as a catchall bedtime aid. You may have heard—accurately—that consuming carbohydrates stimulates the production of that "feel good" hormone serotonin. However, more than a little carbohydrate will cause an energy boost followed by that now-familiar insulin cascade, neither of which is a good idea near bedtime…or ever, for that matter!

Napping: It's Not Just for Cats Anymore

If you are able to obtain all of your requisite sleep at night, there is probably no reason to routinely take naps during the day. On the other hand, if you do have obstacles (job requirements, young children, noisy surroundings, etc.) that prevent you from getting adequate nighttime sleep, napping can help you sustain the focus, energy, and productivity you need for an active life. Many cultures across the world—especially warm weather countries in Latin America, Asia, the Mediterranean, North Africa, and the Middle East—have appreciated nap time throught their history. Furthermore, more than 85 percent of mammals have polyphasic sleep habits, meaning multiple sleep-wake incidents. For proof I needn't look further than my dog, Buddha, crashed out under my desk right now but ready for quick action should the doorbell ring!

Unfortunately, it seems the fast pace of life in the USA (combined, perhaps, with some weird puritanical guilt factors) prevents napping from being a culturally acceptable lifestyle habit. The promo message for Dr. Sara Mednick's book *Take a Nap! Change Your Life* reads:

> Imagine a product that increases alertness, boosts creativity, reduces stress, improves perception, stamina, motor skills, and accuracy, enhances your sex life, helps you make better decisions, keeps you looking younger, aids in weight loss, reduces the risk of heart attack, elevates your mood, and strengthens memory. Now imagine that this product is nontoxic, has no dangerous side effects, and, best of all, is absolutely *free*.

At first glance it might seem like marketing hyperbole, but each exciting claim is well documented with respected studies (research abstracts are provided in the *Primal Blueprint* Resources appendix at MarksDailyApple.com).

Because the rhythm of sleep cycles is so critical to brain and body restoration, brief naps can produce remarkable benefits by helping you catch up on non-REM sleep cycle deficiencies, shortcutting you into the

> *A nap of 20 to 30 minutes will recalibrate your brain's sodium: potassium ratio, a critical factor to recover from nervous system fatigue and wake up feeling refreshed.*

deep sleep cycles characterized by theta brain waves. Many experts recommend a nap period of 20 to 30 minutes. This time frame is believed to be sufficient to recalibrate your brain's sodium:potassium ratio, a critical factor to recover from nervous system fatigue and wake up feeling refreshed. However, a 20- to 30-minute nap is not too long to produce the unpleasant grogginess you might experience from a prolonged siesta. Notable nappers throughout history include Winston Churchill, John F. Kennedy, Napoleon, Albert Einstein, Thomas Edison, Leonardo da Vinci, and Paris Hilton.

Primal Blueprint Law #7: Play

Few would argue the importance of play, yet compliance among many health-minded people is low in this area. We have been so heavily socialized into regimented, technological, industrialized life that scheduling time for play (now there's an oxymoron!) is a big challenge. I don't know about you, but I don't think the word *playdate* existed when I was a kid. Oh, we had playdates in my neighborhood, all right—365 of them, to be exact. They lasted from the final school bell till the dinner bell, not deterred by mud, rain, sleet, or snow (no kidding, I'm from Maine!). We didn't need our moms making transportation arrangements via e-mail or cell phone. We just needed air in our lungs, bike tires, and basketballs.

> *Art is older than production [making things for practical use] for us, and play older than work. Man was shaped less by what he had to do than by what he did in playful moments. It is the child in man that is the source of his uniqueness and creativeness.*
> —*Eric Hoffer*
> *American social writer and philosopher (1902-1983)*

As the challenges and responsibilities of making a living or managing a family accumulate in our adult years, we collectively adopt the belief that play is for youth. The truth is that play is for everyone, particularly those absorbed in the incredible complexity and breakneck pace of modern life. Regular play—time away from work, home duties, school, and other scheduled and unscheduled responsibilities—helps quench your thirst for adventure and challenge (physical and mental), improves health, relieves stress, strengthens your connection with friends and community, and simply enhances your enjoyment of life.

Learning disability specialist Dr. Lorraine Peniston enumerates many research-proven psychological benefits of play, including:

- Perceived sense of freedom, independence, and autonomy
- Enhanced self-competence through improved sense of self-worth, self-reliance, and self-confidence
- Better ability to socialize with others, including greater tolerance and understanding
- Enriched capabilities for team membership
- Heightened creative ability
- Improved expressions of and reflection on personal spiritual ideals
- Greater adaptability and resiliency
- Better sense of humor
- Enhanced perceived quality of life
- More balanced competitiveness and a more positive outlook on life

There is plenty of evidence attesting to the fact that we can be more productive when we carve time for play into our busy schedules. A New Zealand study reported that people were 82 percent more productive following a vacation and enjoyed enhanced quality of sleep—but that 43 percent of Americans had no vacation plans in 2007 due to work pressures (and it's probably worse since the economic collapse). A 2006 study published in the *Sunday Times* (England) noted that the percentage of married couples citing lack of quality time due to overwork as the basis for divorce has more than tripled in recent years, even while the traditional leading divorce reasons, such as violence and infidelity, have dropped sharply. Australian research suggests that frequent breaks from a sedentary workday produce numerous health benefits, including weight control and favorable blood levels of triglycerides and glucose. A study published in the *New York Times* suggests that enjoyable leisure activities boost immune function even more powerfully than stressful events suppress it.

4-Hour Workweek author Tim Ferriss contends that we work more quickly and efficiently when faced with a deadline or other time constraints than when we slog through extended workdays and imbalanced lives. What if you only had to work four hours a day, with the other four devoted to leisure activities of your choice? Can you conceive of the possibility that you might be just as—or more—productive? Think your prioritization skills would improve? How about your tendency to be distracted by off-topic diversions (e-mail jokes and videos, poor discipline for phone or personal work interruptions, etc.)? If you could arrange your schedule accordingly, could you be more productive by opting out of unnecessary meetings or deciding to telecommute when appropriate, instead of burning hours and gas on the road simply for the decorum of showing up?

Seeing that we're talking about play, you need not follow any directives from me or anyone else about the particulars of what, how, or when. Generally speaking, you'll enjoy things that you excel at—or have a passionate desire to excel at. While such sedate activities as drawing trees in the park or reading for pleasure technically qualify as recreation, I believe best results come when you play outdoors, in fresh air and sunlight, with an adequate level of physical exertion. If you are one of the few who live a lifestyle of extensive physical exertion, quiet leisure time might indeed be the ticket. For the majority of us who move far less than we are genetically programmed to, busting out of the confinements of modern life for some exhilarating play will produce the best physical and psychological benefits.

My favorite activity of the week is a regular Sunday-afternoon pickup Ultimate game with my son and several other families at the park. It is a great sport, requiring diverse athletic and strategic skills, and is fun for players of all ages and ability levels. I'd say it's a "safe" sport, too, except for my freak accident that resulted in a serious knee injury in 2007…possibly attributed to my 17-year-old athletic mentality directing a 54-year-old body to get some big air for a circus catch! Most importantly, my enjoyment of playtime has prompted me to reframe my main reason for exercising: I train Primally so I can play hard at whatever I want whenever I choose to, whether it's at Ultimate, snowboarding, soccer, stand-up paddling, or golf.

> *We don't stop playing because we grow old; we grow old because we stop playing.*
> *—George Bernard Shaw, Irish playwright and political activist (1856-1950)*

If you can take the spirit of this message to heart, you can make something happen that will change your life. Let's be clear that I'm not advocating selling the shop and becoming a surf rat. All work and no play makes for a dull boy, but all play and no work makes for a foreclosure. Balance is important in all areas of life, and it's up to you to define your level of work-play balance. It might help to keep this popular sentiment in mind: "No one ever said, 'I wish I'd spent more time at work' on their deathbed."

Primal Blueprint Law #8: Get Adequate Sunlight

While the dangers of excessive sun exposure are well recognized and heavily promoted by today's medical community, it's important to challenge Conventional Wisdom's blanket statement to shun the sun—or lather up with tons of sunscreen as do English Channel swimmers with their lanolin. Adequate exposure to sunlight helps our bodies manufacture vitamin D, which helps regulate growth in virtually every cell of our bodies and prevent a variety of diseases. Vitamin D is essential for healthy teeth, bones, and nails; eyesight; the absorption of other key nutrients, such as calcium and vitamins A and C; and immune function. Vitamin D has also been shown to play a role in the prevention of breast, prostate, and colorectal cancer; cardiovascular disease; diabetes; autoimmune diseases; and inflammatory conditions, such as arthritis.

Perhaps the most exciting revelation about vitamin D has to do with its critical action on Gene P53—the "proofreader" gene. P53 acts as a spell-checker during each of the hundreds of millions of cell replications that occur each day, informing the cell when something has gone awry and instructing it to make necessary changes. Many scientists believe P53 is an important first line of defense against the kinds of mutations that can develop into cancers. The bottom line is that regular sunlight is essential to excellent health and the *prevention* of skin cancer.

Early humans spent hundreds of thousands of years absorbing powerful equatorial rays over their entire bodies every day. As we migrated farther away from the equator, genetic adaptations occurred (the lightening of skin pigment and hair over many generations) to help us continue to absorb sun optimally even when it was less plentiful. Just as we've suffered devastating health consequences from the relatively recent shift in the human diet away from hunter-gatherer to grain-based, the same dynamic holds for our sun exposure—except this lifestyle alteration has been even more severe. Only in the last couple of centuries of industrialization have millions of people in the civilized world gone for long periods of time with little to no direct sun exposure. Consequently, there has been an alarming increase in health problems related to vitamin D deficiency.

The symptoms of vitamin D deficiency are not as overt as the disturbing image of scurvy-stricken sailors staggering around lacking vitamin C (which was, ironically, partly a result of their high grain consumption), but the health consequences are devastating nonetheless. The risk increases for those with confined lifestyles (spent in the home, office, or auto—witness Ken Korg), those with dark skin living distant from the equator, children with vitamin D–deficient mothers, the elderly, or people who are house- or hospital-bound. Recent research suggests that vitamin D levels are also low in those with obesity and Metabolic Syndrome.

Internet and television health advisor Dr. Joseph Mercola (mercola.com) states:

> The dangers of sun exposure have been greatly exaggerated and the benefits highly underestimated. Excess sun exposure is not the major reason people develop skin cancer (many believe poor diet, exposure to other environmental toxins such as swimming pool chlorine, and insufficient sun are more significant risk factors). [A study from the Moores Cancer Center at UC San Diego suggested that] 600,000 cases of cancer could be prevented every year by just increasing your levels of vitamin D.

Granted, the "fell asleep covered with baby oil at the beach" burn-and-peel ordeals are indeed bad news. Medical experts say that even a few severe sunburn episodes in your early years (who hasn't fallen asleep on a beach or chaise lounge as a teenager?!) can generate sufficient ultraviolet radiation damage to lead to the development of melanoma in later decades. But there is a happy medium between too much sun and too little.

Regular *brief* daily exposure to sunlight remains the primary way to obtain an ample amount of vitamin D so critical to good health. While vitamin D is found in small quantities in fatty fish (salmon, sardines, and mackerel), meat (particularly liver), eggs, fortified foods, and dietary supplements, most ingested sources are insufficient to ensure adequate vitamin D levels (e.g., without sun, you'd need some 40 glasses of milk a day to get enough D). It is also possible to overdose on vitamin D with supplements but not with sunlight, because excess vitamin D is destroyed by the sun itself. Blood tests are available to determine how your vitamin D levels compare to recommended levels.

For most people, a slight tan indicates that you are obtaining adequate vitamin D exposure, while a burn is, of course, unhealthy. It's important to observe the critical variable of your skin pigment and moderate your exposure accordingly to make absolutely sure that you never burn your skin. In most of North America or countries of comparable latitude, 20 minutes per day is adequate for health benefits and yet brief enough to prevent damage from overexposure.

The variables of season, climate, and skin tone are substantial and should be carefully considered on a daily basis to ensure you obtain adequate sunlight while avoiding risk factors of excessive exposure. Those with very fair skin may obtain adequate vitamin D exposure with just five minutes of direct sunlight on the face and arms, outside the peak sun intensity hours of 11 A.M. to 4 P.M. in the summertime. Solarly challenged folks (say, someone of African heritage living in Scandinavia or scientists on a winter research project at McMurdo Station, Antarctica) have to make a major effort to soak up enough sun to attain sufficient vitamin D levels. In the event that natural sunlight just isn't available, there are some new forms of artificial tanning lights that have been proven to increase vitamin D levels safely. Information on the latest "approved" versions can be found at MarksDailyApple.com.

Unfortunately, there is little conclusive research about just what constitutes ideal sun exposure times to synthesize adequate vitamin D. My position here is that we have generally exhibited a knee-jerk, fear-based reaction to skin cancer dangers by viewing the sun as evil. I believe that you should obtain between 10 and 30 minutes every day (weather permitting and working up to longer exposure periods as the sunny season progresses) of direct sunlight exposure to at least 40 percent of your body. Just like with calories, your body is adept at soaking up rays and storing vitamin D for prolonged utilization when seasonal and climatic circumstances compromise your sun exposure.

How to Screen Your Opponent

If you find yourself spending more time than the general range required for healthy vitamin D synthesis, you should have a protection plan. Unfortunately, Conventional Wisdom lets us down again by touting sunscreen as a fail-safe method. Credible research has shown that most sunscreens have historically not blocked the UVA rays that cause melanoma. This may have resulted in millions staying in the sun too long simply because their skin wasn't burning from the blocked UVB rays. Had they used no sunscreen at all, at least they would have known enough to get out of the sun when they got a little pink. And in the case of skin cancer susceptibility, genetics does play a significant role. Those with fair skin, red or blond hair, and light eyes or those with numerous moles are six times more likely to develop melanoma than those with darker features. Some researchers even believe that excessive exposure of the skin to swimming pool chlorine is a bigger risk factor for melanoma than ultraviolet sunlight.

Furthermore, many of the popular agents used in sunblock products may have toxic properties, especially when you consider the standard recommendation to reapply these synthetic chemicals frequently to your porous skin. Octyl methoxycinnamate (OMC), a chemical contained in 90 percent of sunscreen products, could damage living tissue if it penetrates your outer layer of dead skin. Titanium dioxide, another popular sunscreen compound, has been named a "potential occupational carcinogen" by the U.S. government due to unclear toxic danger.

Hence, if you must be out in the sun for extended periods of time, it is far preferable to use clothing, especially technical fabrics touted as providing extra sun protection, to minimize your exposure to harmful UVA rays—and to prevent burning. There are numerous apparel brands touting enhanced SPF (sun protection factor) effectiveness; search the Internet or visit a high-quality specialty sports store to find some. If you are partial to good ol' cotton, realize that it, too, will offer significant SPF effectiveness. Examining your skin after a day in the sun to make sure it's not burned will reveal just how well your clothing protects you. As a backup to clothing protection, use a premium sunscreen that protects against UVA, UVB, and the newly described UVC rays, such as Neutrogena's Helioplex or an opaque zinc-based cream that blocks all rays entirely.

If you are concerned about getting overheated by clothing, it's interesting to note that participants in the Badwater 146-mile footrace across Death Valley in the middle of summer (definitely a non-*Primal Blueprint* approved event!) dress from head to toe in loose-fitting white garments. While it might take a little getting used to, light white clothing has been scientifically proven to keep your skin and core temperature cooler than letting your skin glisten in the sun.

Look on the Bright Side

Beyond exposing yourself sensibly and being careful always to use protection (can you believe I slipped that line past my editors?!), the high antioxidant values obtained when you eat *Primal Blueprint* style, combined with the use of potent antioxidant supplements, can also go a long, long way toward reducing or eliminating any damage caused by sun exposure.

> *The high antioxidant values obtained when you eat Primal Blueprint style, combined with the use of potent antioxidant supplements, can go a long, long way toward reducing or eliminating any damage caused by sun exposure.*

On the flip side, a bad diet could be an even more profound risk factor than sun exposure for skin cancer. Research published by the National Academy of Sciences indicates that a healthy dietary omega-6:omega-3 ratio is critical to skin cancer prevention. As we have already learned, eating a diet heavy in processed foods can produce obscene ratios of 20:1 through 50:1, instead of the 4:1 or less omega-6:omega-3 ratio that can be achieved with a *Primal Blueprint* eating style of natural animal meats, vegetables, and fruits—and some prudent omega-3 supplementation. As we also learned previously, an unhealthy imbalance of fatty acid ratios in your diet has been known to exacerbate the growth of tumors and other inflammation-related health conditions.

Reflecting on the big picture of genetics, lifestyle practices, and corresponding health risks, we are sometimes led astray from common sense by looking at isolated examples of people who defy the odds and experience unpredictable results—both positive and negative. Yes, there are health freaks eating optimal diets with good family histories who will inexplicably get cancer, but this is not a logical argument against living a clean life. Also, upon deeper examination, sometimes "inexplicable" becomes clearer. A dark-featured person who avoids sunlight yet contracts skin cancer might be a victim of vitamin D deficiency and an imbalance of fatty acids in the diet more so than simply random bad luck. What about the hard-living, inactive characters who make it to a ripe-old age on processed foods, tobacco, and alcohol? Could it be that they simply got enough sunlight and handled stress particularly well?

In summary, make a concerted effort to obtain a sensible amount of sunlight every single day. If your pigmentation or environment makes you particularly sensitive to the dangers of excessive sun exposure, cover up your skin with protective clothing after you obtain direct rays to a significant percentage of your body (and eat lots of fruits and vegetables!). Sunburned skin is your benchmark to avoid excessive exposure.

Primal Blueprint Law #9: Avoid Stupid Mistakes

Despite common Fred Flintstone-like depictions, early man was far from a numbskull. Grok was most certainly attuned to his surroundings and was skillful in his ability to avoid making mistakes or getting into situations likely to endanger health. This common faulty assumption that our hunter-gatherer ancestors

> *I drive way too fast to worry about cholesterol.*
> —**Author Unknown**

lived "solitary, poor, nasty, brutish and short" lives (as described in the "state of nature" theory advanced by 17th-century English philosopher Thomas Hobbes, when he argued for the need to have government structure in civilization instead of living off the land hunter-gatherer style) has always bugged me.

Research suggests that Grok and his family were actually generally healthy (robust is the apropos term), productive, and so appreciative of their lives that they felt the need to express themselves through art. There may even have been a selective benefit within tribal units for grandparents—meaning that getting older may have actually had an evolutionary advantage (babysitting or the transfer of important knowledge and history, for example) far past procreating.

So, if they were so robust and if our genes truly evolved to allow us—and possibly even encourage us—to live long lives, then why was the average life span relatively short? I had always assumed that it was things like deaths during childbirth, infections, accidental poisoning, even tribal warfare that brought the average life span down. But then I got a real-life experience of what might have affected life span more than anything else. Far from nasty and brutish, it was the mundane lapses in judgment, even minor ones, that likely spelled doom for many primal humans.

My unusually bad dive during an Ultimate match in September 2007 resulted in a torn quadriceps muscle, displaced kneecap, ruptured prepatellar bursa, and smashed nerve. An X-ray revealed no other tendon or ligament damage, and my orthopedist said the soft-tissue injury would heal in 12 weeks. He advised me to use pain as my guide and come back slowly. Because I had no pain at all (smashed nerve, remember?), I felt like I was recovering quickly. I even resumed my beach sprints in early December, followed by a snowboarding trip over Christmas break. But despite wrapping the knee every day and taking it fairly easy (wink, wink—and again no pain), I came home with a very swollen, black-and-blue knee. By the end of the week, I was unable to bend it more than a few degrees. An MRI revealed a large organized hematoma over the quad and kneecap that needed to be removed surgically. During surgery, it was discovered that the original torn quad muscle had never repaired itself and was leaking blood into the space, causing the hematoma. So my surgeon removed the hematoma and stitched the quad back to the patellar tendon.

Here I was, 54 years old, with the body of a 25-year-old and the mind of a 17-year-old, looking forward to living well past 100, but I was effectively incapacitated for more than four months by an injury caused by a random fall. (Truth be told, I had second thoughts as soon as I jumped.) Of course, I had the luxury of modern surgical procedures to repair the damage and eventually recovered fully. Had this happened 10,000 years ago, my inability to run away from a predator might well have spelled the end for me—all because of a momentary lapse of judgment. Even today, a small accident that active younger folks barely sneeze at (e.g., a fall from a ladder while hanging the holiday lights or turning an ankle on a staircase) can mean something entirely different for someone elderly and sedentary (such as a fatal case of pneumonia contracted while "recuperating" in bed).

The Darwin Awards—Long Live Natural Selection

As society continues to modernize exponentially, we arguably exhibit less and less common sense in avoiding stupid mistakes. I believe part of the reason is that deep down, we know we can afford to make them. Our intricate system of safety nets in modern society has compromised our capacity to take responsibility for our role in the "accidents" that occur and are chronicled by the news media seemingly every single day. Look no further than YouTube or Jackass television reruns to confirm that we are actively inviting unnecessary struggle and suffering into our lives—all in the name of expressing the youthful sense of adventure that has been stifled by the constraints and predictability of the modern world. The "Darwin Awards" satirical book and Web site annually bestow special distinction on those who, with particular brilliance, "improve the gene pool by removing themselves from it." Here are some of my favorite recent winners:

Hot Rod: A Texas motorist spilled a gas can in the back of his car. While searching for the can at night, he flicked on a cigarette lighter to get a better view, igniting the vehicle.

Nacho Libre: A Pennsylvania man was critically injured when he crashed his motorcycle into a telephone pole—distracted by a plate of nachos on his lap.

CSI—Alternate Ending: A police officer in Illinois was trying to show another patrolman how a fellow officer had accidentally killed himself. While reenacting the shooting from the previous week, he forgot to unload his gun and shot himself in the stomach. While driving himself to the hospital to seek treatment, he was killed in an auto accident.

Up, Up, and Away: A Catholic priest in Brazil attached a lawn chair to dozens of helium balloons and launched his homemade craft. Winds picked up and he drifted out to sea.

Well prepared for this potential adversity, he fired up his satellite phone to call for help but could not figure out how to operate his GPS unit to provide an accurate location for rescuers. Rescuers were unable to locate him—ever…although bits of balloon were found later on mountains and beaches.

Off the Falls: A man attempted to pilot a rocket-boosted jet ski off the side of Niagara Falls. The idea was for the rocket to launch the jet ski beyond the danger of the falls and then deploy a parachute and float to safety. The damp air caused both the rocket and parachute to fail as he rode off the edge of the falls. Miraculously, he survived the 160-foot drop but drowned because he didn't know how to swim and was not wearing a life jacket.

Stupor Hero

A book I read recently, *Survive!: My Fight for Life in the High Sierra*, may hit closer to home than the more preposterous aforementioned examples. The story dramatizes a familiar modern paradox: we possess vast intelligence and technology to extricate ourselves from all kinds of trouble but lack the common sense to avoid it in the first place.

The book relates the story of author and pilot Peter DeLeo crashing his small plane during a winter sightseeing trip over rugged mountain terrain in the California Sierra. DeLeo left his two seriously injured comrades at the crash site and hiked 50 miles in 13 days to reach civilization—despite a broken leg, a torn shoulder, broken ribs, no food, and no navigation equipment. His survival instincts on the journey, which included several days of blizzard conditions, were remarkable. Each evening, he scavenged materials to bury himself in an elaborate shelter and then conducted intensive breathing exercises for hours to ward off potentially fatal hypothermia. He timed his hiking efforts by the weather, starting before sunrise to ensure crusty snow and ending at midday to allow adequate time to dry his clothes in the sun and avoid dehydration from overheating. DeLeo's awareness of his surroundings, expert risk management, and leveraging of natural resources would have made Grok proud.

Unfortunately, upon closer inspection, his heroics were severely tainted by scathing criticism from experienced pilots and wilderness experts. The official NTSB crash investigation concluded that pilot error was the cause of the accident (countering DeLeo's claim of "freak wind shears"). Lacking proper navigation charts aboard the plane (strike one if you're keeping score at home), he flew into a box canyon with an insufficiently powered plane (strike two), necessitating a forced crash landing. He had failed to file a flight plan at takeoff (strike three) or inform anyone of even a general travel plan (strike four), and he failed to have a fully functional emergency transmitter aboard the plane (strike five, you're out—even in T-ball!). These oversights critically delayed the rescue effort; DeLeo's two friends were dead when he led rescuers back to the craft two weeks later.

Speaking of Darwin and the gene pool, DeLeo's brother participated in the rescue effort by impulsively jumping on his motorcycle and heading into the Sierra from Los Angeles. Gunning up a mountain pass, he snuck past a ranger who had ordered him to turn back, lifted his bike through the "closed for winter" barricade, and continued on until the road was impassable because of snow. He ditched his bike and wandered around on snowshoes looking for his brother for a while and then returned down the treacherous pass. During his descent, he slid on a patch of ice and was nearly pancaked by oncoming traffic.

> *Funny how some guys always find a way to crash and others [namely Armstrong] always find a way to win.*
> —*Martin Dugard*
> *Tour de France journalist*

Extending the lens wider, each of us must admit that we have brought various levels of misfortune and trauma into our lives from lapses in concentration or critical thinking. As we attempt to reflect on these stupid mistakes, often we default to blaming bad luck instead of reenacting the chain of events with a deep, honest assessment of our accountability. In fact, the concept of taking responsibility seems to have all but disappeared from modern life. If we truly deconstruct those times we have been the victim of circumstances, it's quite likely we can discover that exact moment when we were distracted, made a poor choice, or ignored the clear warning signal that might have helped us to avoid the entire incident.

Hypervigilance and Risk Management

As those who aspire to peak performance accumulate self-help libraries full of books on achieving financial freedom, implementing the latest winning management techniques, or mastering complex hobbies (e.g., golf, sailing, triathlon, or oil painting), it makes sense to add hypervigilance and risk management to the list of skills that require careful honing. These are innate skills that we all possess, and like any other skill—or muscle—we have to use and develop them or they will atrophy. Unfortunately, the obsessive effort society makes to diffuse all forms of risk and danger suppresses the use of these natural instincts: endless warning signs on roads and in public venues, warning labels on every consumer product, and sensationalized news reports about the dangers of shampoo, financial scammers, and kids' pajamas catching fire. Furthermore, continued technological innovations in the name of comfort and convenience collectively push us toward running on autopilot, often to our detriment, through various mundane elements of daily life.

In driving through Europe, I'm amused to note how few warnings and safety precautions are on the roadways. You can drive on narrow roads over treacherous alpine passes and find no guardrails, minimal road striping, and only an occasional small sign designating a tight turn, an avalanche danger, or a reduced speed zone. You have utter chaos in many big cities with raw aggression routinely winning out over traffic lights, signage, or the use of turn signals—but cars still seem to reach their destination safely. In contrast, take a spin through the canyons near my home and you will see miles upon miles of sturdy guardrails and endless diamond-shaped yellow signs with admonitions and icons warning you of assorted dangers that lurk around every corner. Nevertheless, every year tragedy strikes our local community with fatal accidents (typically induced by alcohol and/or speeding) on these obsessively protected roads.

Meanwhile, the historic traffic fatality rates in France, Germany, Great Britain, Switzerland, and Scandinavia—per capita and per vehicle miles driven—are significantly lower than those of the United States. Interestingly, some progressive traffic engineers, in the U.S. and abroad, are popularizing the concept of "shared space" as a tool to reduce accident rates. The concept relies on human instincts, such as eye contact, in favor of traditional traffic signals and signs (e.g., the removal of bike lane striping on a roadway may actually make cycling safer by increasing driver vigilance). This seemingly counterintuitive concept speaks to the power of nurturing our natural instincts to navigate potentially hazardous situations effectively when we are not pacified by excessive safety measures.

Bart Knaggs, close friend and business manager of Lance Armstrong, was once asked what qualities set Lance apart from the competition. While many have read about Armstrong's superhuman cardiovascular system or superior killer instinct, Knaggs chose something more esoteric to highlight, calling attention to Lance's hypervigilance and risk-management skills in the context of the incredible complexity and strategic nature of Tour de France racing. On the bike, Lance's hypervigilance enables him to identify those competitors around him who zone out, even for a moment, and to attack (increase pace to break away from the pack, usually in the mountains) at the exact right times for success (over the course of Lance's seven Tour victories, the total time of these attacks amounted to mere minutes out of hundreds of hours of total competition time). Furthermore, Lance and his teammates' ability to constantly assess risk and manage it moment to moment prevent his competitors from turning the tables on him in a similar fashion.

One of Lance's most dramatic Tour moments came on a dangerous descent in 2003. Lance's chief rival crashed heavily and broke his hip. Lance, riding a few seconds behind, averted the crash site by swerving off the road, cutting across a steep hayfield, dismounting to jump over a ditch, and remounting beyond the crash site to carry on! Years later, Tour de France chronicler Martin Dugard wrote in an account of how a rider had suffered an improbable solo accident while wearing the yellow leader's jersey for the first time: "Funny how some guys always find a way to crash and others [namely Armstrong] always find a way to win."

As we strive to "find a way to win" in the game of life, we must respect the importance of holding that steering wheel and resisting the urge to flick the switch to autopilot. We must also be willing to take personal responsibility for our actions instead of defaulting to speed-dialing a personal injury attorney whenever we come to misfortune. If you were to get hit by a motorist running a red light, it would most certainly be his fault, but you may fare better on the road if you remember to fasten your seat belt and look for oncoming traffic before hitting the gas when your light turns green. Every time I encounter a dicey driving situation, I realize something upon further reflection when things calm down: whenever I mumble "asshole" to someone who has just cut me off, I should really be saying it to myself, too—for being in a rush, being too aggressive or impatient, or diverting my focus from the road momentarily. Maybe the motorists who incur my wrath deserve a little choice feedback, but I can find something I bring to the table most every time.

I can't remember if an errant throw or overly aggressive defensive play was involved in my Ultimate accident, as I prefer to focus on the fact that I hurled myself through the air irresponsibly and then tried to come back into action too quickly afterward. When I take responsibility for my actions, my misfortune becomes a growth experience—an appealing alternative to feeling like a victim or placing any importance on the notion of bad luck.

This theme also works in a discussion about dietary habits. You can blame lousy food options in airports, your distressing family medical history, or the limitations of your budget, but in each case you may be better served to accept some personal accountability. Take the extra time to pack healthy snacks for your travel. View your family history as a catalyst to cultivate hypervigilance and risk-management skills instead of as a curse. Take a deeper look at your lifestyle priorities, make some compromises, and stretch your food budget a bit to choose the very best of everything. In this way you can turn negatives into positives and create excellent leverage to be the best you can be, regardless of "bad luck" or other figments of your imagination that are vying for your attention. As my wife, Carrie, says, "They're all choices you can make whenever you want."

> *Everybody gets so much information all day long that they lose their common sense."*
> *—Gertrude Stein*
> *American author and French art patron*
> *(1874-1946)*

Primal Blueprint Law #10: Use Your Brain

Perhaps no other *Primal Blueprint* behavior has been as fundamental to the success of the human race as a devoted reliance on complex thought—working the brain just like a muscle. Hunter-gatherers all around the world developed language, tools, and superior hunting methods independently. Combined with optimum dietary choices (including high levels of healthy fat and protein), humans experienced a rapid increase in human brain size over just a few thousand generations (it should be noted that brain size has actually declined steadily in our recent history, something experts theorize was exacerbated by the dietary changes caused by the advent of agriculture and grain-based diets).

As discussed in the Avoid Stupid Mistakes section, we are experiencing some unfortunate regression in the simple, powerful *Primal Blueprint* behavior of using your brain. While the modern world features plenty of complex thought and a constant and rapid progression in human innovation—technological and otherwise—our overstimulated lifestyles compromise our ability to use our brains with maximum effectiveness. Even Albert Einstein was reputed to have once said, "I don't know my phone number because I can look it up easily in the phone book."

The fact that we are able to outsource brain function is not necessarily bad, but it does reveal that we are having trouble keeping up with today's information overload. In the workplace, the mismanagement of information overload from personal digital assistants (BlackBerry, iPhone, etc.), instant chat, and the like can stifle creativity and innovation, not to mention our levels of energy, motivation, and health. Consequently, many of us operate in a reactive mode, constantly and often futilely trying to keep pace with the information with which we are bombarded. In Mark Bauerlein's book *The Dumbest Generation*, he blames digital technology for compromising the intellectual development of young people. "When we were 17 years old, social life stopped at the front door. Now [via MySpace, Facebook, instant chat, texting, etc.] peer-to-peer contact…has no limitation in space or time," observes Bauerlein. Hence, time to read, daydream, free-associate, or gain an adequate understanding of current events, history, and other mainstays of cultural sophistication goes by the wayside.

The fallout from this cultural shift is difficult to quantify, but the story of our pilot friend offers an intriguing perspective. During his ordeal in the Sierra, DeLeo exhibited magnificent brain use; if he had shown anything short of brilliant creativity, innovation, gross and fine motor skills, mind-body connection, risk management, and hypervigilance, he would not have survived. However, his performance must be placed in the context of the incredibly poor brain function he exhibited to get himself into that mess in the first place. Similarly, we collectively do an exemplary job at consumerism, multitasking, and leveraging technological innovations, but the development and refining of these skills comes at the extreme cost of an unhealthy, imbalanced lifestyle.

If we examine the true definition of *stress* as "stimulus," it's clear that we require a certain amount of daily stress to thrive, prosper, and be happy. "Evolutionary Fitness" advocate Art Devany, Ph.D. (arthurdevany.com) draws a compelling link between exercising our minds and our genetic nature as free, independent, adventurous human beings. "Modern life leaves our minds restless and under-utilized because we are confined, inactive, and comfortable," Devany argues. "We cannot be satisfied with more and more, because we are evolved for another lifeway in which material goods do not matter. The result is that we are deeply unsatisfied with modern life and don't know why." It seems like our genes don't know what to make of all our "stuff."

At first glance, few might agree that our minds are restless and underutilized. Many of us end our days running on fumes, feeling like our minds will explode if we send or receive any more e-mail. Our minds are indeed overstressed, yet technically underutilized, because we lack the balance that creative intellectual outlets, play, healthy diet, exercise, sleep, and other winning behaviors promote. Eight hours of brain power is probably a sensible limit to devote to your daily work efforts. However, engaging your mind with things that stimulate your creativity in other ways and that you have a passion for is critical to mental health and overall well-being.

As we collectively pursue overly stressful, imbalanced lifestyles, the façade of retiring to a life of leisure has become entrenched in our society. Granted, no one would argue with the benefits of having financial independence versus trying to make ends meet every month, but beyond our economic circumstances we must consider what is truly healthy for our minds. A life of true leisure and ease does not represent the highest expression of your talents and therefore is psychologically unhealthy.

Robert Frank's book *Richistan—A Journey Through the American Wealth Boom* chronicles the challenges that trust-fund kids have navigating life with the unearned wealth that many experts argue is a disadvantage. Challenges with motivation, substance abuse, lack of connection or role modeling from busy/famous parents, and protecting or adding to their passive wealth are commonplace, thanks to the lack of perspective or compelling reason to apply themselves to the familiar challenges of obtaining an education and career through the competitive free market.

What if you won the lottery and had all the money you would ever need? How would your life change? I'm not talking about the observable change in your credit card balances or new toys in the driveway. I'm asking how you would spend your time. Would you really kick back on the beach in Maui for months on end? Would you cast aside your plain, average friends in favor of a new, exciting blue-blazered crowd from the country club? Or, when push came to shove, would you perhaps drift very close to what you are doing now—working with cherished colleagues, volunteering in school and community, and pursuing simple, inexpensive passions with family and friends?

Those who are content to punch the clock and skate along at bare minimum effort would be well served to look at what has happened to those who rest on their laurels throughout history. From failed ancient civilizations to today's too-comfortable middle manager or cocky eleventh grader dragging his heels on SAT prep and college applications, those who fail to exercise their creativity, imagination, and awareness will likely suffer not only from the high drama of defeat, failure, or physical trauma but also from that "restless mind" syndrome discussed previously.

> *A life of true leisure and ease does not represent the highest expression of your talents and therefore is psychologically unhealthy.*

Chapter Summary

1. Get Adequate Sleep: Despite being a critical component of good health and stress management, sleep is regularly compromised today due to the pull of technology and hectic schedules. Insufficient sleep can lead to numerous health problems and declines in cognitive function. Tips for optimum sleep include having a clutter-free bedroom, a calm, low-stimulation transition into bedtime, having consistent bed and wake times, and eating minimally (and consuming the right foods) in the hours before bed. Furthermore, occasional naps can produce many health benefits, including reduced risk of disease plus improvements to mood, concentration, and physical performance.

2. Play: The regimented nature of modern life leaves many adults—and even kids—deficient in play. The profound psychological benefits of play are integral to healthy cultures, communities, and individuals, including a direct relationship to work productivity. Pursue unstructured play opportunities—preferably physical play, which counters the negative effects of sedentary, technological existence—on a daily basis to manage stress and be happy.

3. Get Adequate Sunlight: A reasonable amount of daily sun exposure (depending on numerous variables, including skin pigment and climate) can produce numerous health benefits and alleviate many health risks, because it enables your body to synthesize optimal levels of vitamin D. The dangers of sun exposure are overdramatized and many even suffer from sun deficiency today. Risks of skin cancer are greatly minimized if you avoid sunburn and eat a high-antioxidant diet. Clothing is the best protection, as sunscreens have some health objections and may be less effective than advertised.

4. Avoid Stupid Mistakes: Avoiding stupid mistakes was a critical survival factor for Grok, because margin for error was much lower. Today, modern life attempts to shield us from all manner of danger, yet—possibly desensitized by all these protection mechanisms—we still seem to find a way to invite trauma and tragedy into our lives by making stupid mistakes. We must practice our hardwired, evolution-perfected skills of hypervigilance and risk management to navigate successfully through even the seemingly mundane elements of daily life to avoid unnecessary suffering and ensure longevity.

5. Use Your Brain: Human innovation and overstimulation have compromised our ability to use our brains to maximum effectiveness. We must exert great discipline to leverage technology to our advantage instead of fall victim to it by spacing out, burning out, or otherwise misusing our greatest weapon as human beings: complex thought. Pursue new challenges, such as music, language, hobbies, or adventures, that stimulate your brain and allow you to depart from your daily routine.

CHAPTER 8

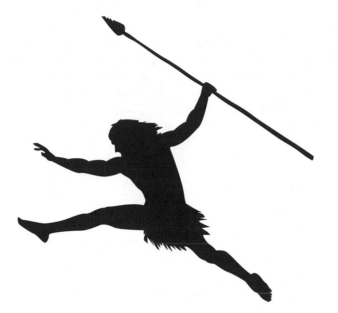

A Primal Approach to Weight Loss

"A Primal Breakfast, a Primal Lunch, and a Sensible Primal Dinner"

In This Chapter

I provide a detailed step-by-step process for losing an average of one to two pounds of body fat per week. You'll learn how to target protein, carb, and fat intake specifically in order to ramp up fat metabolism, maintain high dietary satisfaction levels, and avoid the risk of depleting muscle tissue and suffering from the typical rebound-rebellion effect of severe caloric restriction. I discuss how deregulating food intake and fasting intermittently can be effective calorie-restriction tools and how exercise can support and accelerate progress toward your body composition goals.

I review two weight-loss case studies (Ken and Kelly Korg, naturally!), calculating their average daily caloric expenditure and optimal daily intake of each macronutrient—*Primal Blueprint* style—to produce effortless fat loss. We'll examine a daily food journal for each of them, featuring delicious, nutritious Primal meals. The journals contain detailed caloric analysis' and macronutrient breakdowns for each meal plus daily totals. The case studies result in a loss of eight pounds for Ken and 7.75 pounds for Kelly in a single month. Finally, I provide troubleshooting tips for possible setbacks and plateaus that arise for people when trying to lose weight in the real world.

I asked the clothing store clerk if she had anything to make me look thinner, and she said, "How about a week in Bangladesh?"

—**Roseanne Barr**

These are the critical elements of the *Primal Blueprint* weight-loss approach:

Minimize carb intake to control insulin production and enable stored body fat to be burned for energy.

Optimize protein intake to preserve energy levels and maintain or increase muscle mass while you exercise.

Optimize fat intake to achieve high satiety levels, provide energy, and eliminate hunger.

Engage in occasional Intermittent Fasting (I.F.) and deregulated meal habits to produce accelerated caloric deficits that lead to greater fat loss.

Engage in a Primal Blueprint–style exercise program that fine-tunes your fat metabolism, builds/tones lean muscle, and accelerates body composition improvements without exhausting you.

Avoid excessive regimentation or results obsession in favor of a long-term perspective. Assess results monthly and don't worry about daily calorie counting or frequent scale measurements.

Lose a pound or two of fat a week just by following the incredibly reasonable, flexible, and simple *Primal Blueprint* laws detailed in this book—can it be this easy? Let's not mince words here. The science of reducing stored body fat requires you to burn more calories than you consume. Unless you plan to lose water and muscle tissue (and I know you don't), losing one to two pounds of fat per week (your personal maximum rate within this range depends on your existing body weight, metabolic rate, and activity level) means an average daily deficit of 500 to 1,000 calories. It's just unrealistic to lose weight safely any quicker than that without depleting muscle mass or becoming fatigued.

It's also a truth of homeostasis and evolution combined with the abundance of modern life that it's easier to pack on excess weight than burn it off. (We've fine-tuned our Grok-like ability to store excess calories!) So, now that you know the science of how the body stores and/or burns fat, it's a simple matter of executing the right strategy.

The good news here is that when you do reach your desired body composition, all you have to do to maintain it is reasonably control carbohydrate intake to average 100 to 150 grams per day. Then, even if you consume excess protein and fat calories, your body will simply ramp up its metabolism enough to burn off extra fuel. This will happen in numerous ways. Your brain, enjoying stable blood sugar levels and optimal hormone balance, will inspire you to be more active, both consciously (through more spirited workouts, for example) and subconsciously (with a generally more energetic pace through your day). Your core temperature will rise slightly (through increased internal cellular activity), and you will even experience increased energy dissipation in the mitochondria within each of your cells.

Primal Blueprint–style eating allows you to eat more calories than a restrictive diet yet be far more successful losing body fat. This seemingly illogical claim has played out in numerous studies where control groups ate the same number of calories and had the same activity level but ate different kinds of foods. The disparate results achieved were attributed to what scientists call a *metabolic advantage* provided by eating certain foods (namely, those that moderate insulin production).

The idea is to hit the sweet spot where carbs have been reduced just enough so that your body prefers to burn fats and a moderate amount of ketones instead of relying so much on glucose. This carbohydrate sweet spot is 50 to 100 grams per day for most people, with the range depending on your size, age, sex, and metabolism. Consume more carbs than that (up to 150 grams a day) and you'll maintain weight quite easily without gaining, but you'll have to work a little harder to burn it off. On the other hand, it's certainly healthy to take in less than 50 grams per day of carbs once in a while (as I discussed in Chapter 3, you could live on zero carbs for a long time), but the idea is to stay just on the fringe of ketosis. In the sweet spot, you will maintain high energy levels (no more insulin crashes), you can exercise (including regular intense sessions) and recover without getting exhausted, and you won't exhibit any of the unpleasant byproducts of severely carb-restrictive diets that put you in full-on ketosis. These include the annoying "ketone breath," insufficient vitamin/mineral intake (due to the severe restriction of vegetables and fruits), and poor compliance due to the deprivation and inconvenience involved in trying to bottom out on carb intake.

Weight-Loss Macronutrient Plan

For those of you seeking detailed, quantifiable guidelines for your caloric intake, you can follow this simple formula that begins with obtaining a calculable level of protein sufficient to preserve lean muscle mass, strictly limiting carbs to an average of 50 to 100 per day, and using fat as the main variable to obtain your daily caloric needs.

To ensure your success and comfort during the fat-reduction period, please make an extra effort to have appropriate Primal snacks available at all times. These include low-glycemic carbs (e.g., berries or crunchy vegetables) and foods high in protein and/or fat (nuts, seeds, trail mix, meat, cheese, etc.). If you experience some difficulty transitioning over from a carb-dependent diet to *Primal Blueprint* eating, grabbing a handful of nuts, a stick of beef jerky, or a hard-boiled egg when you get hungry can make all the difference in the world.

Protein

As you learned already, you need an average of 0.7 to one gram per pound of lean body weight per day to repair, build, and/or maintain lean muscle mass effectively and to adequately support numerous other metabolic functions dependent upon dietary protein. I like to calculate the average over a time period of at least four days (this is easy to do with an online calculator, such as found at FitDay.com) to account for the natural variance of your daily eating habits and activity level.

For an active female (1.0 factor) with 100 pounds of lean body mass, this is only 400 protein calories per day. For an active male with 150 pounds of lean body mass, this amounts to only 600 protein calories per day. Coupling protein minimums with our strict limitations on carbohydrates (at 50 to 100 grams per day during the fat-loss phase, even the male is under 1,000 calories per day before considering fat intake), it's easy to see how you can reduce body fat at an accelerated rate. Furthermore, you can lose weight aggressively without the deprivation commonly associated with weight-loss efforts. With the *Primal Blueprint* weight-loss approach, you can sensibly enjoy rich, satisfying high-fat foods that will eliminate the slightest feelings of deprivation. While the "eating fat is okay for weight loss" idea might seem contradictory at first glance, it is valid; without insulin, eating fat will not make you fat!

Keep in mind I'm not asking you to undergo an expensive underwater body composition test to pinpoint your lean body mass and then carry around a calculator to nail your exact protein requirements every day. Your appetite will guide you effectively to meet your protein requirements, just as your thirst does for hydration requirements. That said, if you experience low energy or a reduction in muscle mass, you may want to delve further into just what you are eating to be sure the levels are in proper range. Jot down everything you eat for a few days, and then use a food calculator to determine how many grams of the various macronutrients you are consuming. I've provided some suggested meals with detailed nutrient breakdowns in this chapter to give you a feel for how healthy and satisfying the *Primal Blueprint* weight-loss plan can be.

Carbohydrate

Limiting your average carb intake to 50 to 100 grams per day will effectively moderate your insulin production and optimize your fat-burning process. At this level of carbohydrate intake, your body will be stimulated to burn more stored fats and manufacture a little extra glucose in the liver through gluconeogenesis. In this case, however, dietary protein will provide the substrate for gluconeogenesis instead of your precious muscle tissue, which I have discussed as a bad thing in the context of the fight-or-flight response (triggered by Chronic Cardio or a protein-deficient extreme diet).

As an added benefit of this process, your liver will generate a moderate level of ketones that will help spare muscle tissue and provide added fuel for cells that might otherwise require glucose. Hence, limiting your carbs to well under 100 grams per day will put you in a very mild (and desirable, because you'll be burning fat like crazy) state of ketosis. If your batting average drifts above 100, your blood glucose levels will start to redirect energy pathways more toward glucose burning. I'm not asking you to split your carrot sticks down the middle nor to skimp on salad portions to stay under 100 grams. As you can see from this chapter's examples, you can still enjoy abundant servings of vegetables and ample servings of fruit (nutrient-dense foods that are particularly important to consume when you are restricting calories and exercising diligently) and land in the optimum range for insulin control and weight loss. The key to meeting this seemingly strict guideline effortlessly is to virtually eliminate processed carbs from your diet—then it's truly a breeze.

Really, It's All About the Carbohydrate Curve

As you learned when the Carbohydrate Curve was introduced in Chapter 3, your body composition success is overwhelmingly dependent on controlling your carbohydrate intake and, hence, your insulin output. Exercising correctly, managing your stress levels, and genetics are minor factors in the equation. Your failure to maintain desirable body composition may be related to one of several things—unlucky genetics, an overly stressful exercise program, insufficient sleep, self-destructive eating and lifestyle behaviors, a sedentary existence, and more—but an excess body fat condition almost always includes excessive carbohydrate intake.

Limit your carbohydrate intake to 100 to 150 grams per day (depending on size and gender) and you will not store more fat (unless you have a severe overeating problem…but even then it will be hard!). Limit your carbohydrate intake to 50 to 100 grams or less per day and you will begin to lose stored body fat. Your rate of fat loss will also be affected by your exercise efforts, sensible eating of healthy fats and protein, and, lastly, genetic factors. Here again is the Carbohydrate Curve and the general effects that various levels of average daily carbohydrate intake have on your body.

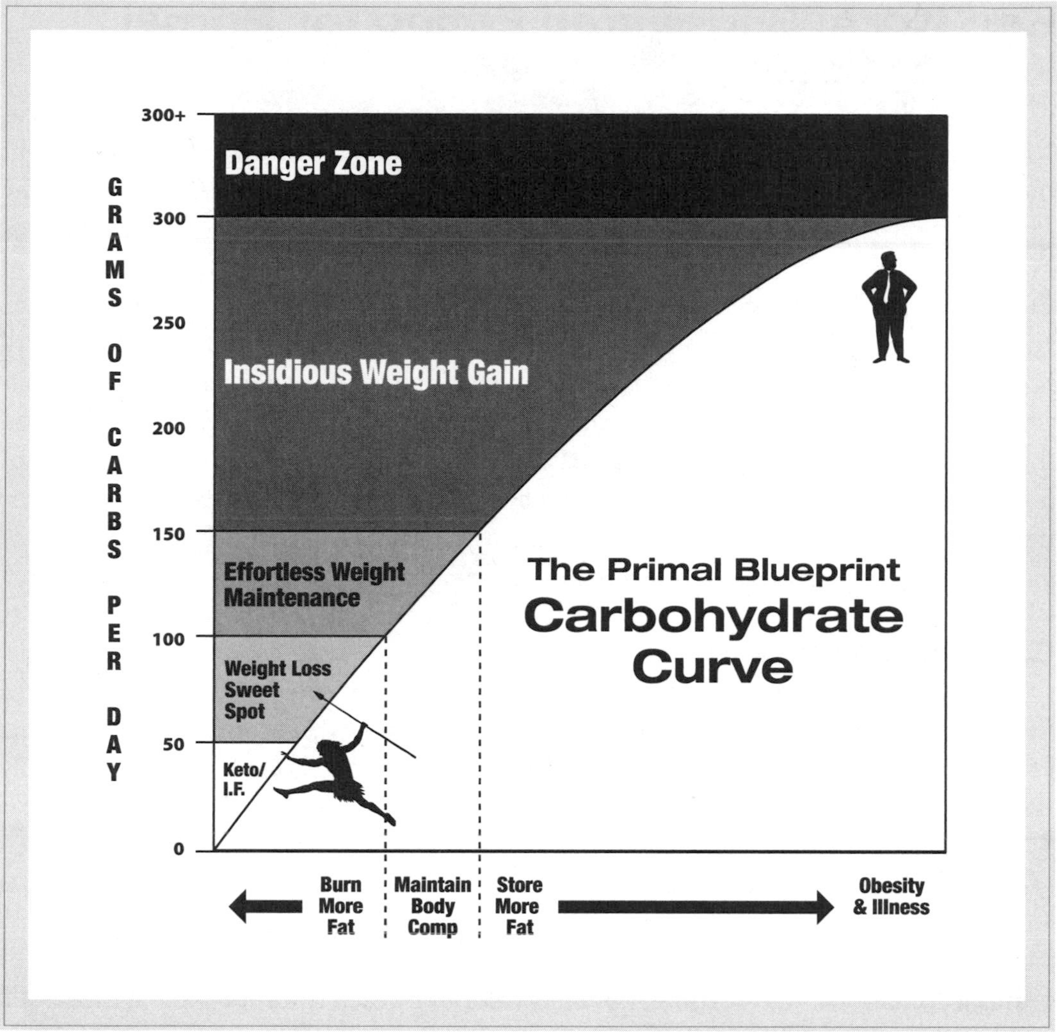

300+
Danger Zone
GRAMS OF CARBS PER DAY
300
250
Insidious Weight Gain
200
150
Effortless Weight Maintenance
100
Weight Loss Sweet Spot
50
Keto/ I.F.
0
The Primal Blueprint
Carbohydrate Curve
Burn More Fat
Maintain Body Comp
Store More Fat
Obesity & Illness

Fat

The variable for your energy needs and total calorie consumption is fat. If you are committed to success, you will make a concerted effort to eat only what you need to feel satisfied and energized. Because fat has such a high satiety factor, a little will go a long way. Even something like a handful of nuts can sustain you for hours when you skip meals or need an easy snack to keep you going. With the right meal choices and healthy snacks around, your intensive weight-loss experience will not involve the typical struggling and suffering of a "diet." After you reduce the amount of body fat you desire, you can consume even more liberal amounts of fat without worrying about gaining weight.

Ken Korg: Suggested Eating for Primal Weight Loss

Let's look at a case study of our old friend Ken Korg, a 40-year-old, five-foot-eleven, 197-pound, moderately active male with 25 percent body fat who wants to lose weight aggressively (near the maximum suggested rate of two pounds per week) following the *Primal Blueprint*. We'll calculate Ken's estimated daily caloric expenditure and suggested macronutrient intake based on *Primal Blueprint* guidelines. Then, I'll present a list of suggested meals and snacks with accompanying macronutrient analysis. The day's example will show how Ken can enjoy sensible, satisfying meals and snacks and still achieve a dramatic improvement in body composition by meeting the average macronutrient guidelines for a single month. Throughout these examples, remember to focus on the concept of *averages*. While it's instructive to examine a detailed daily example of both expenditure and intake to understand how we can properly achieve caloric deficits, in reality you will have days where you exceed your carb limit, fall short of your protein limit, and exercise more or less than the averages in our calculations.

Caloric Expenditure

The basal metabolic rate (BMR) estimates were derived using a BMR calculator (many are available on the Internet, such as one at bmi-calculator.net). BMR factors your age and weight to estimate the number of calories your body burns if you simply stay in bed all day. An Activity Factor adding additional calories to the daily estimate is derived using the Harris Benedict Formula (also available at bmi-calculator.net), which takes into account various typical levels of activity. You can input your personal variables and generate similar estimates for total daily caloric expenditure.

1. **Basal Metabolic Rate:** Number of daily calories burned to support basal metabolic functions = 1,923.

2. **Activity Factor:** Harris Benedict Formula for additional calories burned when "moderately active." This represents a *Primal Blueprint* exercise routine of two hours per week of low-level cardio; one or two intense workouts of 10 to 30 minutes each, strength or sprinting, per week. BMR × 0.55 = 1,057.

3. **Total Average Daily Calorie Expenditure:** BMR (1,923) + Activity Factor (1,057) = 2,980

Macronutrient Calculations

- 197 pounds at 25 percent body fat = 148 pounds of lean body mass
- Moderately active = 0.7 factor for protein intake per pound of lean body mass
- 148 pounds × 0.7 = 104 grams of average daily protein intake (Combine this with a carb intake target of 75 grams, and you have only 716 calories before considering fat intake.)
- Goal of losing 8 pounds per month = 932 calories per day average caloric deficit
- Desired average caloric intake per day = 2,048 (2,980 average caloric expenditure less 932 deficit)
- Desired protein grams = 104 (416 calories)
- Desired carb grams = 75 (300 calories)
- Desired fat grams = 148 (1,332 calories)

You can see right away that the diet will not be difficult for Ken to follow, as that number of fat calories will provide ample energy and extensive satiety at each meal, while the number of protein grams will ensure that his body recovers from exercise stress and continues to burn at the average caloric expenditure of 2,980 calories—or higher. In his past dieting efforts, Ken tried to cut back on calories in general, slightly reducing normal intake of fat, protein, and carbs. More likely, he probably made a little extra effort to cut back on fatty foods but was not nearly diligent enough with carbs and possibly compromised some lean body mass (depending on how devoted his efforts were) by falling short of protein requirements.

Each time he tried to lose this way in the past, Ken's energy and exercise level declined slightly but insulin was still prevalent to drive consumed calories into fat cells. Hence, his body fat percentage has drifted upward for years to reach the current 25 percent, despite repeated half-hearted and misguided efforts to reduce. Let's see how the results can differ when eating *Primal Blueprint* style.

Food Journal

Breakfast

"Mark's Primal Omelet"
Eggs (three medium) with cream (1 ounce) and shredded cheddar cheese (1 tablespoon)
Chopped mushrooms, red onions, and red peppers (1/4 cup of each)
Topped with sliced avocado (2 ounces) and fresh salsa (2 tablespoons)
Fresh blueberries (1/4 cup)
Cup of black coffee

FitDay.com Analysis
Total Calories: 463
Protein: 23 grams, 89 calories (19 percent)
Carbs: 22 grams, 82 calories (18 percent)
Fat: 33 grams, 292 calories (63 percent)

continued

Food Journal (continued)

Lunch

"Mark's Primal Salad"
Mixed salad greens (2 cups)
Chopped onions, carrots, jicama, red peppers, and cherry tomatoes (2 ounces each)
Chopped or shredded chicken (3 ounces)
Sesame seeds (1/3 ounce)
Chopped walnuts (1/2 ounce or 7 halves)
Oil-based dressing (2 tablespoons)

FitDay.com Analysis
Total Calories: 585
Protein: 31 grams, 124 calories (21 percent)
Carbs: 30 grams, 120 calories (21 percent)
Fat: 38 grams, 341 calories (56 percent)

Dinner

Salmon and Vegetables
Broiled wild salmon (6 ounces)
Steamed asparagus and zucchini (6 ounces each) with butter (1 tablespoon)
Red wine (5-ounce glass)

FitDay.com Analysis
Total Calories: 560
Protein: 39 grams, 157 calories (28 percent)
Carbs: 16 grams, 63 calories (11 percent)
Fat: 26 grams, 232 calories (41 percent)
Alcohol: 16 grams, 108 calories (21 percent)

Snacks

Hard-boiled egg
Macadamia nuts (1-1/2 ounces or 17 nuts)
Venison jerky (one 4-inch strip)

FitDay.com Analysis
Total Calories: 437
Protein: 14 grams, 58 calories (16 percent)
Carbs: 8 grams, 32 calories (7 percent)
Fat: 41 grams, 347 calories (79 percent)

Daily Totals

Calories: 2,045
Protein: 107 grams, 428 calories (21 percent)
Carbs: 78 grams, 297 calories (15 percent)
Fat: 139 grams, 1,212 calories (59 percent)
Alcohol: 16 grams, 108 calories (5 percent)

Caloric deficit from average daily expenditure (2,980) = 935
Projected net fat loss over 30-day period: **8 pounds**

To make up for the caloric intake deficit, Ken will derive his additional 935 daily calories from stored body fat, thanks to Grok passing that ability on to him. He is now using the same fat-burning mechanism as his primary means of getting through the day, instead of his previous roller coaster of carbs, caffeine, insulin, cortisol, fatigue, and insufficient exercise.

You Won't Believe What's Primal!

The diary entries for Ken and Kelly illustrate the concept that *Primal Blueprint* weight loss does not have to be a Spartan exercise of weighing and measuring bland food, choking down powdered replacements for real food, or otherwise engaging in repetitive, restrictive eating habits. While the rules of *Primal Blueprint* macronutrient intake are clear-cut, there is tremendous opportunity for flexibility within these guidelines. At MarksDailyApple.com, we have hundreds of recipes, shopping tips, and detailed meal-planning strategies that will help you actually enjoy the process of eating healthy, perhaps to an even greater extent than you did your pre-Primal dietary habits. Take a glance at this list of recipes that are posted on the site—yep, they're all *Primal Blueprint* approved!

> *Ken is now using fat metabolism as his primary means of getting through the day, instead of his previous roller coaster of carbs, caffeine, insulin, cortisol, fatigue, and insufficient exercise.*

Arugula Endive Salad with White Wine Vinaigrette

Spicy Thai Coconut Soup

Broiled Halibut with Garlic Aioli and Steamed Broccoli

Crustless Quiche with Spinach and Scallions

Baked Mahimahi with Pesto and Tomatoes

Grilled Flank Steak with Sauteed Beet Greens and Creamy Horseradish Beets

Smoked Salmon with Asparagus and Poached Egg

Spicy Korean Seaweed Salad with Shrimp

Sauteed Broccoli Rabe with Sundried Tomatoes and Pine Nuts

Kelly Korg: Suggested Eating for Primal Weight Loss

Now let's examine a program Kelly Korg, our 40-year-old, five-foot-four, 148-pound, very active female with 27 percent body fat, would follow using the *Primal Blueprint*. While her goal of losing nearly eight pounds of body fat in a single month is ambitious for a female, she is fit enough to tolerate a pretty ambitious exercise schedule and create substantial caloric deficits with sensible *Primal Blueprint* meals. She will actually reduce her total weekly exercise hours and corresponding calories burned in favor of a more sensible program with slower-paced cardio, more rest, and shorter-duration intense workouts.

Caloric Expenditure

1. Basal Metabolic Rate: Number of calories burned to support basal metabolic functions = 1,411.

2. Activity Factor: Harris Benedict Formula for additional calories burned when "very active." This represents a *Primal Blueprint* four hours per week of low-level cardio; three intense workouts of 10 to 30 minutes each, strength or sprinting, per week BMR × 0.725 = 1,023.

3. Total Average Daily Calorie Expenditure: BMR (1,411) + Activity Factor (1,023) = 2,433

Macronutrient Calculations

- 148 pounds at 27 percent body fat = 102 pounds of lean body mass
- 1.0 factor for protein intake per pound lean body mass (due to high stress levels and history of exhaustive exercise requiring more protein per pound than a moderately active person like her husband)
- 102 pounds lean mass = 102 grams of average daily protein intake
- Goal of losing 7.66 pounds of body fat per month = 894 per day average caloric deficit
- Desired average caloric intake per day = 1,539 (2,433 average caloric expenditure less 894 deficit)
- Desired protein grams = 110 (408 calories)
- Desired carb grams = 79 (316 calories)
- Desired fat grams = 91 (816 calories)

You can see right away that the diet will be much more pleasant for Kelly to follow than were her previous efforts to severely restrict calories interspersed with inevitable carb binges. The fat calories will provide extensive satiety at each meal (missing from her last diet, which featured heavily processed, insulin-stimulating liquid shakes). The protein calories will ensure that her body recovers from exercise stress and also maintains and even builds some attractive lean muscle tissue and that her metabolic rate stabilizes at 2,433 calories daily.

Food Journal

Breakfast

Steak and Fruit
Flank steak (4 ounces)
Blueberries (1/2 cup)
Peach (1/2 of whole)
Green tea (1 cup)

FitDay.com Analysis
Total Calories: 238
Protein: 25.0 grams, 106 calories
  (44 percent)
Carbs: 15.7 grams, 56 calories (24 percent)
Fat: 8.5 grams, 76 calories (32 percent)

Lunch

Chicken Club Lettuce Wrap
Lettuce (3 large leaves)
Diced cooked chicken (4 ounces)
Sliced red pepper (1/2 cup)
Plum tomato (1 medium)
Avocado (1/2 of whole)
Mayonnaise (1 teaspoon)

Total Calories: 397
Protein: 38.5 grams, 159 calories
  (40 percent)
Carbs: 17.2 grams, 62 calories (14 percent)
Fat: 20.5 grams, 176 calories (44 percent)

Dinner

Beef Stir-Fry
Sliced beef steak (4 ounces)
Olive oil (2 tablespoons)
Sliced zucchini (1 medium)
Sliced mushrooms (1 cup)
Spinach (1 cup)
Sliced bamboo shoots (1/2 cup)
Sesame seeds (1/4 ounce)

FitDay.com Analysis
Total Calories: 611
Protein: 37.6 grams, 150 calories
  (25 percent)
Carbs: 9.5 grams, 35 calories (6 percent)
Fat: 48.1 grams, 426 calories (70 percent)

Snacks

Hard-boiled egg (1 large)
Apple (1 large)
Almond butter (1 tablespoon; spread
  on apple)

FitDay.com Analysis
Total Calories: 283
Protein: 9.3, 35 calories (13 percent)
Carbs: 33.1 grams, 121 calories,
  (43 percent)
Fat: 14.8 grams, 127 calories (45 percent)

Daily Totals

Calories: 1,529
Protein: 110.4 grams, 450 calories (29 percent)
Carbs: 75.5 grams, 274 calories (18 percent)
Fat: 91.9 grams, 805 calories (53 percent)

Caloric deficit from average daily
expenditure (2,433) = 904
Projected net fat loss over 30-day
period: **7.75 pounds**

How to Lose Like a Winner

You cannot realistically (or safely) lose any more than a pound or two a week of body fat. This is evident when you consider that one pound of fat contains 3,500 calories and adults only burn between 1,500 to 3,000 total calories per day. What about the "Biggest Losers" glorified on the television program, or in before-and-after magazine contests, who alter their body composition dramatically in a short time (and do so "safely" under professional supervision)? These results are achieved with a combination of incredibly intense exercise coupled with severe caloric restriction, an approach that is simply inhumane and impossible to follow long-term.

Any extreme stress (including a crash weight-loss program) prompts a fight-or-flight response in your body. Buzzed on adrenalin, you can triumphantly complete your six-, eight-, or twelve-week program (particularly when the bright lights of television and monetary incentives are there to motivate you). At some point afterward, you are likely to collapse in exhaustion when the fight-or-flight response wears off and your body's energy reserves are depleted. In this "post-traumatic stress" state, many become sedentary (or much less active, in any case) and tend to overeat—a genetically programmed reaction to an ordeal perceived as a starvation threat. Lo and behold, the "before-and-after" ideal typically becomes a "before, after and back-to-before…and then some" reality. There is absolutely no reason to have to struggle or suffer to achieve your body composition and health goals. In fact, if you are, I can guarantee that your approach is flawed and will come back to haunt you in the future. I say the same thing to fervent endurance athletes who train too hard, "feel great" (since they are bathed in cortisol) and inevitably crash and burn later.

Before the disappointment of hearing "only a pound or two a week" gets etched onto your face, understand that if you proceed with a *Primal Blueprint* lifestyle, you can transform your physique in a few short months. (Dropping 10 to 15 pounds of body fat and maintaining or adding a few pounds of lean muscle is nothing short of a transformation; believe me, you will know by the frequency of flattering comments!) Furthermore, your sensible approach will allow you to continue a steady march toward your ideal body composition and then let you maintain that ideal composition indefinitely without major deprivation or stress. For someone who's currently obese, a fat loss of even 100 pounds a year is safe and achievable using this method.

It's essential to reject the ridiculous prevailing mentality that weight loss can be achieved quickly with extremely severe measures. You want to lose 10 pounds in just a few hours? I've done it—at the 1973 Boston Marathon. The intensity of the competition at the world's most prestigious marathon coupled with an unseasonably humid day left me totally depleted and dangerously dehydrated at the finish. I'll never forget roaming around in a daze in the finishers' area (an underground parking garage) and passing by a full-length mirror. I paused, locking eyes with the gaunt image in the mirror (he seemed to recognize me as well…), and asked, "Hey, how did you do?"

Weight-Loss Exercise Plan

While my view that 80 percent of your body composition success is determined by your diet is difficult to prove scientifically, the anecdotal evidence is overwhelming. Go to the starting line of a major marathon or ironman triathlon and take note of the surprising level of excess body fat sported by many of these very highly trained athletes. The same goes for the droves of gym rats and aerobics queens with flawed diets and physiques that belie their tremendous devotion to fitness. There's no better proof that regardless of how many calories you burn, consuming excessive processed carbohydrates ultimately inhibits your ability to access and burn stored body fat efficiently around the clock. Instead, all that arduous training results in an increased appetite, again thanks to insulin-driven sugar cravings from poor food choices combined with, or as a consequence of, overly stressful workouts. Unless you are a gifted, extremely devoted endurance athlete, it's a vicious cycle that you cannot escape no matter how hard you exercise.

While it's true that exercise moderates the insulin response (i.e., a sugary energy gel consumed during a tough workout will be burned quickly and not prompt an insulin release like it would if you sucked it down at your desk), burning lots of calories (particularly with Chronic Cardio) and eating lots of carbs throughout the day will simply make you carb-dependent for energy. Invariably, left to its own devices, your body will want to overcompensate by tempting you to eat slightly more than you need to refill the tank, as if it's actually thinking, "What if this clown decides to do this again tomorrow? I'd better be ready!" Chronic Cardio folks have programmed their genes over the years to battle recurring depletion and fatigue with an increased appetite.

The bottom line is that you will not lose fat effectively with exercise-driven weight-loss efforts unless your eating habits moderate insulin production. Of course, a sensible exercise program will improve your health, sense of well-being, and muscle tone and somewhat minimize the negative effects of the high-carb diet, but it won't get rid of that spare tire. On the flip side, I have been able to maintain my ideal body composition effortlessly, even working out only one-tenth as much as I used to, since I evolved to eating very low-carb *Primal Blueprint* foods (getting increasingly observant over the past 10 years and eventually reaching "very strict" Primal beginning in 2002). During my recovery from knee surgery in 2007, I was able to maintain my exact weight and 8 percent body fat on zero exercise for a month and very limited exercise for a few more months after that.

> *The bottom line is that you will not lose fat effectively with exercise-driven weight-loss efforts unless your eating habits moderate insulin production.*

Of course, we all have genetic differences that create the reality of "results may vary." Regardless, you must focus on the concept of triggering the ideal expression of your own genetic potential through the combination of *Primal Blueprint* diet and exercise behaviors. Consider an age when you were pleased with your fitness level and physique. It *is* possible to approximate your appearance and energy levels at age 18 or 21, reversing years or even decades of suboptimal diet and exercise practices, in a relatively short time.

Be content with uninterrupted gradual improvement in your body composition and a wholehearted enjoyment of the process. This improvement may not be a linear "pound or two a week" experience. Instead, you may have some months, or seasons, when you will really lean out. At other times you will experience inevitable plateaus, which I'll discuss how to handle shortly. With the mind-set that you are taking care of your health and constantly progressing toward your goals (at a speed you determine, mainly by controlling your carb intake), your motivation and compliance levels will be strong even years down the line.

By the way, you are welcome to pursue weight loss with more enthusiasm and discipline to produce accelerated results, but you must align your efforts with your fitness level. A serious athlete who has added a few pounds in the off-season can ramp up training easily and return to ideal weight relatively quickly. An old-time pro triathlete I coached was once asked how long it took to drop the typical seven pounds gained over the off-season after resuming training: "'couple long rides," he deadpanned. On the other hand, a novice unaccustomed to regular exercise must follow a more patient approach to avoid burning out. Following are some Primal exercise recommendations to turbocharge your weight-loss efforts.

> *Be not afraid of growing slowly, be afraid only of standing still.*
> —*Chinese Proverb*

Ramp Up Low-Level Activity

As discussed previously, when you exercise at moderate heart rates, you run little risk of fatigue or burnout. Increase your daily activity level in every possible way—walking or cycling instead of driving for nearby errands, taking the stairs, parking at the edge of the lot, strolling the neighborhood after dinner, and enjoying leisurely hikes on the weekends. One friend of mine makes business calls while walking briskly on a treadmill (a great icebreaker, by the way: "Hey, what's that hum in the background?"). Considering that the average American watches 28 hours a week of television, we could possibly cure obesity if we all casually pedaled stationary bikes during our viewing time (and of course regulated our insulin production by eating Primally)!

Make Your Hard Workouts Harder

Focus on intense strength training and sprint sessions, ensuring that you are well rested and fully recovered between efforts. Remember, it's not frequency of your intense workouts that matters as much as quality. When you exercise a muscle to short-term exhaustion at 12 reps or deliver a max effort for 10 pull-ups, you'd be surprised what your body can do two minutes later if you repeat the effort. If you think you've pushed it to the limit at your typical 25-minute intense workout, take a five-minute water break and then go back out there for another 15 minutes of high intensity. If you pat yourself on the back after your typical eight sprints, rest five minutes and go back and do a few more!

Chill Out and Break Through

I cannot emphasize strongly enough how important it is for you to reject the Conventional Wisdom mind-set toward weight loss that obsesses on daily calories burned, strictly controlled portion sizes, and other anal-retentive nonsense. If you are hungry, eat (the right stuff). If you are motivated, exercise (the right way). And if you are tired, rest! When you are dragging, your energy is going toward rebuilding broken-down muscles and energy systems. Pushing a fatigued body through exercise will only lead to depletion, burnout, and undesirable sugar cravings.

The key to the exercise component of weight loss is in expertly balancing stress and rest to allow for peak efforts to be reached in conjunction with adequate recovery and rebuilding. With my athletes, I call these peak efforts *Breakthrough Workouts*—sessions that are difficult and challenging enough to help you "break through" to a higher fitness level (or, in our context here, stimulate a reduction in body fat). Whether you want to reduce your 10k time or drop 10 pounds, it comes down to directing optimal gene expression, primarily through diet, and secondarily through an effective workout plan with occasional Breakthrough sessions. From our understanding of the selection pressures of evolution, it's clear that taking fat off is more difficult than packing it on. Only by harnessing your energy with careful attention to stress management and the occasional bouts of brief, very intense, good old-fashioned hard work can you expect something different than the "same ol' same ol'": scale numbers, clothing sizes, race times, and so forth.

Sisson's Six-Pack Secrets

"How to have washboard abs on a high fat diet, no cardio and no ab exercises" was the title of one of my most popular MarksDailyApple.com posts ever. (In the weeks after the post, my shirtless photo accompanying the article was "tagged" and spread all over Facebook, necessitating my taking a crash course on the amazing technology of cyber social networking in order to protect my name and likeness!) While a "six-pack" is the universal hallmark of a lean, fit, well-toned man or woman, getting there following Conventional Wisdom protocol (grueling crunches and sit-ups to the point of nausea, burning endless calories on a treadmill, and then obsessively limiting what you take in—especially those high-fat foods so reviled by diet and fitness personalities) is too daunting to be a realistic goal for all but the most devoted gym rats. The truth is, we all have washboard abs…underneath whatever fat might currently be obscuring them.

Remember, 80 percent of your body composition success comes from how compliant you are with *Primal Blueprint* eating. A possible genetic predisposition to storing extra belly fat might indeed limit your ultimate potential to land on a magazine cover, but I'm willing to bet many times the price of this book that you can bring to the surface impressive ripples you never knew existed (or at least haven't seen since your college intramural days) by hitting the sweet spot with your carb intake and naturally engaging your abs throughout daily life. In fact, washboard abs can be considered an effortless side effect of living Primally.

Grok had to have a great set of abs in order to be an effective thrower, climber, runner, jumper, crawler, and lifter. Not that abs themselves lift, throw, catch, or push—but the whole complex of abdominals (rectus and transverse abdominis, internal and external obliques, and pyrimidalis) provides the foundation for nearly every athletic and everyday movement you do. Thus, they are part of today's popular "core" training—the ultimate functional muscle group. But rather than isolating them on some fancy $4,000 machine or getting rug burns on your butt from doing a bazillion crunches in your living room (you know who you are), the best way to work your abs is to involve them in routine functional movements and brief focused engagements throughout the day.

When you do push-ups, you should make a concerted effort to tighten your abs (pressing the navel toward the spine); the same is recommended during pull-ups, squats, lunges, curls, and other complete body exercises. Raking leaves, carrying your toddler, reloading the bottom drawer of the copy machine, lugging groceries out of the trunk and onto the kitchen counter, and infinite other daily activities—including simply sitting at your desk or in your car—can all be considered opportunities for a mini abs workout. I bet I did more than a thousand of these efforts sitting at my desk writing this book!

When you are engaged in basic movement, sitting or walking, you should tighten your belly as if you are going to be punched in the gut while blowing out the candles on your birthday cake. Hold it for 10, 20, or more seconds a few times every hour. Now do it while slightly tilted to one side. Repeat for the other side. For even better results and a stronger core, you can also simultaneously contract your buttock muscles. Do these short exercise bursts while you are watching TiVo or driving to pick up the kids. After a while, it will become second nature to squeeze your abs spontaneously. I do some of my best abs work while bent over doing sprints on the stationary bike. It's really all about squeezing, tightening, and trying to isometrically shorten the distance between your sternum and your pubic bone. Engage your abs, eat Primally, you'll soon notice improved muscle tone in your core. Furthermore, a strong, functional set of abs will help you avoid back problems as well as perform all outdoor activities safely and with less risk of injury.

Suggested Exercise Week Schedule

Walk, walk, walk. Hike, hike, hike. Move, move, move. This might seem like strange advice to help you get lean and ripped like our primal role model. However, by now you should have a clear understanding of why ill-advised frequent moderate- to high-intensity workouts simply burn glucose and increase appetite and that your exercise program on the whole is only dealing with the 20 percent slice of the weight-loss pie. After all, walking around the block or hiking up to the water tower doesn't burn enough calories to contribute notably to weight loss. However, increasing your daily movement will build you from the inside out—toning muscles, joints, and connective tissue to enable you to thrive on the high-intensity workouts that strongly influence body composition.

Coupled with *Primal Blueprint* eating habits, your active lifestyle will refine your fat-burning skills so that you become an efficient fat-burning machine around the clock and easily reach your ideal weight in a matter of weeks or months, as seen with the Korgs' case studies. Best of all, as you scan the suggested daily meal plan (earlier in this chapter) and the weekly exercise plan (next), you'll see that it's easy to eat and exercise in a Primal manner for the rest of your life. Here's a sample of what Kelly and Ken can do to "go Primal" with their exercise program:

Sunday: Two-hour hike at low intensity. (The Korgs can do this together and enjoy quality time as well.)

Monday: Easy 45-minute spin on stationary bike and 15-minute walk after dinner.

Tuesday: 30-minute intense strength-training session. Go for an 8 to 10 effort on a 10 scale. Choose gym routine, body resistance routine, or Grok workout from the *Primal Blueprint* Strength Workout Suggestions appendix at MarksDailyApple.com. 15-minute walk after dinner.

Wednesday: Rest.

Thursday: Easy 45-minute stationary bike ride or hike.

Friday: Sprint session at grass field, school track or even the beach. You can also sprint indoors on a treadmill, elliptical or stationary bicycle. Duration, including warm-up and cool-down, is about 20 minutes. Choose from the recommended sessions based on ability level from the *Primal Blueprint* Sprint Workout Suggestions appendix at MarksDailyApple.com.

Saturday: 10-minute intense strength-training session. Go for a 7 effort on a 10 scale.

Mark's Exercise Week Analysis

Total Calories Burned: Who cares! Enough to accelerate fat reduction and get in shape without suffering.

Muscle Groups Exercised: Arms, legs, core, and everything in between or attached.

Total Scenery Enjoyed: A ton more than someone on a treadmill or in a Spinning class.

Total Fun Had: Lots! What a far cry from Kelly Korg's exhausting regimen of predawn high-intensity workouts, mundane malnutrition shakes replacing real meals, and the resulting fatigue, energy-level swings, and sugar cravings.

Kelly on the *Primal Blueprint* plan could wake up leisurely with the rest of the family and enjoy herself with comfortable exercise sessions (possibly including some of her less than optimally active family members?). Instead of suffering several mornings a week, she could pick her spots with high-intensity Breakthrough Workouts that leave her exhilarated and accelerate her fat reduction. In three months' time, she'll have shed nearly 24 pounds of body fat and likely have added a few pounds of well-placed, lean, toned muscle tissue. She'll be happier and more energetic and she'll look better than she has in decades, with less effort and less struggle than before.

Meanwhile, Kelly's neighbor Wendy (remember her, the peppy network marketing enthusiast who dropped eight pounds in two weeks?) will almost assuredly weigh the same or more than she did when she started her cleansing diet six months prior. Furthermore, because 99 percent of network marketing participants lose money (from a survey of the largest and most reputed network marketing operations—after considering all expenses and inventory purchased from the company for resale), she'll probably have a lot of cleansing diet kits gathering dust on the garage shelves.

I.F. You Want to Lose Even More Fat, Try It!

As we reflect on the tidy examples of Ken and Kelly Korg nailing their daily caloric deficits with delicious, fulfilling meals, I must stress once again the concept of averages and expanding your timeline for measured progress out from a day or week to at least a month-by-month view. The meal diaries for Ken and Kelly obviously represent a good—make that perfect—day. In real life, your ability to optimize your meal choices and caloric intake will be more difficult than the examples (they were based on some of my own favorite meals!) printed here. I realize there will be days, and even longer periods, when you slip away from ideal.

However, you can get back on track and even make up ground easily because of the metabolic leverage you create with *Primal Blueprint* eating habits. When your insulin production is moderated and your fat metabolism is optimized, you have a greatly reduced need to snack or even eat regular meals. As you'll see from my 72-hour personal journal sidebar in the next chapter, my own day-to-day caloric intake frequently varies by 250% or more! When your body has reprogrammed gene expression to be able to get energy from fat whenever it wants, hunger tends to subside, and blood sugar and energy levels stabilize. Why not tap into this new "skill" and take full advantage? You can not only easily make up lost ground when you slip a little, but you also accelerate the process of fat reduction to virtually whatever speed you want (up to the maximum mentioned previously) by engaging in a classic Primal strategy called *Intermittent Fasting* (I.F.).

Your choices of just when and how to practice I.F. should fit with your personality, lifestyle schedule, and unique habits and preferences. Both meticulous planners and spontaneous types can succeed with these varying styles. I suggest trying a mixture of unplanned meal skipping combined with structured fasts of 12 to 24 hours, or even longer for devoted and experienced fasters. There are few rules or strict guidelines to follow with I.F. Most readers will be well-served to simply break free of their habituation (does that sound nicer than "addiction"?) to regimented mealtimes and other cultural traditions, such as always having dessert after dinner, eating until you are stuffed, or freaking out if you skip a meal.

Numerous studies show that I.F. offers a multitude of benefits, including lowered blood pressure, improved insulin sensitivity and glucose uptake, loss of body fat (obviously), a decrease in oxidative damage, and even a kick start for tissue repair. These benefits are achieved when certain genes are "turned on" to repair specific tissues that would not otherwise be repaired in times of surplus. One could surmise that this genetic adaptation allows certain cells to live longer (as repaired cells) during famine because it's energetically less expensive to repair a cell than to divide and create a new one. That might help explain some of the phenomenal longevity results produced by studies on animals eating restricted-calorie diets. With mice, longevity continues to improve as calories are restricted by 10 percent, 20 percent, and even 50 percent of normal.

I.F. has also been shown in animal studies to reduce spontaneous cancers, possibly by decreasing oxidative damage or increasing immune response. Pockets of research around the globe strongly suggest that deregulated meal timing and generally moderated caloric intake produce many health benefits (particularly for those who are overweight) and promote longevity with virtually no negative side effects. How about that for an alternative to the zillion-dollar pharmaceutical and agricultural industries?

Whatever method of caloric restriction you engage in, the net effect is to send signals to your genes to up-regulate fat burning and down-regulate glucose burning, as well as to turbocharge your body's calorie processing system. It's a similar dynamic to that invigorating feeling you get from a splash in cold water, an afternoon nap, or an intense workout. Your body likes to be stimulated and challenged with these brief *natural, positive* stressors that fine-tune gene expression and numerous other functions and evolutionary skills. In contrast, your body rebels and weakens from chronic *artificial* stressors such as jet travel, working long hours indoors, pushing through frequent, long, uncomfortable cardio workouts, or eating till you are full three times a day for your entire life. Here is a quick overview of some ways you can achieve I.F.:

> *Your body likes to be stimulated and challenged with brief natural, positive stressors that fine-tune gene expression and numerous other functions and evolutionary skills.*

Skipping Meals: With heightened awareness, you may discover that you're not always hungry when your regular mealtimes come around. Take advantage of this occasionally and skip a meal or two. You will learn to appreciate food even more when you use it to truly nourish and energize yourself, instead of habitually shoving stuff down the pipe just because it's six o'clock or because everyone else is partaking at the alumni mixer.

Condensed Eating Window: Condense your daily food intake into a set period of four to seven hours, based on your preferences. This allows for a sustained fasting period until the next day when you factor in sleep time.

Early and Late: Enjoy an early-morning meal and a late-afternoon/early-evening meal. This is a good option for people who have stressful jobs or otherwise have difficulty carving out a relaxed time period for lunch in the middle of the day.

Planned Fast: Enjoy dinner and then fast until the following evening (24 hours), or continue to fast until the next morning (about 36 hours). Many have success doing this once weekly. You may want to start by trying it once a month and work up to more frequently. For a deeper cleansing effect, you can try an occasional alternating day fast that lasts for a week. You can drink water, tea, or small amounts of juice on your fasting days and eat normally—or slightly less than normal—on your alternate days.

Regardless of what approach you use, be sure that you don't overeat when your fast ends. After a skipped meal or fasting period, you will be especially attuned to your body's hunger signals and satisfaction levels. Overeating is a largely psychological response to the anxiety of altering a familiar routine. Expert fasters typically ease out of their fast with several sparse meals to gently reengage the digestive system.

By seamlessly integrating I.F. into your *Primal Blueprint* eating routine, you will prove to your conscious brain that you can survive quite nicely without constantly needing food. This is easy to handle when you control insulin production with *Primal Blueprint* foods and really, really hard when you are entrenched in a typical American diet with lots of carbs and insulin highs and lows. If you have tried fasting or skipping meals in the past but (as with Kelly Korg) concurrently ate a diet moderate to high in carbs, you can likely relate to becoming irritable and exhausted when you miss even a single meal.

In my days as an endurance athlete, I burned so many calories (and relied so heavily on carbohydrate to repeatedly fill the glycogen stores I drained on a daily basis), I'd feel like I was on the verge of a hypoglycemic coma if I did so much as skip breakfast or otherwise failed to stuff my face several times a day. Now I marvel at how often I forget to eat—and the fact that doing so has no impact on my energy levels.

If you take a moment to reflect on the principles of evolution and homeostasis, it's clear how messed up our modern eating culture is. It should not be this hard for humans to sustain daily energy levels and optimal body composition—we just make it hard by constantly pumping our bodies with foods that we are not adapted to eat. If you give I.F. a try while strictly observing *Primal Blueprint* food choices, I promise that you will experience this epiphany: that you are eating the way evolution designed you to (perhaps for the first time since you were an infant) and that it's easy and fun and leads to incredible breakthroughs in fat loss and long-term weight management.

> *Intermittent fasting is easy to handle when you control insulin production with Primal Blueprint foods and really, really hard when you are entrenched in a typical American diet*

Weight-Loss Troubleshooting

If you are making a sincere effort to drop body fat with the *Primal Blueprint* and not satisfied with your results, here are some suggestions to alter your routine and issues to investigate further that might be tripping you up.

Get into the Sweet Spot and Stay There!

When you limit your carbs to 100 to 150 grams per day, you can pretty much maintain your weight and body composition indefinitely. You will probably even experience a gradual and sustained reduction of body fat if you come from eating a typical Western diet of double or triple that many carbs and carry a bit, or a lot, of excess fat.

However, if the fat is not coming off quickly enough after a month or two of Primal weight loss efforts, the best remedy is to tighten up the reins even further with your carbohydrate intake and stay in the sweet spot for several weeks.

While you may experience difficulty adjusting to the severe reduction of dietary "staples" (e.g., grains and pleasure foods including sweetened beverages and snacks), your body will quickly adapt to an eating style that is aligned with your genes. Yes, I know, getting your carbs down to 50 to 100 grams a day is easier said than done. It is on this issue that many people get stuck in the mode of "trying" to cut back instead of making a firm commitment to modify their habitual intake of certain foods and replace them with ample servings of foods that are more nutritious and technically more satisfying to your body than your favorite carb treats. For what it's worth, paleo biologists believe Grok's average daily intake of carbs was as low as 80 grams per day for months on end—and he thrived on that!

Keep in mind that there are days when you will go well above 100 or even 150 grams, thanks to the reality of prevalent carb choices and cultural traditions that can entice you away from a strict *Primal Blueprint* eating style. It will require great discipline to maintain an average of 50 to 100 grams (remember, most of us are accustomed to throwing down 300 grams per day or even more), but you only have to do it for a short time—say a month or two—depending on your starting point and how ambitious your goals are. By "great discipline" I'm not talking about suffering with a cloud of anguish and anxiety hanging over your head; it's more like "Eat reasonably generous amounts of eggs, meat, chicken, fish, nuts, and seeds, plus all the vegetables you want and fruits (with a little bit of restraint and selectivity), and stay away from all grains and processed foods."

If you find yourself struggling to meet your weight loss goals, I strongly recommend using an online food calculator to know exactly where you stand instead of "guesstimating." I find the mere act of having to write down everything I eat for one, two, or five days increases my awareness of dietary habits and provides an effective check and balance against idle grazing or overeating when awareness is low. Chart everything you eat for a few days and then enter the results at a site like FitDay.com or TheDaily-Plate.com to get a truly accurate indication of where your carb intake is. Even today, with what I consider a pretty decent knowledge of the macronutrient content of many foods, I continue to be surprised at some of the results that the online calculators spit out when I input my data.

Moderate Stress Levels

Body fat reduction simply doesn't work well when you are skimping on sleep, working too hard, or experiencing high levels of emotional and psychological stress. Scientific research is validating the connection between things like lack of sleep and hormone irregularities that hamper fat metabolism or increase appetite. To succeed long-term with changing your body composition, you must have the time, energy, and patience to devote great attention and care to the topic. Rushing through meals or reaching for sweet foods when you are stressed is not aligned with the simple lifestyle of the *Primal Blueprint*.

While the insulin control and intense sprint sessions might be the more exciting elements of the *Primal Blueprint* weight-loss plan, you should not discount the importance of the supporting lifestyle elements that can make or break your success. Getting enough sleep (including naps, which trigger positive hormone flow, balanced appetite, more energy for and faster recovery from exercise), sunshine (vitamin D enhances all cellular function, including fat metabolism), and even taking the time to play regularly will greatly assist your weight-loss goals. It's time to start walking your talk, stop burning the candle at both ends, and make the right choices to allow your genes to express themselves optimally. When you follow the laws of the *Primal Blueprint*, the weight you want to lose will come off naturally.

Adopt a Positive Mind-Set

I believe there is a bigger picture to observe that involves optimism, positive thoughts, and enjoyment of the process when you pursue body composition changes. The subject of body composition is laden with failure, deprivation, restriction, self-limiting beliefs ("I have the fat gene"), and superficial judgment from society (here's a sampling of *Shape* magazine article teasers: "Cellulite Solution," "Firm Your Trouble Spots," "Simple Ways to Age-Proof Your Body from Head to Toe"). It's critical to approach the subject with a positive attitude and an appreciation for the process. Your primary motivation must be to enjoy a higher quality of life and better health. The by-product of a change in body composition is not something to obsess about, measure, and judge as success or failure each day or each week, but instead to experience effortlessly as a consequence of lifestyle change driven by higher ideals than wanting to look good in a bikini for your summer vacation in Hawaii.

Accept Your Plateaus, Then Carry On—Primally

After a few months of progress, you often arrive at a frustrating point where the weight stops coming off, the sustained run of high energy levels fizzles a bit, or you stop building extra muscle. That makes sense from an evolutionary perspective, because the body is so well-tuned to adapt to any situation. Even with carefully restricted carb intake, your body may react to a sustained period of fat loss by taking subtle actions to drift closer toward homeostasis. For example, genes could "down-regulate" insulin receptors and other metabolic systems in the interest of preserving fat – a crucial survival mechanism for millions of years.

Accept that plateaus are going to happen and exercise a little patience. Weight loss does not happen in a linear manner—there are simply too many variables and homeostatic forces at work. When I say you can "average a pound or two a week" of fat loss, I'd like you to consider this statement with a four-month or six-month timeline attached. I know we are conditioned to a "what have you done for me lately" mentality, but we are dealing with lifestyle change here, not journal entries of happy faces or frowns based on your scale numbers or food calculator graphs and charts.

I guarantee you that making some elementary Primal changes (e.g., eliminating grains from your diet to regulate your carb intake to average less than 100 grams per day; adjusting your exercise program to refrain from Chronic Cardio and add some brief, intense sessions to the mix) will result in a certain amount of "effortless weight loss", as I promise on the cover. Clearly, there is a range of outcomes based upon individual factors (e.g., compliance rate as I'll discuss in the following sidebar, life stress levels, and how long and how severely you have diverted from *Primal Blueprint* laws before embarking on this journey). A female might effortlessly go from 185 pounds to 152 in six months, at which point, she might long to drop into the 140s and find the process a bit more difficult.

One of my favorite sayings—whether it has to do with business, fitness, or balancing the varied demands and responsibilities of daily life—is, "If it were easy, everyone would be doing it." There is a reason you don't see 80 percent of American adults sporting single-digit body fat nor dozens of runners flying by in the park at a pace of six minutes per mile. If you are unsatisfied with your results after months of devoted effort, revisit the following sidebar and this Troubleshooting section and consider making an increased commitment to achieve superior results. Rest assured that there are no mysteries involved here, nor even much genetic "good luck" that we are so conditioned to believe is important. It's all up to you, and how you can direct your genes to do the right thing.

Avoiding the Three Biggest Reasons for Weight Loss Failure

1. Lack of awareness and/or lack of commitment to actually moderate your carb intake to "sweet spot" levels. If it turns out from your online pie graph results that you have been a little loosey-goosey here, I promise you that even a few days of Primal-style low-carb eating will cause noticeable changes in your appetite and an increase in your energy level—and lead you on the path to the promised land. Start your day tomorrow with a Primal Omelet and notice how your inclination to snack in the hours afterward is eliminated. Keep the momentum going with a Primal Salad for lunch, followed by a meat and vegetable dinner, and you'll see how these (and many other) *Primal Blueprint*–approved meals leverage one another to get you off the carb-insulin-stress response-sugar craving cycle and into round-the-clock fat burning.

2. Failure to stock up on Primal Blueprint–approved foods. Dropping from several hundred grams of carbs down to 50-100 range essentially means you must eliminate the foods that once served as major energy sources (albeit very poor, quick-burning sources) throughout your day. If you have no logs around (filling, nutritious, long-burning food) and your flame is petering out, your reaction might naturally be to fan the flames with wads of newspaper (cheap carbs). Make absolutely sure that you stock your home, office, car, and backpack with *Primal Blueprint*–approved snacks, such as my favorites mentioned in the Chapter 4 sidebar. (The Primal Approved - At a Glance sidebar at the end of the book summarizes healthy eating choices and also what foods to avoid.) Reach for them any time you need an energy boost or feel a sugar craving coming on.

3. Lack of awareness/commitment to Primal Blueprint–style exercise program. Many exercisers are unaware of their working heart rates and the effect they have on metabolic rate and stress levels. Because the perceived exertion of aerobic exercise (75 percent or less of maximum heart rate) is extremely moderate, most exercisers (again, misguided by Conventional Wisdom) push too hard; equating suffering—with getting in shape. Walk through the room of a typical Spinning or Step class or along the window lineup of cardio machines at an urban health club and note the suffering etched on the faces of the participants. For the most part, America's devoted exercisers—a culturally elite anomaly in the world's fattest, most sedentary nation—are burning sugar and tiring themselves out from their well-meaning efforts. While I still favor an intuitive approach over a mechanical one, many exercisers have benefitted from purchasing a heart rate monitor and using it for several months to get a clear picture of what 75% feels like. This practice will help you develop the discipline to keep your cardio efforts in the optimal range.

Chapter Summary

1. Primal Weight Loss: You can lose one to two pounds of body fat per week on the *Primal Blueprint* program by targeting optimal intake levels of each daily macronutrient, fasting intermittently, doing *Primal Blueprint*–style workouts and approaching the challenge with a positive, process-oriented, big picture attitude.

2. Macronutrients: Adequate protein intake (0.7 to one gram per pound of lean body mass, depending on activity level) will preserve muscle tissue (and metabolism) during calorie-restriction efforts, avoiding the "crash and burn" effect of most diets. Maintaining the "sweet spot" of 50 to 100 grams of carbohydrates per day will moderate insulin production and allow stored body fat to be your primary energy source. Fat intake will be the main variable to ensure you are satisfied and nourished at each meal, making your weight-loss efforts effective, realistic, and even enjoyable.

3. Korgs: Ken and Kelly Korg can achieve their ambitious fat-reduction goals eating delicious, nutritious *Primal Blueprint*–style meals. When the carb intake sweet spot is observed and protein requirements are met, ample amounts of fat will provide a high satiety factor at meals but will not result in excess fat storage thanks to low insulin levels.

4. Exercise: Exercise can complement the main variable of optimal nutrient intake to support and accelerate weight-loss success. Increase low-level activity, make hard workouts even harder, and understand that the commitment to changing your body requires focus and dedication.

5. Intermittent Fasting: I.F., whether deliberate or as a natural course of fluctuating mealtimes (now that stored body fat instead of ingested carbs is your preferred energy source), will create caloric deficits that lead to fat reduction and effortless long-term maintenance of ideal body composition. You can engage in I.F. by skipping meals, eating in a condensed window of time, eating morning and night but not in between, or engaging in planned fasts lasting for 24 hours or more.

6. Troubleshooting: If your progress slows, try being more diligent in hitting the carb intake sweet spot (using an online nutrient calculator to know exactly where you stand), moderating your life stress levels (utilizing the *Primal Blueprint* lifestyle laws), adopting a positive mind-set, and realizing that plateaus in your progress rate are natural and acceptable, thanks to our bodies' innate desire for homeostasis.

CHAPTER 9

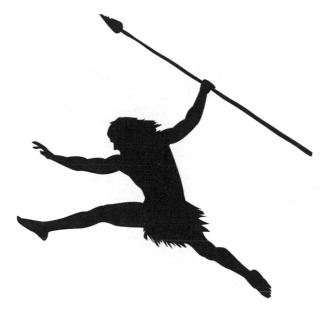

Conclusion

Time to Party like a Grok Star!

A person will sometimes devote all his life to the development of one part of his body; the wishbone.

—Robert Frost

As we near the end of the book, I want to call attention to the special place in my heart that Chapter 2, "Grok and Korg," occupies. I've been fascinated by the "Primal" concept for nearly two decades. (I self-published my *Training and Racing Duathlons* book using the name Primal Urge Press in 1988!) As an athlete and a coach, I've reflected on the Primal theme constantly—inspiring athletes to balance the unnatural act of endurance training with proper recovery and lifestyle support and to temper our competitive human instincts with common sense to avoid burnout.

My work in the fields of nutrition and personal training and my immersion into the health community on the Internet have enlightened me about the realities of everyday modern life for the masses. While we are making progress in some ways, I am increasingly disturbed by the seemingly inexorable drift farther and farther away from natural, healthy, evolutionary behavior in the technological world.

As my staff and I worked through the stages of Chapter 2—conceptual, research, first draft, editing, soliciting external feedback, and revisions—I finally had the chance to print a fresh copy, sit on a lounge chair in my yard, and truly "read" the material for the first time. I have to admit I was downright horrified. I questioned whether people would think the commentary was sensational or unrealistic and be turned off accordingly. I returned to my computer, reviewed all the references, connected more research, and generally made darn sure this was an accurate and realistic picture of modern life.

Unfortunately, the draft withstood my own devil's advocate scrutiny as well as that of numerous health, medical, nutrition, psychology, and sociology experts. Family and career men in their 40s and 50s take prescriptions left and right, families frequently feel that life is too hectic and stressful to align with the broad definition of *health*, and teenagers often feel overpressured and disconnected from parents. Today's kids have too much body fat and too little physical fitness. We eat too much beige stuff and not enough green stuff. We avoid exercise and sit at desks all day staring at a screen in the name of increased productivity. We go home at night and stare at a bigger screen in the name of relaxation. We stay up too late and then awaken to the stressful screech of an alarm clock. We are stressed by bills, traffic, air, noise, digital pollution, the future, and all kinds of anxiety we manufacture in our restless minds. Our first line of defense when our genes react as they are programmed by these lifestyle habits is prescription drugs, which treat symptoms quickly but, over time, weaken our natural ability to achieve homeostasis.

As we bombard our genes with these lifestyle risk factors, they respond the only way they know in an often futile attempt to maintain homeostasis and a desperate effort to keep us alive in the short term—with inflammation, early cell death, insulin resistance, atrophy, and so on. If you are an "above-average" American family, you can congratulate yourselves while remembering that "average" is actually borderline obese (64 percent of American adults are classified as overweight, of which one-third are classified as obese). In California, 40 percent of 10-year-old schoolchildren failed to attain a bare minimum aerobic conditioning performance standard known as the Healthy Fitness Zone (established by the Cooper Aerobics Institute), meaning that hundreds of thousands of "average" kids in California (what I consider to be a progressive, fair-weather state with a population arguably fitter than found in the United States as a whole) are technically classified "at risk" to develop serious health problems related to inactivity. *40 percent!* Take a big fat zero off that figure and you'd approximate the relevant statistic during the time of my youth.

> *Today, peak physical and intellectual performance and self-discipline are no longer requirements for survival. Man has become self-indulgent and has reverted to behaviors that provide short-term gratification.*

As we reflect on how far we have drifted from Grok's simple lifestyle and ponder how we can better honor and reprogram our genes by following the *Primal Blueprint*, it is critical to proceed with a clean slate and a deep conviction that you are doing the right thing. This is not an easy task. Numerous elements of the *Primal Blueprint* flat out oppose mainstream dogma that government espouses or that big Agra and big Pharma promote with billions of advertising and marketing dollars.

One must also wonder how society has strayed so egregiously far from healthy living that Grok has devolved to the carb-overdosed, pill-popping, overfed, overweight, overstressed Ken Korg. How can Conventional Wisdom that you have believed for years and decades, read in respected publications, or been handed down from trusted elders be wrong and even dangerous? The truth is, human nature is to blame. Just like Grok, we have programmed into our genes a desire to manipulate and rule our environment for our benefit—to pursue a more advanced, more comfortable life. Our indomitable human spirit has accomplished many great things but has also created tremendous fallout from our constant quest for "progress."

Man has conquered the world. As a species, he is the fat cat. He is on top of the heap. Yet now, peak physical and intellectual performance and self-discipline are no longer requirements for survival. Man has become self-indulgent and has reverted to behaviors that provide short-term gratification. Like the miners who stripped and poisoned the land and water during the gold rush, we have done similar to our bodies in the name of making life easier, more convenient, and more productive. In Eric Schlosser's *Fast Food Nation*, he reveals how the fast-food phenomenon exploded in popularity because fast food made life easier: No more cooking or lengthy waits for expensive meals! Now everyone can live the good life by dining out on delicious food! Unfortunately, the fare served up was disastrous not only to the human body but to the human spirit—destroying a centerpiece of family fabric that was the shared home-cooked meal.

When there is interest and demand to make life easier, profit seekers often swarm in and exploit this element of the human spirit. Nowhere is this more evident than in my own field of health. While I am all in favor of capitalism and making a profit, it seems that where health is concerned, we have allowed forces to run amok to the extent that today we must question the approach, motives, and trustworthiness of some of the traditional pillars of health and expert medical knowledge.

We must admit that doctors, despite their extensive knowledge, training, and loyalty to the Hippocratic Oath, are focused on treatment rather than prevention. As with drugs, it's wonderful to have extensively trained and prepared doctors standing ready when we need them. The sad reality is that most of their business comes from dealing with symptoms—not causes—of easily preventable conditions (as evidenced by the remarkable comment from a solo family practice doc I know, who lamented that his "business was down" due to America's 2008 economic recession!). The fact that doctors receive little or no training in nutrition is nothing short of abysmal.

Our government's laws, subsidies, and diet education efforts (flawed USDA food pyramid, anyone?) are seemingly driven more by lobbyists for the beef, grain, and dairy industries than by unbiased scientific evaluation and concern for human health. In the media, the historical checks and balances provided by the impartial investigative journalist have been pushed aside by giant ratings-driven corporations. Salacious stories that elicit fear, anger, or other strong emotions are what sell, regardless of their legitimacy. Even our educational community experiences free market influences that potentially bias the objectivity and even the premise of many studies.

The Korg Komeback

Let me reiterate my distaste for a perfectionist mentality toward diet, physical appearance, lifestyle change, and even school, career, and competitive athletics. Respecting the broad definition of health and the legacy of the simple lifestyle that our ancestors lived, we need to reject the measuring and judging forces of society and pursue fun and peace of mind in conjunction with health and fitness goals.

Admittedly, the comprehensive and emphatic nature of the *Primal Blueprint* might seem intimidating, and your efforts to go Primal will possibly require some serious departures from and adjustments to your comfortable modern existence. If you feel overwhelmed or take occasional exception to my strong positions (e.g., "Everything in moderation, including moderation"), keep in mind my 80% Rule as well as the suggestion to take one step at a time.

While the Korgs seem quite far down a disastrous road, they can also easily turn things around, step by step. No, they are not going to be perfect anytime soon, but they will be happier, healthier, and fitter with minimal pain, suffering, negativity, or disruption of the things they love to do in life. If Ken modifies his late-night activities by snacking on walnuts instead of cheesecake and enjoying a focused TiVo-assisted evening of television entertainment that ends at 10:30 p.m. instead of midnight, he'll fall asleep more easily and wake up refreshed the next morning, without having to rely on Ambien. This means more quality time with the kids, including walking young Cindy to school. If he brings the walnuts and a couple of pieces of fresh fruit to work and chooses lunch wisely at the supermarket deli, he'll maintain stable energy levels all day long, increase his productivity, and better handle workplace stress. Ken will leave the office at 6 p.m. feeling ready to enjoy and appreciate the leisure and family time options that await.

By reducing the stress of her exercise program and eating delicious, satisfying *Primal Blueprint* meals, Kelly will get her blood sugar and energy levels under control and tap into her stored body fat for a steady, reliable source of energy. With a few sensible and consistently enforced limits on digital entertainment and bedtimes, Kenny can reconnect with the family, focus better in school, and consider the option to eliminate his medication.

Talk about little things making a big difference! There is no better example to illustrate this maxim than the momentum (particularly the unbridled increase in physical energy) created by healthy lifestyle changes begetting further healthy lifestyle changes. If all you do after reading this book is cut way back on grains, you will dramatically improve your health. With more stable energy levels and better immune function, your dietary alteration could trigger an increased interest in exercise. If all you do after reading this book is simply back off your taxing jogs and Step classes in favor of long neighborhood walks and the occasional sprint workout, you'll have more energy and less cravings for carbs, which will likely lead to improved dietary habits and general health. Forget diet and exercise for a moment; if you took only four letters of the entire book to heart and added more *play* to your busy life, this could still stand as one of the most important, life-changing books you ever read.

On Your Own

Opening our eyes to the direction the bullet train carrying modern society is heading is sobering to say the least. In my opinion, the heaviest realization of all is that *you are on your own.* The imagined safety net of government, modern medicine, or the food or pharmaceutical industries looking after your health is a façade. Oh sure, you'll be cared for very, very well if something catastrophic happens (that is, if you have good medical insurance), whether it's a high-risk childbirth, serious injuries from a car accident, or one of the small fraction of cancers that are not lifestyle related. But when it comes to eating healthy, getting in shape, avoiding stupid mistakes—even building a career and a nest egg—the world can lead you astray and separate you from your cash (and other assets, such as health, sanity, etc.) in the blink of an eye, à la Matt Damon's deft pickpocket character in *Ocean's Eleven.*

A discernable pattern emerges when I relate the story of Grok to friends and casual acquaintances. After first expressing disbelief that Grok was leaner, stronger, and healthier than modern humans, most are captivated by the story of his uncomplicated life and the 10 surprisingly simple behavioral laws that dictated his (our) evolution. After a few moments of silence to absorb the information, people then commonly call attention to the most unpleasant aspects of Grok's life, a surreptitious way of asserting their superiority over some vulnerable, primitive caveman.

It seems we are scared of what's beyond our comfort zone of comfort foods, Conventional Wisdom, "Chronic" workouts, culturally glorified fitness goals that are too extreme, and the rest. I've discussed previously the tendency we have to get in our own way, manufacturing self-limiting beliefs and knee-jerk defense mechanism reactions ("Yeah, but didn't cavemen, like, die when they were like 30 years old—before they could even get heart disease?") when confronted with our frailties or the prospects of lifestyle change.

The Elitist Race

Recently, I read with amusement a blogger's critique of the *Primal Blueprint* eating style, something to the effect of "This is an elitist diet—too expensive [eschewing inexpensive grains and switching from conventional animals and plants to the natural, organic variety] and impractical for the average person to follow. Furthermore, there are not enough wild animal products or organic produce to sustain our society at its current population." My gut reaction was, "You're damn straight it's an elitist diet!" Expensive? Depends on your perspective. Eating *Primal Blueprint* style for the rest of your life is much cheaper than long-term prescription drug regimens or extensive doctor visits or hospital stays for cardiac bypass surgery or cancer treatments.

My evolutionary theme pops into mind here. Our increasingly comfortable modern life disguises the fact that the concept of survival of the fittest still permeates our being. Competition is everywhere in the world, with human nature programmed for "*Citius, Altius, Fortius*"—the Olympic Games motto (in Latin) meaning "faster, higher, stronger." Make no mistake, we are in a competition to achieve good health and prosperity with a massive number of entrants worldwide. Economically, you need only glance through Fareed Zakaria's *The Post American World*, to see the writing on the wall for the world's leading superpower. America is heading steadily down the pop charts while larger, hungrier, more strategically-minded societies, such as China and India, will soon catch and surpass our economy. (Poor investment in education and technology in favor of billions spent on military are some key reasons for our impending downfall, according to Zakaria.) Now imagine if all the money recently spent on bank bailouts had been channeled into diet, fitness, and health education!

Over the past century of rapid technological progress, we've figured out how to manufacture and package food and mass-produce animals, producing huge profits without regard to the health, humane, or green consequences. Stepping back for a moment to grab a wide-angle view of the wide angles in the buffet line at a Vegas casino, it's evident how ridiculously out of control this situation has become. No offense, but America looks like one giant yard of fattened cattle ready for slaughter, complete with a significant percentage of "downers" (a term for sick cattle that can't stand up; they are dragged with forklifts to slaughter).

The global macroeconomic example offers an interesting parallel with your own health. The emerging countries parallel those like you and I who challenge Conventional Wisdom and the consumerism "pack mentality" to seek the truth about healthy living. The military waste and economic bailout parallels the Western medicine approach to treat disease instead of pursue wellness—or, in this analogy, peace and economic stability. The annual harvest of wild salmon in Alaska is indeed limited, and it can run 20 bucks or even more per pound. In contrast, there is an abundant supply of farmed salmon that I've seen at big-box stores for as low as three-something per pound. Ditto for the heavily sprayed, genetically modified fields of corn and soybeans that will feed the masses for years to come versus the relatively few organic baskets of vegetables your local grower schleps out of his pickup at the weekly farmers' market. There will also be plenty of prescription drugs and hospital beds available (although you might deplete your life savings, but I digress...) to help you overcome the health problems that ensue from a lifetime of consuming processed foods.

In comparison, being "elitist" doesn't seem bad at all. Theoretically, if everyone wanted wild salmon and organic strawberries, we would indeed run out in the short term (however, demand would also stimulate increased production, thereby changing the world one person at a time through the power of our wallets). Right now, the race is on and you are welcome to participate. So suck it up and pop for the organic meat, eggs and leafy greens, especially if you are pregnant or have a two-year-old in his most crucial brain-development stage. Come to think of it, make that especially if you are *not* pregnant; are age 20, 30, 40, or 80; and have an interest in enjoying a long, healthy, happy life.

While you can clearly discern my passion throughout the book for the Primal way of life, I don't wish to be judgmental and assert that there is a right or wrong way of life for you. We live in an age of abundant freedom and choices for how to spend our time, raise our families, and fill our plates with food. While I have dedicated my career to promoting health and being a motivational force in people's lives, I want to temper my enthusiastic message with the understanding that I'm simply presenting you a specific blueprint of choices (hopefully very compelling!) and explaining the benefits of choosing them or the possible ramifications of disregarding them.

If you make it through this book and then do nothing to diverge from the path of the typical modern human, it's quite likely you will still lead a reasonably happy, productive, and comparatively healthy life. We've certainly come a long way in the last few hundred years with regard to health and enjoyment of life. As you read this, folks are working hard to develop new drugs and medical advancements intended to alleviate the devastating impact of today's prevalent diseases, most of which are due to lifestyle. Granted, this "indulging in modern comforts and benefiting from medical advancements" is a bit far removed from the *Citius, Altius, Fortius* component of our genome for my taste. But again, I'm merely presenting choices to you. There is no right or wrong answer. If you are drawn to a life of inactivity, big-screen TVs, lavish desserts, and microwaveable meals, we can still be friends. But you can bet I'll bend your ear now and then when the opportunity presents itself!

Furthermore, I'm sometimes more concerned about the adverse effects of fanaticism than I am about mediocrity, as I mention with my own endurance background and the Conventional Wisdom about Chronic Cardio. For example, if you simply cannot do without dietary indulgences that you believe greatly enhance your enjoyment of life, you can take solace in Deepak Chopra's commentary about the dietary habits of centenarians across the globe. Chopra explains that a *psychologically pleasing* diet contributes in a quantifiable and very meaningful way to their overall state of health, even if their daily pipe or other indulgence is clearly "unhealthy." Now that you are clear that the choice is yours, we can proceed to the next section about taking action!

> *"When it comes to eating right and exercising, there is no "I'll start tomorrow." Tomorrow is disease.*
> *—V. L. Allineare"*

Taking Action

Perhaps you are concerned about the hassles of the new eating guidelines and restrictions, whether they're too extreme or whether you have the ability to stick to them in the long term. Don't get tripped up by the common mistake of thinking you have to plunge, all-or-nothing style, off a towering cliff into the *Primal Blueprint* world. It goes without saying that the amenities of modern life are substantial and that you deserve to enjoy them. You can bet that Grok himself would have indulged in a big slice of the Cheesecake Factory's namesake dessert or settled into his seat at the Regal Cineplex to enjoy some big-screen entertainment (he would have particularly enjoyed *Crocodile Dundee*, eh, mate?). When it comes to getting in shape, you don't need to plunk down for an expensive gym membership if that's not your thing. All you need is an open road or athletic field to get a simple, fun, intense Primal workout.

The foods of the *Primal Blueprint* diet are within easy reach virtually anywhere on the civilized globe, including many outstanding Internet resources for those in remote areas or lacking good local options. You can also plant some seeds and grow your own food. In fact, you may be minimizing or getting rid of more stuff than you need to acquire to get Primal, such as clearing your cupboard of offensive processed foods, reducing your total hours of exercise in favor of a more focused and balanced program, eliminating nonessential prescription and over-the-counter medications from your medicine cabinet, and powering down your alarm clock, computer, or BlackBerry in favor of a less stressful, more natural existence. Minimizing might also extend to reconsidering expensive consumer purchases—even leisure items, such as that new boat or tropical vacation—that require more working time and energy to pay for. Perhaps the following tips will make your transition a bit more manageable—and more inviting, especially if you're a "slowly slip your way into the pool" type of person.

> *You may be minimizing or getting rid of more stuff than you need to acquire to get Primal, such as clearing your cupboard of offensive processed foods, and reducing your total hours of exercise in favor of a more focused and balanced program.*

Rome Wasn't Built in a Day: Not everyone needs or wants to ease into it, but it's a viable option to avoid being overwhelmed by new diet, exercise, and lifestyle practices. On the other hand, if you're up for diving in, particularly if you're facing a major health complication (e.g., arthritis, diabetes, or obesity), a fast and furious beginning can reap major health benefits quickly and even be psychologically more comfortable to your personality than a gradual approach.

For some aspects of the *Primal Blueprint*, such as the reduction in dietary carbohydrates, slow and steady may have definite benefits. If you feel sluggish or foggy cutting back on carbs (particularly if you've been eating 400 or more grams a day, like many), take your time cutting these foods back and even hold steady at 150 grams per day for a while if needed. Simply eliminating grains will get you most of the way there. Use your time in this holding pattern to ramp up efforts toward other lifestyle changes. If you find you're having a hard time adequately recovering from strength training or sprint workouts, reduce their frequency and severity and allow your body to adapt over a more comfortable time frame. Progress is rarely a smooth, uninterrupted trajectory for anyone. The point is to do what's necessary to keep your general momentum and motivation going.

Divide and Conquer: Sometimes it's easier to tackle one aspect of a project (or a lifestyle) at a time than to attend to all of them at once. If you're trying to cut carbs and kick a nasty caffeine habit, it might behoove you to take on one at a time or at least take one slowly and focus on the other. Although all the elements of the *Primal Blueprint* work together (and actually make other efforts easier), there's nothing wrong with homing in on a few select areas first. Make a commitment to total health, put yourself in the center, but take on only what you feel is manageable for now. If you keep the rest in sight, chances are you'll begin gravitating toward those other changes anyway. Healthy choices have a way of begetting other healthy choices.

Track Your Day-to-Day Practices and Progress: Keep a free-form food, exercise, and stress management journal. Input your food intake diary into an online macronutrient calculator, such as the free tools offered at FitDay.com and TheDailyPlate.com. In addition to documenting the actual foods and exercises themselves, make some observational notes on how you feel, what you are able to accomplish, and where you feel challenged. Looking back on your notes will give you a sense of how far you've come. Your notes can also serve as a reminder of how you made it through challenges in the past. Remember that the *Primal Blueprint* isn't about temporary fixes or fad gimmicks. Overarching lifestyle change takes time, care, and an ever-evolving commitment to align your behavior with your genes and goals for health, fitness, and fun.

> *I put a dollar in one of those change machines. Nothing changed.*
> —*George Carlin*

Around the World (or at Least to Dallas and Back) in 72 Hours

My MarksDailyApple.com posts describing my personal experiences, daily diet, and exercise and lifestyle practices tend to elicit the most commentary and interest. I'm often asked to reveal my "secrets" to interested readers. The truth is, I'm short on secrets but big on guidelines and practical tips that will help you successfully navigate the particulars of your daily life, including the innumerable challenges to being Primal that we face in the modern world. Because the *Primal Blueprint* is a blueprint and not a regimen, what I do has less relevance to your success than *what you like to do*. That said, I hope my real-life experiences give you some perspective that I'm a regular guy trying to raise a family, make a living, achieve peak health and fitness levels, forage Primal foods in a modern world, and, most of all, enjoy the heck out of my life.

The exercise of keeping an accurate journal for 72 hours to produce this sidebar helped me realize that even the times when I slip from optimum are no big deal. When "stuff happens" to take you off track, it's a great opportunity to develop your "go with the flow" skills, staying positive and relaxed instead of stressed. Consider the following example from my Tuesday journal where my son called me, begging for a ride to the valley for a social opportunity while I was en route to the gym for a precious final workout before a business trip. My 30 minutes of captive teen audience time in the car was a far more valuable experience than yet another workout.

Furthermore, when I was driving home after dropping Kyle off, I realized that the concept of *hormone manipulation* supersedes the need to cover all your bases on food choices and workout goals every day. When you direct insulin, glucagon, cortisol, testosterone, growth hormone, and other agents in the correct pathways by following the *Primal Blueprint*, you can easily handle the unexpected because you have built a healthy, efficient foundation. A little sugar here, a few missed workouts there, or an occasional deficient sleep night can be effortlessly righted with, respectively, low-carb follow-up meals, a maximum-intensity workout, and a power nap! Likely you can attest to the phenomenon of returning from an extended exercise absence (due to illness, vacation, or whatever) and picking up right where you left off—or performing even better, thanks to the rest.

The *Primal Blueprint* message that you can achieve robust health and ideal body composition without obsessive calorie restriction or exhausting exercise is the best takeaway lesson I can offer from sharing my routine. I regulate my carb intake naturally by simply avoiding sugars, grains, and other processed foods. It's no trouble, because by all measures I enjoy a satisfying—you could even say indulgent—diet. I engage in an average of a few brief, intense exercise sessions per week that deliver the precise signals my body needs to stay strong and lean, with minimal time commitment. I also have occasional extended stretches where I do embarrassingly little—and nothing bad happens! And then there are weeks when my body and mind are geared up to exercise many consecutive days in a row—when I am enjoying every minute of being in the gym, sprinting on the beach, or hiking the trails.

I follow the *Primal Blueprint* lifestyle laws naturally, thanks to a lifelong appreciation of the outdoors, a stimulating career, and a positive attitude—one that I've worked hard to cultivate over the years. I've seen the alternatives and traveled a long, long way down that marathon road to nowhere—the vicious cycle of a carb-based, sugar-burning, fat-storage diet, the struggle-and-suffer approach to fitness goals and the inevitable anxiety and disappointment that comes from such a tenuous approach. Here then are my journal entries for a three-day stretch from January 2009, featuring a business trip to Dallas bookended by typical weekdays at home in Malibu.

Tuesday—Travel Day

6:30 a.m.: Wake up and drink large cup of strong coffee with heavy whipping cream. Read paper (almost finish *LA Times* crossword puzzle—Law #10, natch!). Move to desk and answer e-mails, blog, and pack for afternoon flight to Dallas.

10:15 a.m.: Down protein shake (water, a banana, and 1.5 scoops of Responsibly Slim protein powder). Head to the gym for quick workout.

10:30 a.m.: En route to gym, son Kyle calls my cell, begging for a ride to the valley (gotta love winter break!). Return home, pick up Kyle.

11:30 a.m.: Return from valley trip with no time for workout or lunch. Depart for LAX and 2:00 p.m. flight to Dallas. Can you say, "Been there, done that?" I've flown this route 150+ times in the last 10 years. Destination: a suburban television studio (I've never once been to downtown Dallas; I hear it's nice) to tape regular appearances on my friend Doug Kaufmann's show—*Know the Cause*—a nationally distributed daily cable talk show on health and nutrition.

8:00 p.m.: (6:00 p.m. PST): Check into hotel, enjoy leisurely dinner at Outback Steakhouse (flank steak with asparagus and red wine—hold the potato).

11:30 p.m.: Time change contributes to late bedtime. Elapsed time stuck in metal boxes today = about six hours (counting drive to and from valley, to airport—featuring traffic jam on Pacific Coast Hwy—shuttle bus rides, and three-hour flight).

Tuesday Micronutrient Calculations

Coffee, heavy whipping cream
Protein shake
Granny Smith apple
Flank steak (6 ounces), asparagus, red wine

FitDay.com Analysis
Total Calories: 774
Protein: 88 grams, 352 calories (41 percent)
Carbs: 56 grams, 224 calories (24 percent)
Fat: 22 grams, 198 calories (22 percent)

Around the World in 72 Hours (continued)

Wednesday—Dallas Day

7:00 a.m.: Wake-up call comes after not sleeping well (hate when that happens). Turn on early news and conduct short, intense Primal routine (one-minute rest between exercises): 3 × 60 pushups, 3 × 35 squats, 3 × 25 abbreviated dips between armchair and coffee table, 3 × 60-second abs planks. Elapsed time from first effort to stepping in the shower: 17 minutes.

8:00 a.m.: Breakfast of four-egg chile-chicken omelet at IHOP. Extra sour cream and Cholula hot sauce. Try as they might (and they try hard), they still can't get me to take the pancakes (or toast or English muffin) that come free with the order. Coffee with cream and packet of sugar.

9:00 a.m.: Arrive at studio for four to five hours of taping. Drink a couple bottles of water—the most water I drink all week!—to keep my vocal chords lubed.

2:30 p.m.: Late lunch with the production team. All the ribs you can eat (which isn't all that much) and iced tea at a local rib joint. I'd prefer a salad bar, but this is where the crew wants to eat and we are in Texas…who am I to say no? Skip the mashed potatoes, potato salad, corn, cornbread, applesauce, and bug juice, thus sparing my system of well over 200 grams of carbs in one fell swoop.

4:00 p.m.–5:00 p.m.: Walk the Irving Mall (low-level aerobic activity) and make phone calls the whole time. Head to airport.

6:00 p.m.: Dinner at TGI Friday's (in the terminal)—pecan crusted chicken salad and a glass of cabernet. One of my favorite travel meals. Board plane, fly home.

Wednesday Micronutrient Calculations

Coffee with cream and packet of sugar
Chile-chicken omelet
Ribs (6 ounces) and iced tea
Chicken salad and glass of cabernet

FitDay.com Analysis
Total Calories: 2,087
Protein: 153 grams, 612 calories
  (29 percent)
Carbs: 92 grams, 368 calories (17 percent)
Fat: 123 grams, 1,107 calories (50 percent)

Note: this was a long day of hard work, but even with the three sit-down meals, I ate fewer calories than I normally do. I often use traveling as a great opportunity to engage in Intermittent Fasting. Tuesday's busy schedule contributed to my consuming only around 30 percent of my normal daily caloric intake. Because the food options on the road are generally inferior or difficult to find, I hone my foraging skills and look for nothing but protein and vegetables.

Thursday—Malibu Day

7:30 a.m.: Wake up and shake off the effects of jet lag with a quick plunge in the pool (I'd estimate mid-60s temp) and a coffee with cream. Head to desk to catch up.

10:00 a.m.: Down Primal Omelet with four eggs, sprinkled mozzarella cheese, sliced mushrooms, and green peppers, topped with sliced avocado and a scoop of fresh salsa. Back to desk.

11:00 a.m.: 11:00 a.m.: Head to gym for "pull and sprint day". Intense 30-minute gym workout (cable rows, wide grip pull-ups, inverted rows, cable curls). Jog to car, drive to beach to catch low tide. Commence 10 barefoot sprint sets (jog 10 strides, transition 12 strides, all-out sprint 15 strides). Easy cooldown jog, brief Grok Squat stretch, quick plunge in ocean. Gym and beach total time: 50 minutes. Head home and shower.

1:00 p.m.: Make my world-famous Primal Salad (check video at MarksDailyApple.com) with 15 veggies and a scoop of canned salmon, drenched in olive oil–based dressing. Nothing to drink. Granny Smith apple for dessert. Back to work in the office.

4:00 p.m.: Big handful of almonds and break from desk to throw tennis ball to a very old, very slow yellow lab named Buddha. En route back to desk, a challenge is issued by my son, Kyle. Detour from office to garage for a battle royale championship match on Wii Rock Band. Obtain perfect score of 100 on Rock Band vocals to reign supreme in Sisson family (Law #7, Play).

7:30 p.m.: Grass-fed steak (10 ounces), three cups of steamed broccoli dripping in real butter, glass of merlot. Okay, one more. Doesn't get any better than that!

8:30 p.m.: Watch TiVo replay of one of our favorite 30-minute sitcoms, followed by 60-minute ESPN SportsCenter broadcast. Watch both broadcasts in only 52 minutes total.

10:00 p.m.: Five-minute outdoor walk with Buddha, retire to bed for some pleasure reading. Lights out, and out like a light, at 10:30 p.m.

Thursday Micronutrient Calculations

Coffee with cream
Primal Omelet
Primal Salad
Granny Smith apple
Big handful of almonds
Steak and broccoli
Two glasses of merlot

FitDay.com Analysis
FitDay.com Analysis
Total Calories: 2,676
Protein: 168 grams, 672 calories
  (25 percent)
Carbs: 108 grams, 432 calories (15 percent)
Fat: 170 grams, 1,530 calories (57 percent)

Average Over Three Days
Allows for rounding margin of error

Calories: 1,842
Protein: 136 grams, 544 calories (38 percent)
Carbs: 86 grams, 344 calories (18.5 percent)
Fat: 106 grams, 954 calories (51 percent)

Rethinking Your Goals

You may have noticed in the tips throughout the book that I emphasize the long-term approach and the enjoyment of the *process* of healthy lifestyle change. In discussing weight loss, I take great pains to position this eventuality as a *by-product* of healthy eating, exercise, and lifestyle habits. We must reflect on the importance of this distinction because we are so conditioned to approaching lifestyle goals with a short-term, results-oriented approach.

Bookstore shelves are stocked with a dizzying array of self-help, financial success, and weight-loss titles; the sum total of the exhortations to do this and do that to be happy are truly overwhelming. Ditto for the level of negative cultural programming I have been exposed to working with my personal training clients. We have essentially been programmed to attach our happiness to our achievements, possessions, personal appearance, position of influence in career or community, and other superficial factors. I contend that setting and pursuing goals is screwing us up more than it's helping. That's right, I'm going to suggest you lay down what you might think is the most important weapon in your arsenal to "succeed" with lifestyle change—the determination and pursuit of specific and quantifiable goals.

We live in a superficial world where everything we do is measured and judged, and success (and often happiness) is thus defined by what we accomplish and accumulate, rather than what kind of character we have. For athletes, the world hits us with, "How far did you run?" "What was your time?" "What place did you take in the race?" "Did you beat your previous time or your opponent?" All these interrogations typically come before the only relevant question we ever need to ask ourselves or anyone else about a workout or race: "Did you have fun?"

We use computer technology to provide objective data about whether we are reaching our goals—or failing. We use elaborate training logs to record every possible bit of information about our workouts (such as time, distance, strength-training reps, calories burned—even "shoe mileage!" Me, I used to determine my useful shoe life by noticing when the sole started to peel off...). We strain, struggle, and suffer to obtain predetermined times, paces, and distances of our workouts, thinking that our bodies and spirits will actually appreciate a robotic approach to fitness.

Throw it all out the window. Take it from me, because I have been a long, long way down the road, and it leads nowhere. My fervent desire to achieve my athletic goals—run in the Olympic trials, average 100-mile weeks, beat my training partners—ruined my physical health and my running career. When I returned to competition as a triathlete, I had a more relaxed attitude. I enjoyed the challenge of a new sport and pushing the limits of human endurance, just for the heck of it. Gun-shy from my injury history, I adopted a more relaxed approach. I listened to the signals from my body and backed off when energy levels declined or aches and pains crept up. I enjoyed longer, slower bike rides into the mountains, connecting with nature and enjoying a sense of adventure in exploring new routes. I built my fitness in a comfortable manner and felt refreshed, energized, and inspired about my training—a far cry from the out-and-out suffering I endured from recurring intense running sessions with a fit pack of training partners.

Lo and behold, with my casual approach I became the fourth fastest Hawaii Ironman triathlete in the world one year, avoided injuries, and had a great time. After retiring from professional racing and pursuing a "real" career, I continued competing just for kicks on the amateur level, well into my late 30s. I had no goals, structured training program or logbook. I was just having fun, inspiring my personal training clients, and mixing with the professional athletes that I coached at the time, but I was ranked among the top racers in the world in my age group. Often I would see the "game faces" worn by others on race morning—tense, anxious, snapping at their loved ones, looking like they weren't having much fun. I'll never forget American swimmer Rick Carey, visibly distraught as he stood on the podium listening to the national anthem after winning the gold medal in the 1984 Olympics—because he failed to break the world record en route to his gold (he later apologized).

It's simply no fun to predicate your happiness on whether you reach your goals. Failing to reach your goals will lead to disappointment and dwindling motivation levels. Even reaching your goals can lead to a dead end and a flawed mentality. Many "winners"—in sports or other competitive arenas, such as business—develop a distorted sense of self-worth, leaving them vulnerable to up-and-coming opponents or negligent in behaving themselves in ordinary society because of our twisted hero-worshipping of winners and the wealthy.

There is a phenomenon in endurance sports known as the post-marathon blues (or post-ironman blues for triathletes)—so common that it's been discussed in psychological journals. It seems on the occasion of the glorious achievement for which they've trained diligently for months or even years, many athletes get that "now what?" feeling that leads to a profound sense of letdown. Ideally, we would use our physical accomplishments as catalysts for continued growth (including perhaps moving on to less extreme fitness pursuits), exploration, and challenge, not an excuse to get depressed and pig out on jelly beans in the weeks after the big event.

We must take a close look at the goal-setting process to avoid these common pitfalls and bring a relaxed, fun-first approach to our diet, fitness, body composition, career, and other lifestyle pursuits. The primary reason for switching to a *Primal Blueprint* eating style should be enjoyment—eating foods that taste great, stabilize your energy levels, optimize the function of all the systems in your body, provide long-lasting satisfaction, and alleviate the psychological stress of regimentation and deprivation that accompany many diets. Yes, you will look better, become stronger, have more energy, avoid illness, disease, and obesity, and enjoy other quantifiable results, but these motivators pale in comparison to the instant gratification you get at every single meal from eating the foods that your body was meant to eat. The primary reason for your exercise should be for enjoyment as well—with the typical goals of weight management or competitive aspirations coming as a by-product. That's right, even a world champion athlete such as Tiger Woods competes primarily because it's fun, not because he's driven by money or glory. If the latter were true, he would have quit, or at least lost a little of his legendary focus, early in his career, when fame and fortune were assured.

If you have any psychological stress about your diet, reject it flat out and start eating foods and meals that make you happy, drawing upon the long list of foods and minimal logistical restrictions of the *Primal Blueprint* eating style. Do whatever you need to do to enjoy your life, including indulging once in a while with a clear conscience and a big smile. If you are not having fun with your current workout regimen, junk it and figure out other endeavors that will turn you on. Instead of struggling and suffering to keep pace (with your peppy group exercise instructor or your training partners), adopt the *Primal Blueprint* suggestions to make your sustained workouts comfortable and energizing so they become fun again. Throw in some fun fast stuff occasionally to get you excited about pushing your physical limits and enjoying tangible breakthroughs including weight loss, more energy, and peak performance. Play once in a while. Forget the notion of consistency in this context and align your exercise program comfortably with your energy level, mood, and life responsibilities. Push yourself when you are rested and motivated and rest when you are tired.

> *It's certainly okay to aspire to specific results, but you must never lose sight of the concept that the rewards come from the chase, not from reaching the finish line.*

When you discard unnecessary goals that are mentally and emotionally stressful, you can focus your attention on process-oriented goals. Goals such as having fun, aligning workout choices with energy levels, and tackling new endeavors should define your exercise mentality. That said, great champions like Tiger Woods have an esteemed ability to blend a process-oriented approach with a strong competitive drive to achieve measurable results. It's certainly okay to aspire to specific results (e.g., losing 10 pounds or completing a 10k, marathon, or triathlon), but you must never lose sight of the concept that the rewards come from the chase, not from reaching the finish line. You can lose 10 pounds very quickly via any number of ill-advised methods (remember that skeletal guy at the Boston Marathon?). The true joy from changing your physique comes not from a surgeon's knife, a brutal calorie-restriction diet coupled with an exhaustive workout routine, nor even accolades from the cocktail party crowd. The most lasting rewards come from the positive, fun lifestyle changes you implemented to make it happen.

This is essentially what I did by accident as a triathlete. I was still the same driven, competitive athlete that had once run himself into the ground; I had simply reframed my perspective to approach competition with a more enlightened attitude. Believe me, it still hurt just as much to swim 2.4 miles, bike 112 miles, and run 26.2 miles through the steamy lava fields, but my purpose was grander than the uptight athletes who have their self-esteem attached to their finish time or place.

It is time for you to accept the grand purpose of the *Primal Blueprint* and reject other motivators that are confusing, petty, or contradictory to your health and well-being. To get more connected with the ideal represented by Grok, we have to pare down, not accumulate. The power and the magic are in the simplicity—a refreshing break from the complexity of modern life, the sordid influence of the ego on your endeavors and emotional state, and the dizzying admonitions on the bookstore shelves that can easily make you feel like a loser if you aren't as tight as the beautiful person on the cover. Grok did not traffic in any of this nonsense. Granted, he was preoccupied with survival, and we surely don't need to regress to that point to adjust our mentalities. What we *can* do is leverage the *Primal Blueprint* laws in our daily lives to become healthier, fitter, happier, and more connected with our basic nature as human beings. Make it your goal to honor your genes and your destiny to make the most of your life on earth, without attachment to any outcome.

What are you waiting for? Let's get Primal!

Primal Approved - At a Glance

Diet

Beverages: Water (in moderation according to thirst), unsweetened tea.

Coffee/Caffeine: Enjoy in moderation (cream and minimal sweetener okay); don't use as an energy crutch.

Dairy: Enjoy in moderation (only if able to digest comfortably). Raw, fermented, high-fat and organic products (including cheese) are preferred.

Eggs: Organic preferred for high omega-3 content. Yolks especially!

Fats and Oils: Coconut, dark roasted sesame, first-press, extra virgin, locally grown olive, hi-oleic sunflower/safflower, marine (supplements), palm, high omega-3 oils (borage, cod-liver, krill, salmon, sunflower seed, hemp seed). Refrigerate and use quickly. Animal fats (chicken fat, lard, tallow), butter, and coconut oil are best for cooking.

Fish: Wild-caught from remote, pollution-free waters. Small, oily, cold-water fish best (anchovies, herring, mackerel, salmon, sardines).

Fruits: Locally grown, organic, (or wild) in-season preferred. Berries are premier choice. Go strictly organic with soft, edible skins. Moderate intake of dried fruit and those with higher glycemic/lower antioxidant values. Wash thoroughly.

Fruit/Vegetable Juice: Fresh-squeezed only, in moderation. Home-juiced with organic produce preferred.

Herbs and Spices: High-antioxidant, anti-inflammatory, immune-supporting, flavor-enhancing.

Indulgences: Dark chocolate (high cocoa content), alcohol sensibly (red wine best choice). If forced under duress to have dessert, select premium-quality, high-fat (low-sugar) options and enjoy guilt-free.

Meat and Fowl: Organic, free-range, grass-fed/grass-finished, hormone-free designation is critical. If you must eat conventional meat, choose the leanest possible cuts and trim excess fat to minimize toxin exposure.

Nuts, Seeds and Their Derivative Butters: High omega-3, nutritious, filling snack. Refrigerate and use butters quickly (cold-processed, organic if available.)

Snacks: Jerky, celery with cream cheese or almond butter, cottage cheese with nut or fruit topping, canned tuna or sardines, berries, hard-boiled eggs, nuts, seeds, olives, trail mix and other high-fat and/or high-protein, low-carb Primal foods.

Starchy Tuber Vegetables: Enjoy yams and sweet potatoes (instead of white or brown potatoes) in moderation. Good choice for athletes needing extra carbs.

Supplements: Multivitamin/mineral/antioxidant formula, omega-3 fish oil capsules, probiotics, protein powder. Choose premium quality to supplement healthy diet.

Vegetables: Locally grown, organic, in-season preferred. Go strictly organic for large surface area (leafy greens) and soft, edible skins (peppers). Wash thoroughly.

Wild Rice: Enjoy in moderation (instead of white or brown rice).

Exercise

Low-Level Cardio: Two to five hours (or more) per week of walking, hiking or other exercise at 55 to 75 percent of max heart rate.

Schedule: Vary workout type, frequency, intensity, and duration, always aligned with energy levels. Make it fun!

Shoes: Gradually introduce some barefoot time (in low-risk activities) to strengthen feet and simulate natural range of motion. Choose shoes with minimalist design (Vibram, Nike Free) to prevent cuts and other injuries. Ease into it!

Sprinting: All-out efforts lasting 8 to 60 seconds. Total workout duration under 20 minutes. Conduct every 7 to 10 days when fully energized.

Strength Training: Brief, intense sessions, always under an hour, and often just 7 to 30 minutes. Full-body, functional exercises that promote balanced, **"Primal and Fitness."**

Stretching: Full-body, functional stretches to transition from active to inactive: *Grok Hang* and *Grok Squat*.

Lifestyle/Medical Care

Medical: Medication and invasive care for serious or acute conditions. If on prescription medication, combine with aggressive lifestyle modification in pursuit of drug-free health. Request additional blood tests for CRP, Lp2A, A1C, fasting blood insulin levels, and vitamin D.

Play: Change attitude – it's not just for kids! Enjoy daily, outdoor physical fun to enhance work productivity and manage stress.

Sleep: Consistent bed and wake times, calm evening transition, "empty room" environment, and sensible evening eating. Strive to awaken naturally without alarm. Take twenty-minute power naps when necessary.

Stupid Mistakes: Cultivate hyper-vigilance and risk-management skills (e.g. - "green light = look around, confirm it's clear, *and only then proceed*" mentality).

Sunlight: After adequate exposure (for vitamin-D), use clothing (or approved sunblock) to protect from burning.

Use Your Brain: Engage in fun, creative intellectual pursuits to stay sharp and enthusiastic for all of life's challenges.

Primal Avoid - At a Glance

Diet

Beverages: Avoid sweetened "energy drinks" (Red Bull, etc.) and "teas" (Snapple, Arizona, etc.), soft drinks, powdered drinks, and performance drinks used outside of workouts (Gatorade, etc.).

Coffee/Caffeine: Avoid excessive use, or using as energy crutch in place of adequate sleep and healthy lifestyle habits.

Dairy: Limit or avoid GMO or conventional products due to hormone, pesticide, antibiotic, allergenic and immune-suppressing agents.

Eggs: Limit eggs from chickens commercially raised in cages, and fed with grains, hormone, pesticides and antibiotics. Go organic first!

Fats and Oils: Avoid all trans and partially hydrogenated, canola, cottonseed, corn, soybean, all other high polyunsaturated (safflower, sunflower, etc.) oils, margarine, vegetable shortening, and deep-fried foods.

Fast Food: Avoid chemically treated, deep-fried, insulin-stimulating fare that is devoid of nutritional value: French fries, onion rings, burgers, hot dogs, chimichangas, chalupas, and all the rest.

Fish: Avoid fish from farms, polluted waters, or from top of marine food chain (shark, sword, and others that might have more concentrated levels of contaminants).

Fruits: Limit or avoid GMO, remote grown, or conventionally grown with soft, edible skins. Find local or organic alternatives.

Fruit/Vegetable Juice: Avoid juices with added sugar or that are heat processed, or from pesticide-laden produce. Limit total consumption, even for good juice.

Grains: Avoid wheat, rice, corn, oats, cereals, breads, pasta, muffins, rolls, waffles, pancakes, croissants, baguettes, crackers, donuts, swirls, Danishes, tortillas, pizza, other grains (barley, millet, rye, quinoa, amaranth, etc.), and other baked or processed high-carb foods. Even avoid whole grains due to higher levels of objectionable phytates, lectins and gluten. Everyone is allergic to grains at some level!

Indulgences: Avoid high carbohydrate (sugar or flour based), heavily processed treats: cookies, cake, pie, brownies, candy, candy bars, ice cream, donuts, popsicles and other frozen desserts.

Legumes: Limit or avoid alfalfa, beans, peanuts, peas, lentils and soybeans due to high insulin response and lectin content.

Meat and Fowl: Limit or avoid commercially grown, grain-fed ranch animals (with concentrated hormones, pesticides and antibiotics). Limit or avoid smoked, cured, or nitrate-treated meats (hot dogs, salami, etc.).

Processed Foods: If it comes in a box or a wrapper, think twice!

Snacks: "Energy" bars, granola bars, pretzels, chips, puffed snacks (Cheetos, Goldfish, popcorn, rice cakes, etc.), and all other grain-based snacks.

Sugar, Soda, and Grains: The less you consume, the less you'll want! Get off the "high-low, high-low" carb-insulin-stress response cycle to regulate your energy and improve your health.

Supplements: Avoid cheap, bulk-produced vitamins and supplements with additives, fillers, binders, lubricants, extruding agents, and other synthetic chemicals.

Vegetables: Limit or avoid GMO, remote grown, or conventionally grown with large surface areas or edible skins (leafy greens, peppers).

Exercise

Chronic Cardio: Avoid a consistent schedule of sustained cardio workouts at medium to high intensity (above 75 percent of max heart rate). Occasional sustained hard efforts are okay; allow for sufficient recovery.

Chronic Strength Training: Avoid prolonged, repetitive workouts conducted too frequently (e.g., hour-plus sessions featuring exhausting, non-functional, isolation exercise sets).

Schedule: Avoid consistent workout type, frequency, intensity, and duration (compromises health, energy, and motivation levels).

Stretching: Avoid stretching "cold" muscles, prolonged sessions (either before or after exercise), or isolated muscle group stretches, except by professional reccomendation for injuries/imbalances.

Lifestyle/Medical Care

Medical: Limit or avoid prescription medication for minor health problems easily corrected by lifestyle changes. Reframe "fix it" mentality into a "prevention" mentality.

Sleep: Don't burn the candle at both ends. Avoid excessive evening digital stimulation, morning alarms after insufficient sleep, or fighting off a much-needed nap with caffeine.

Stupid Mistakes: Avoid multi-tasking, zoning out, or trusting that the world will keep you safe (e.g., *"Green light = Go!"* mentality). Don't blame others for your stupid mistakes.

INTERNET APPENDICES

I've taken advantage of the infinite capacity of the Internet to augment the *Primal Blueprint* with continually updated supporting material to make this not just a book but a starting point for a complete lifestyle movement. I encourage you to visit MarksDailyApple.com and explore our conveniently organized appendices, featuring *Primal Blueprint* text references and suggested reading, extensive Q&A with deeper insights about book content, and detailed strength and sprinting workout suggestions—not to mention daily diet and fitness insights, recipes, videos and more, "with a side of irreverence" at MarksDailyApple.com. Following are the *Primal Blueprint*-related categories published at MarksDailyApple.com when this book went to print.

Primal Blueprint Text References, Resources, and Suggested Reading

Primal Blueprint Q&A: Everything You Always Wanted to Ask...but Were Afraid to Know

All About Grok
- Dispute About Recent Human Evolution
- Details About Genes Directing Cellular Function
- Reconciling Evolutionary Rationale with Religious Beliefs
- Grok and Korg Nicknames

Diet
- Differing Scientific Conclusions
- Insulin-Balanced Meals
- Fiber
- Diet Sodas

Exercise
- Compliance for Low Body Fat Athletes
- Cortisol
- Natural vs. Synthetic Human Growth Hormone and Testosterone

Lifestyle
- Getting Kids' Buy-In
- Prescription Drugs

Primal Blueprint Comparisons to Popular Diets

Atkins Diet
Low-Fat Diets (Ornish, MacDougall, Pritikin)
Metabolic and Blood-Typing Diets
Paleo Diet
South Beach Diet
Vegetarian Diet
Zone Diet
Primal Blueprint (Pre-emptive strike...because it's my book!)
The Biggest Losers

Law #4: Lift Heavy Things—Workout Suggestions

Grok Workout
Quick Bodyweight Routine

Law #5: Sprint Once in a While—Workout Suggestions

Novice Sprint Workouts
Advanced Sprint Workouts
Cycling Sprint Workouts

INDEX

A

acidity, 111
activity. *See also* exercise
  insulin and, 68
    in Primal Blueprint exercise
      routine, 228
  ramping up, 236
adaptation, genetic, 19–20
ADHD, 53, 59
adolescents
  lifestyle of, 52–54
  sleep needs of, 44–45, 58
advertising, of foods, 149–150
aerobics
    conditioning performance
      standard, 252
    slow-movement pace and,
      26–27, 179–180
Agile Gene, The (Ridley), 39
aging, organ function and, 169–170
agriculture
  in human history, 16, 17, 151
  life expectancy and, 57
  origin of, 35
  primal families and, 39
alcohol, 137, 268
alkalinity, 111
Allen, Mark, 179
allergies
  to grains, 153, 155
  to peanuts, 126
almonds, 126, 127
Ambien, 44, 58
animal fats, 118–119, 133
animal foods, 23–24, 109, 117–125
antibiotic-free meats, 119, 121

antibodies, 45
antioxidants, 63, 77, 109
  list of vegetables, 112
  Metabolic Syndrome and, 82
  sun exposure and, 210
  supplements as sources, 139–140
  vitamin C as, 72
approved foods, 268–269
Armstrong, Lance, 215–216
arterial plaque, 78
artificial sweeteners, 58
atherosclerosis, 62, 70, 78
  insulin and, 70
athletic goals, specialized, 167
athletic shoes, 191, 269
Atkins diet, 65, 273
attitude, health and, 11–12

B

bacteria, 141–142
barefoot workouts, 191
basal metabolic rate (BMR), 228
Bauerlein, Mark, 217
beef jerky, 127
behavior
  glucose levels and, 72
  modern lifestyle and, 49
benchmarks, establishing, 88-89
berries, 116, 127
beta-carotene, 111
beverages, 114
  approved, 268
  to avoid, 270
  carbonated drinks, 114
bicycle. *See* cycling
binge eating, 46

Biology of Belief, The (Lipton), 11
blood glucose (blood sugar), 24–25
blood insulin. *See* insulin
blood-typing diets, 273
body composition, 183, 224
  diet determination of, 110
body fat, insulin from diet and, 66
body mass, 86–87
body mass index (BMI), 43
body size, population density and,
  11
borderline obesity, 252
bottled water, 136
brain. *See also* intellectual ability
  size of early vs. modern humans,
    39
breakfast, 202
  in Kelly Korg eating plan, 233
  in Ken Korg eating plan, 229
Breakthrough Workouts, 237
breast-feeding, 40, 45
breathing, during weight training,
  184–185
B12 vitamin, 153
Bush, Reggie, 168
butter(s), 129, 133, 268
  from seeds and nuts, 125–126

C

caffeine, 50–51, 59, 129, 270
calories
  from animal sources, 117
  Conventional Wisdom on, 85,
    87–88, 237

F

fads, fitness, 161–193
family life
    comparison between primal and
        modern-day, 38–55
    financial stress and, 51, 59
    time spent together, 43, 56
farmed fish, 122
fast food, 51–52, 251–253
    avoiding, 269
Fast Food Nation (Schlosser), 51, 95,
    253
fasting
    intermittent (I.F.), 223
    planned, 243
fat(s), 93–95. *See also* oils
    animal, 118–119
    approved, 133
    to avoid, 134
    carbohydrate grams for
        accelerated burning, 91
    chemically altered, 24
    good vs. bad, 93–94
    healthy, 82–83
    metabolism of, 64
    obesity and, 10
    omega-3, 63, 82–83
    omega-6, 83
    optimizing intake, 223
    polyunsaturated, 75
    Primal Blueprint accelerated
        fat-loss program, 97
    roles of, 86
    saturated, 2
    trans and partially hydrogenated,
        156–157
    in weight-loss macronutrient
        plan, 227
fat cells, 68
    insulin resistance and, 69–71
fatigue
    grains and, 155
    mental, 48
fat metabolism, 8, 171
fat weight, losing, 66–67
FDA, 95
feet. *See* shoes

Feinman, Richard, 81
fermented dairy products, 129
Ferriss, Tim, 202
fiber
    Conventional Wisdom on, 3,
        154
    Primal Blueprint on, 3
fight-or-flight response, 27, 42, 44,
    48, 72
    fitness workout and, 189
financial stress, 51, 59
fish, 122–123, 127, 268
    to avoid, 270
    chemicals in farmed fish, 122
fish oil, 133
    in supplements, 140
FitDay.com, daily food consumption
        analysis by, 229–230,
        233, 259
fitness. *See also* workouts
    fads, 161–193
    Primal, 161–193
    sprint workouts for, 187–191
five favorite meals strategy, 102
flavonoids, 109
food
    animal sources of, 23–24, 117–
        125
    approved, 268–269
    availability of, 257
    cholesterol-lowing, 79–80
    choosing among, 108
    to enjoy in moderation, 128–136
    FitDay.com analysis of daily
        consumption, 229–230,
        233
    healthful, 46
    "heart-healthy," 126
    plant sources of, 23–24, 111–116
    Primal, 63, 89
    for primal families, 39
    stocking up on approved, 247
food calculator, online, 244–245
food choices, 102–103
food diary, for weight loss, 229–230
food propaganda, books on, 95
Food Pyramid
    in Primal Blueprint, 110

USDA, 92
footwear. *See* shoes
4-Hour Workweek, The (Ferriss),
    202, 205
fourth fuel. *See* ketones
fowl, 119–121, 268
    to avoid, 270
Framingham Heart Study, 74
Frank, Robert, 218
free range poultry, 121
fresh meats, 121
fruit, 109, 113–116, 268
    to avoid, 270
    to enjoy in moderation, 128
    in Primal Blueprint eating
        strategy, 65
    washing, 113
fruit juice, 268
    to avoid, 270
"Fruit Power Rankings" chart, 113,
    115–116
fuel. *See* carbohydrates; energy;
    fat(s); ketones; protein

G

genes, 7–8
    antioxidants and, 109
    attitude and, 11–12
    healthful lifestyle habits and, 33
    optimal expression of, 22
    reprogramming of, 14, 20–22
    slow movement and, 27
genetically modified organisms
    (GMOs), 114, 115
genetic destiny, 11
genetic drift, 19
GERD (gastroesophageal reflux
    disease), 49
gluconeogenesis, 96
glucose (blood sugar), 24–25
    behavior and, 72
    HFCS and, 159
    insulin resistance and, 69
    ketones and, 96
    minimum daily requirement for,
        95–96

International Network of
Cholesterol Skeptics, 75
Internet resources, 272–273. *See also*
www.MarksDailyApple.com
on Internet
intimacy, lifestyle and, 47, 48

J

Japanese diet, omega-3 and fatty
acids in, 83
jet lag, 201
jogging. *See* running
journal, daily, 260–263
journaling, 89
juices, 114–115
to avoid, 270
fruit/vegetable, 268

K

ketogenic diet, 88–89
ketones, 95–97
ketosis
carbohydrate grams for, 91
defined, 96–97
Keys, Ancel, 94
Knaggs, Bart, 215
Korg family (characters)
daily activities of, 55
lifestyle changes by, 254
modern-day family contrasted
with primal family,
43–55
weight loss case study of Kelly
Korg, 231–233
weight loss case study of Ken
Korg, 228–230, 231
kosher meat, 121
Kustes, Scott, 129

L

lactose, 130
laws. *See* lifestyle; Primal Blueprint
Laws
LDL, 48, 75, 76–77
benign and dense forms of, 79
carbohydrate reduction and, 82

medication to control, 79
oxidation and, 77–79
Primal Blueprint eating plan and,
79
lean body mass, 86–87, 229
lectin, 153
legumes, 158, 269
leisure. *See* play
Lewis, Carl, 187
life expectancy
of primal humans, 17–18, 35, 56
of today's child, 59
lifestyle
changing, 254, 258
elements to avoid, 271
goals of, 264–267
health and, 21–22, 33, 269
heart disease risk factors and, 74
laws for, 195–220
of modern humans, 43–55
of primal humans, 17–18, 39,
40–43
rethinking goals for, 264–265
lifestyle risk factors, 252
lifting, 164
lipid hypothesis, of heart disease,
73, 75
Lipitor, 47
lipoproteins, 75
Lipton, Bruce, 11, 12
liver, insulin and, 69
local produce, 111–114
selecting vegetables, 111–113
longevity, organ reserve and,
169–170
low-carbohydrate diet, 65, 88–89
ketosis and, 96
low-fat diet, 7, 76, 273
low-intensity aerobic movement,
170–171
low-level cardio exercise, 269
low-level exercise zone, 171–172
L-tryptophan, 202
lunch
in Kelly Korg eating plan, 233
in Ken Korg eating plan, 230
Lydiard, Arthur, 178

M

MacDougall diet, 273
macronutrients, 62, 85–95
calculating, 229, 232
carbohydrates, 88–92
fat, 93–95
protein, 86–88
for weight loss, 224–227,
229, 232
magnesium, 131, 202
maintenance range, 91
marathons, 177
margarine, 134
marine oils, 133
massive multiplayer online
role-playing games.
See MMORPG
McGovern, George, 95
meal choices, "Oh, Positive" diet
and, 98–99
meal habits, 223
Conventional Wisdom vs.
Primal Blueprint on, 3
meals
five favorite meals strategy, 102
insulin-balanced, 86
in Kelly Korg food journal, 233
in Ken Korg food journal,
229–230
schedules for, 100
skipping, 242
meat, 119–121, 268
to avoid, 270
fish and, 122–123
red, 117–118
medical care, 269
elements to avoid, 274
medications, 44, 45, 47–48
sleep, 44, 58
Mediterranean diet, 94
Mednick, Sara, 203
melanoma, UVA rays and, 209
melatonin, 44, 197–198, 200, 202
memory loss, 53
men
heart rate for, 172

Primal Fitness for, 167
metabolic diets, 273
metabolic processes, 97
Metabolic Syndrome, 2, 62, 77
   carbohydrates and, 90
   markers for, 81
metabolism
   Chronic Cardio and, 178
   energy and, 46
   of fat, 8, 64, 171
milk, 129
   lactose in, 130
   raw, 135
"mind-body connection," 11
mind-set, positive, 245
minerals, in dairy products, 131
mistakes, 31, 211–214, 269
   behaviors to avoid, 271
MMORPG (massive multiplayer
   online role-playing games),
   53, 59
moderate-use foods, 128–136
modern life, genetic inheritance and,
   18
monounsaturated oil, 132
movement, frequency and speed,
   164, 170–180
multivitamin/mineral/antioxidant
   booster, 139–140
musculoskeletal system, aerobic
   exercise and, 171

N

naps, 41, 203–204. *See also* sleep
   benefits of, 57
natural healing, 41
natural meat, 121
natural selection, 212
Neel, James V., 16
negative thoughts, health and, 11
net carbs, 89
Nexium, 48–49
Nike Free product line, of shoes, 191
non-REM sleep, 200, 203–204
nonsteroidal anti-inflammatory drug
   (NSAID), 49, 84

nutrients. *See* macronutrients
nutrition, diet and, 46
nutritional deficiencies, in grain-
   based diets, 152–153
nutritional value, of fruits, 116
Nutrition Facts, on packaging, 149
nuts and nut butters, 125–126, 127,
   144, 268
   sleep and, 202

O

obesity, 9–10. *See also* weight
   borderline, 252
   childhood, 59
"Oh, Positive" diet, 98–99
oils, 132–134. *See also* fats
   approved, 133–134, 268
   to avoid, 134, 270
   canola oil, 132–133, 134
   olive oil, 132
old age, dying from, 10
olive oil, 132, 134
olives, 127
omega-3 oils, 63, 133
   in fish, 123
   inflammation reduction with,
      82–84
   in nuts, 126
   in organic meats, 120
   in supplements, 140–141
omega-3—Omega-6 ratios, 82, 210
omega-6 oils, 83
   in fish, 123
ORAC report, 112
orange produce, 111
organ function, 169–170
organic foods
   chocolate, 138
   eggs, 124
   meats, 119, 120
   value of, 108, 113–114
   vegetables, 111–113
Ornish, Dean, 76
Ornish diet, 273
outdoors play, 206
"out of Africa" theory, 35

overexercising, 26–27
overweight. *See* obesity; weight
overwork, play and, 205
oxidation
   LDL and, 77–79
   polyunsaturated fats and, 75

P

Paleo diet, 273
Paleo Diet, The (Cordain), 151
palm oil, 133
pancreatic beta cells, 69
partially hydrogenated fats, 156–157
partially hydrogenated oils, 134
pasture-raised or finished meat, 121
peanuts and peanut butter, 126, 127
Peniston, Lorraine, 205
pesticides
   on fruits, 113, 114, 116
   in meats, 119
phenylethylamine, in chocolate, 138
physical effort, bursts of, 28
physique, 166–167
phytates, 152–153
phytonutrients, 109
Pigg, Mike, 179
plants
   in diet, 109
   as food source, 23–24, 111–116
plaque, arterial, 78
plateaus, 246
play, 29–30, 204–206, 269
   Conventional Wisdom vs.
      Primal Blueprint on, 5
poisons (dietary), 24–25, 110
   avoiding, 148–160
   grains as, 150–155
   legumes as, 158
   processed foods as, 158
   sugar as, 159
   trans and partially hydrogenated
      fats as, 156–157
polyphasic sleep habits, 203

polyunsaturated fatty acids (PUFAs), 2, 75, 118–119
polyunsaturated oils, 132–133
population, evolution of, 19
portion control, Conventional Wisdom on, 237
positive mind-set, 245
Post American World, The (Zakaria), 256
potatoes, 135
poultry, free range, 121
power-to-weight ratio, 167–168
prescription drugs. *See also* medications
 Conventional Wisdom vs. Primal Blueprint on, 6
Primal Blueprint. *See also* Primal Blueprint Laws
 adapting primal lifestyle to modern life, 14
 approved lifestyle features, 268–269
 Atkins diet and, 65
 Carbohydrate Curve in, 90, 226, 227
 on carbs and grain fiber, 89
 vs. Conventional Wisdom, 2–6
 costs of following, 124–125
 critique of eating style, 255
 daily journal about, 260–263
 Danger Zone in, 92
 eating in, 61–106, 63–64
 eating style and inflammation, 84
 on eating well, 98–102
 80% Rule and, 101
 Food Pyramid in, 110
 genes and, 7–8
 HDL, LDL, and, 79
 insulin-balanced meals, 86
 Internet resources for, 272–273
 ketones as fourth fuel, 95–97
 ketosis in, 97
 lifestyle features to avoid, 270–271
 maintenance range in, 91
 on meats, 118

 for Metabolic Syndrome, 82
 primal ancestors and, 15–18
 snacks in, 102, 127
 steady weight gain and, 92
 stocking up on approved foods, 247
 Sweet Spot in, 91
 for weight loss, 221–248
Primal Blueprint Laws, 22–33
 Law 1: Eat Lots of Plants and Animals, 23–24, 107–145
 Law 2: Avoid Poisonous Things, 24–25, 147–160
 Law 3: Move Frequently at a Slow Pace, 26–27, 170–180
 Law 4: Lift Heavy Things, 28, 180–186
 Law 5: Sprint Once in a While, 28, 187–191
 Law 6: Get Adequate Sleep, 29, 197–204
 Law 7: Play, 29–30, 204–206
 Law 8: Get Adequate Sunlight, 30–31, 206–210
 Law 9: Avoid Stupid Mistakes, 31, 211–217
 Law 10: Use Your Brain, 31–32, 217–219
Primal Fitness, 161–193
 process for, 166–169
 Pyramid for, 164
 zones for heart rate, 173–174
Primal foods, 89
primal humans
 lifespan of, 35
 lifestyle of, 39, 40–43
Primal Sweet Spot. *See* Sweet Spot
Pritikin diet, 273
probiotics, 141–142
processed foods, 111
 avoiding, 158, 269
 carbohydrates, 8, 24, 65, 78
 eliminating, 65
 as poisons, 24–25

produce
 local, 111–114
 nonorganic, 113
 organic, 111
productivity, leisure and, 205–206
progress, tracking daily, 258–259
propaganda, about food, 94–95
prostate cancer, foods and, 111
protein, 86–88
 burning of, 95
 optimizing intake, 223
 per pound of lean body mass, 87
 in weight-loss macronutrient plan, 225
protein powder, 142
PUFAs. *See* polyunsaturated fatty acids
push-ups, 238
Pyramid
 Fitness, 164
 Food, 92, 110

Q

quality time, 43, 56

R

raw milk, 135
rBGH. *See* recombinant bovine growth hormone (rBGH)
Recent African Origins (RAO) model, 35
Recent Single-Origin Hypothesis (RSOH), 35
recombinant bovine growth hormone (rBGH), 130–131
recreation, for children, 53, 59
red meat, 117–118
red plants, 111
reference points, establishing, 89
regimentation, avoiding, 223
Reid, Daniel, 201
REM sleep, 200
Replacements Hypothesis, 35
reprogramming, of genes, 20–22
resources, on strength training, 185
rest. *See also* sleep

thirst, 135–136
thyroid gland, 70–71
TiVo, sleep and, 199
total fitness. *See also* fitness
    Chronic Cardio and, 178 Tour de
        France, avoiding mis-
        takes on, 215–216
toxic agents, ingesting, 24–25
toxins
    in fish, 122
    in grains, 153
tracking, of progress, 258–259
trail mix, 126, 127
training. *See* exercise; fitness
Training and Racing Duathlons
    (Sisson), 251
trans fats, 134, 156–158
triglycerides, 48, 76–77
Troubleshooting, 244–246
tryptophan-rich foods, 202
tuber vegetables, 135, 268
type 2 diabetes, 77

U
USDA
    Food Pyramid and weight gain
        and, 92
    ORAC report, 112
    organic meat certified by, 119
UVA rays, 209

V
Valtin, Heinz, 135, 136
vegetable juice
    approved, 268
    to avoid, 270
vegetables, 109, 269
    to avoid, 271
    as center of diet, 112
    list of antioxidant, 112
    in Primal Blueprint eating
        strategy, 65–66
    selecting, 111–113
    starchy tuber, 135, 268
    washing, 113
vegetable shortening, 134

vegetarian diet, 273
    animals with, 121
Viagra, 47
Vibram FiveFingers shoe, 191
Vioxx, 49, 84
vitamins
    A, 153
    B12, 153
    C, 72, 153
    D, 30, 131, 153, 207–208, 210
    in dairy products, 131
    in fish, 122
    supplements and, 139–143
VLDLs, 75, 76
volume, of food, 67

W
Waddington, C. H., 21
walking
    by primal families, 40–41
    to school, 58
walnuts, 126
washboard abs, 238–239
washing, of fruits and vegetables,
    113
water, 135–136
    benefits of cold water, 41, 57
website. *See* www.MarksDaily
    Apple.com on Internet
weekly exercise schedule, 239–241
weight, 52. *See also* obesity
    of modern humans, 43
    natural management of, 63–64
    of primal humans, 41–42
    sleep deficit and, 198
weight gain, 92
weight loss, 67
    Chronic Cardio and, 174–175
    Conventional Wisdom vs.
        Primal Blueprint on, 5
    crash programs for, 234
    critical elements of, 223–224
    exercise plan for, 27, 235–241
    food diary for, 229–230, 233
    macronutrient plan for, 224–227
    Primal Approach to, 221–248

    Primal exercise and, 166
    Primal Sweet Spot for, 91
    reasons for failure, 247
    slow and steady, 258
    speed of, 234
    troubleshooting for, 244–246
Weil, Andrew, 98
Western diet, 100
whole grain, 46, 154
wild rice, 136, 269
wine, 77, 118, 135, 137, 202, 268
women
    heart rate for, 172
    Primal Fitness for, 167
Woods, Tiger, 266
workout plan, 8–9, 168–169
workouts, 165. *See also*
        cardiovascular endurance
    cardio, 4, 58, 170–178
    energy levels and, 47
    intense, 178–180
    intensifying, 237
    Internet on suggestions for, 272
    sprint strategy for, 189–190
    for strength training, 180–190
    stressful, 26
    10-minute, 163, 182, 240
work-play balance, 206

Y
yellow produce, 111

Z
Zakaria, Fareed, 256
Zone Diet, 65, 273

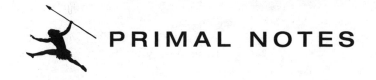

PRIMAL NOTES

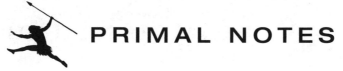

PRIMAL NOTES

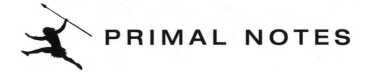

PRIMAL NOTES